T0343202

Antibiotic Resistance: Challenges and Opportunities

Editors

RICHARD R. WATKINS
ROBERT A. BONOMO

INFECTIOUS DISEASE CLINICS OF NORTH AMERICA

www.id.theclinics.com

Consulting Editor
HELEN W. BOUCHER

June 2016 • Volume 30 • Number 2

ELSEVIER

1600 John F. Kennedy Boulevard • Suite 1800 • Philadelphia, Pennsylvania, 19103-2899.
http://www.theclinics.com

INFECTIOUS DISEASE CLINICS OF NORTH AMERICA Volume 30, Number 2
June 2016 ISSN 0891–5520, ISBN-13: 978-0-323-44618-1

Editor: Kerry Holland
Developmental Editor: Donald Mumford

Infectious Disease Clinics of North America (ISSN 0891–5520) is published in March, June, September, and December by Elsevier Inc., 360 Park Avenue South, New York, NY 10010-1710. Periodicals postage paid at New York, NY and additional mailing offices. Subscription prices are $295.00 per year for US individuals, $560.00 per year for US institutions, $100.00 per year for US students, $350.00 per year for Canadian individuals, $699.00 per year for Canadian institutions, $420.00 per year for international individuals, $699.00 per year for international institutions, and $200.00 per year for Canadian and international students. To receive student rate, orders must be accompained by name of affiliated institution, date of term, and the *signature* of program/residency coordinator on institution letterhead. Orders will be billed at individual rate until proof of status is received. Foreign air speed delivery is included in all *Clinics* subscription prices. All prices are subject to change without notice. **POSTMASTER**: Send address changes to *Infectious Disease Clinics of North America,* Elsevier Health Sciences Division, Subcription Customer Service, 3251 Riverport Lane, Maryland Heights, MO 63043. **Customer Service: 1-800-654-2452 (US). From outside of the US and Canada, call 1-314-447-8871. Fax: 1-314-447-8029. E-mail: JournalsCustomerService-usa@elsevier.com (print support) or JournalsOnlineSupport-usa@elsevier.com (online support).**

Infectious Disease Clinics of North America is also published in Spanish by Editorial Inter-Médica, Junin 917, 1er A 1113, Buenos Aires, Argentina.

Reprints. For copies of 100 or more, of articles in this publication, please contact the Commercial Reprints Department, Elsevier Inc., 360 Park Avenue South, New York, New York 10010-1710. Tel. 212-633-3874, Fax: 212-633-3820, E-mail: reprints@elsevier.com.

Infectious Disease Clinics of North America is covered in *MEDLINE/PubMed (Index Medicus), Current Contents/Clinical Medicine, Science Citation Alert, SCISEARCH,* and *Research Alert.*

Contributors

CONSULTING EDITOR

HELEN W. BOUCHER, MD, FIDSA, FACP
Director, Infectious Diseases Fellowship Program, Division of Geographic Medicine and Infectious Diseases, Tufts Medical Center, Associate Professor of Medicine, Tufts University School of Medicine, Boston, Massachusetts

EDITORS

RICHARD R. WATKINS, MD, MS, FACP
Associate Professor, Department of Internal Medicine, Northeast Ohio Medical University, Rootstown, Ohio; Division of Infectious Diseases, Cleveland Clinic Akron General Medical Center, Akron, Ohio

ROBERT A. BONOMO, MD
Chief of Medical Services, Louis Stokes Cleveland Veterans Affairs Medical Center; Professor, Departments of Medicine, Biochemistry, Pharmacology, Molecular Biology and Microbiology, Case Western Reserve University School of Medicine, Cleveland, Ohio

AUTHORS

AMOS ADLER, MD
Clinical Microbiology Laboratory, Tel-Aviv Sourasky Medical Center; Sackler School of Medicine, Tel-Aviv University, Tel-Aviv, Israel

YOSHICHIKA ARAKAWA, MD, PhD
Professor, Department of Bacteriology, Nagoya University School of Medicine, Nagoya, Aichi, Japan

CESAR A. ARIAS, MD, MSc, PhD
Associate Professor, Division of Infectious Diseases, Department of Internal Medicine; Associate Professor, Department of Microbiology and Molecular Genetics, University of Texas Medical School at Houston, Houston, Texas; Director, Molecular Genetics and Antimicrobial Resistance Unit, International Center for Microbial Genomics, Universidad El Bosque, Bogota, Colombia

CHARLES M. BARK, MD
Division of Infectious Diseases, Department of Medicine, MetroHealth Medical Center, Case Western Reserve University, Cleveland, Ohio

ROBERT A. BONOMO, MD
Chief of Medical Services, Louis Stokes Cleveland Veterans Affairs Medical Center; Professor, Departments of Medicine, Biochemistry, Pharmacology, Molecular Biology and Microbiology, Case Western Reserve University School of Medicine, Cleveland, Ohio

STAN DERESINSKI, MD
Clinical Professor of Medicine, Division of Infectious Diseases and Geographic Medicine, Stanford University School of Medicine; Medical Director, Stanford Antimicrobial Safety and Sustainability Program, Stanford Health Care, Stanford, California

YOHEI DOI, MD, PhD
Associate Professor of Medicine, Division of Infectious Diseases, University of Pittsburgh School of Medicine, Pittsburgh, Pennsylvania

DONALD M. DUMFORD III, MD
Department of Internal Medicine, Northeast Ohio Medical University, Rootstown; Division of Infectious Diseases, Akron General Medical Center, Akron, Ohio

ANDREA ENDIMIANI, MD, PhD
Professor, Institute for Infectious Diseases, Faculty of Medicine, University of Bern, Bern, Switzerland

THOMAS M. FILE Jr, MD, MSc
Chair, Infectious Disease Division, Summa Health System, Akron, Ohio; Master Teacher; Chair, Infectious Disease Section; Professor, Internal Medicine, Northeast Ohio Medical University (NEOMED), Rootstown, Ohio

JENNIFER J. FURIN, MD, PhD
Department of Global Health and Social Medicine, Harvard Medical School, Boston, Massachusetts

DEBRA A. GOFF, PharmD, FCCP
Infectious Diseases Specialist, Department of Pharmacy; Infectious Diseases Specialty Pharmacist, The Ohio State University Wexner Medical Center; Associate Professor, College of Pharmacy, The Ohio State University, Columbus, Ohio

MARISA HOLUBAR, MD, MS
Clinical Assistant Professor of Medicine, Division of Infectious Diseases and Geographic Medicine, Stanford University School of Medicine; Associate Medical Director, Stanford Antimicrobial Safety and Sustainability Program, Stanford Health Care, Stanford, California

MICHAEL R. JACOBS, MD, PhD
Professor of Pathology and Medicine, Department of Pathology, University Hospitals Case Medical Center, Case Western Reserve University, Cleveland, Ohio

DAVID E. KATZ, MD, MPH
Department of Internal Medicine 'D', Shaare Zedek Medical Center; Hebrew University School of Medicine, Jerusalem, Israel

KEITH S. KAYE, MD, MPH
Department of Medicine, Detroit Medical Center, Wayne State University, Detroit, Michigan

SEBASTIAN G. KURZ, MD, PhD
Division of Pulmonary, Critical Care and Sleep Medicine, Department of Medicine, Tufts University School of Medicine, Boston, Massachusetts

JIAN LI, PhD
Drug Delivery, Disposition and Dynamics, Monash Institute of Pharmaceutical Sciences, Monash University, Melbourne, Australia

DROR MARCHAIM, MD
Sackler School of Medicine, Tel-Aviv University, Tel-Aviv, Israel; Division of Infectious Diseases, Assaf Harofeh Medical Center, Zerifin, Israel

LINA MENG, PharmD
Critical Care Pharmacist, Stanford Health Care; Critical Care and Antimicrobial Stewardship Pharmacist, Department of Pharmacy, Stanford Antimicrobial Safety and Sustainability Program, Stanford Health Care, Stanford, California

WILLIAM R. MILLER, MD
Fellow, Division of Infectious Diseases, Department of Internal Medicine, University of Texas Medical School at Houston, Houston, Texas

BARBARA E. MURRAY, MD
Professor and Director, Division of Infectious Diseases, Department of Internal Medicine; Professor, Department of Microbiology and Molecular Genetics, University of Texas Medical School at Houston, Houston, Texas

ROGER L. NATION, PhD
Drug Delivery, Disposition and Dynamics, Monash Institute of Pharmaceutical Sciences, Monash University, Melbourne, Australia

KRISZTINA M. PAPP-WALLACE, PhD
Research Service, Louis Stokes Cleveland Veterans Affairs Medical Center; Department of Medicine, Case Western Reserve University, Cleveland, Ohio

DAVID L. PATERSON, MBBS, PhD
University of Queensland Centre for Clinical Research, Brisbane, Queensland, Australia

JASON M. POGUE, PharmD
Clinical Pharmacist, Department of Pharmacy Services, Sinai-Grace Hospital; Detroit Medical Center; Wayne State University School of Medicine, Detroit, Michigan

LOUIS B. RICE, MD
Professor and Chairman, Department of Medicine; Professor, Department of Microbiology and Immunology, Warren Alpert Medical School of Brown University, Providence, Rhode Island

MARION SKALWEIT, MD
Louis Stokes Cleveland Veterans Affairs Medical Center; Departments of Medicine and Biochemistry, Case Western Reserve University School of Medicine, Cleveland, Ohio

THIEN B. TRAN, BLabMed(Hons)
Drug Delivery, Disposition and Dynamics, Monash Institute of Pharmaceutical Sciences, Monash University, Melbourne, Australia

DAVID VAN DUIN, MD, PhD
Division of Infectious Diseases, University of North Carolina, Chapel Hill, North Carolina

JUN-ICHI WACHINO, PhD
Assistant Professor, Department of Bacteriology, Nagoya University School of Medicine, Nagoya, Aichi, Japan

RICHARD R. WATKINS, MD, MS, FACP
Associate Professor, Department of Internal Medicine, Northeast Ohio Medical University, Rootstown, Ohio; Division of Infectious Diseases, Cleveland Clinic Akron General Medical Center, Akron, Ohio

[illegible]

RICHARD R. WATKINS, MD, MS, FACP
Associate Professor, Department of Internal Medicine, Northeast Ohio Medical University, Rootstown, Ohio; Division of Infectious Diseases, [illegible] Center, Akron, Ohio

Contents

INFECTIOUS DISEASE CLINICS OF NORTH AMERICA

FORTHCOMING ISSUES

September 2016
Infection Prevention and Control in Healthcare, Part I: Facility Planning and Management
Keith S. Kaye and Sorabh Dhar, *Editors*

December 2016
Infection Prevention and Control in Healthcare, Part II: Management and Prevention of Infections
Keith S. Kaye and Sorabh Dhar, *Editors*

March 2017
Legionnaire's Disease
Cheston B. Cunha and Burke A. Cunha, *Editors*

RECENT ISSUES

March 2016
Fungal Infections
Luis Ostrosky-Zeichner and Jack D. Sobel, *Editors*

December 2015
Pediatric Infectious Disease: Part II
Mary Anne Jackson and Angela L. Myers, *Editors*

September 2015
Pediatric Infectious Disease: Part I
Mary Anne Jackson and Angela L. Myers, *Editors*

RELATED INTEREST

Clinics in Geriatric Medicine, August 2016 (Vol. 32, Issue 3)
Infectious Diseases in Geriatric Medicine
Thomas T. Yoshikawa and Dean C. Norman, *Editors*

Preface

Antibiotic Resistance in the Twenty-First Century: Current Concepts and Future Directions

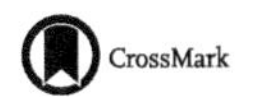

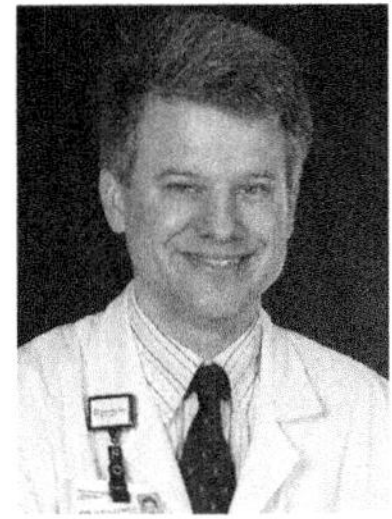

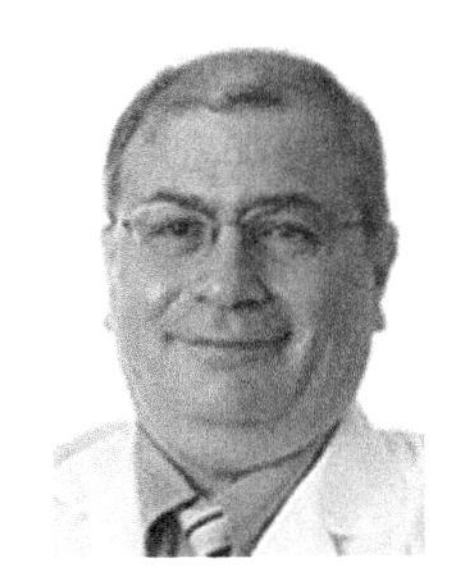

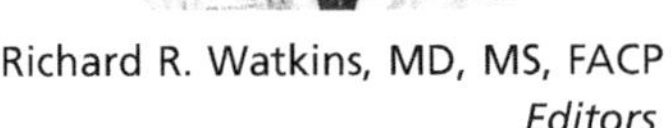

Richard R. Watkins, MD, MS, FACP   Robert A. Bonomo, MD

Editors

Humanity's struggle against infectious diseases was significantly bolstered by the discovery of potent antimicrobial agents in the mid twentieth century. Regrettably, our advantage has been compromised by rising antibiotic resistance. This phenomenon is not new as resistance genes have been present in bacteria for millions of years. However, the spread of antibiotic-resistant pathogens has become an increasing concern because of the potential of untreatable bacterial infections, thus leading to a postantibiotic era. Currently, antibiotic misuse in both agriculture and human medicine is the major modifiable factor driving antibiotic resistance and a crucial threat to global public health. Indeed, some experts have equated the threat posed by antibiotic resistance to be on par with global warming.

For many years, physicians and the public assumed that the discovery of new antimicrobial agents would outpace the ability of bacteria to mutate and develop drug resistance. Yet the development of new antibiotics has not kept up with bacterial evolution, especially since the late 1990s. At that time, a multitude of pharmaceutical companies abandoned antibiotic research because of strong economic disincentives. For example, it is challenging for these companies to recuperate the investment (typically in the hundreds of millions of dollars) made in developing a new antibiotic, which is typically prescribed for a few days, compared to drugs that treat chronic conditions like heart disease or mental illness. This situation has led the US federal government to take a more active lead in addressing antibiotic resistance. Recently, the White House announced an action plan that includes improving surveillance, developing better diagnostic tools, accelerating drug development, and improving global coordination of antibiotic resistance issues. Equally important is the $1.2 billion that has been pledged to fund these efforts.

Infect Dis Clin N Am 30 (2016) xiii–xiv
http://dx.doi.org/10.1016/j.idc.2016.04.001   **id.theclinics.com**

While we await the implementation of new policies, this issue of *Infectious Disease Clinics of North America* brings together leading authorities in the field of antibiotic resistance, who discuss current issues including antibiotic stewardship, the changing role of the microbiology laboratory in determining antibiotic resistance in gram-negative pathogens, the continuing spread of metallo-β-lactamases, extended spectrum beta lactamases (ESBLs) and *Klebsiella* pneumonia carbapenenases (KPCs), antibiotic options for treating resistant gram-negative infections such as colistin and tigecycline, resistance mechanisms and new treatment options for *Mycobacterium tuberculosis*, emerging resistance mechanisms in aminoglycosides, issues with antibiotic resistance in immunocompromised patients, new β-lactamase inhibitors in the clinic, and resistance in vancomycin resistant *Enterococcus* (VRE) and *Staphylococcus aureus*. In addition, combination therapy for resistant gram-negative infections has been advocated by some authorities and the advantages and disadvantages of this strategy are reviewed.

We thank Dr Helen Boucher for inviting us to develop this issue and the editorial staff of *Infectious Disease Clinics of North America* for their assistance. Comments and feedback from the readers are welcome.

Richard R. Watkins, MD, MS, FACP
Cleveland Clinic Akron General Medical Center
224 West Exchange Street, Suite 290
Akron, OH 44302, USA

Robert A. Bonomo, MD
Louis Stokes Cleveland Veterans Affairs Medical Center
Departments of Medicine, Biochemistry, Pharmacology
Molecular Biology and Microbiology
Case Western Reserve University School of Medicine
10701 East Boulevard
Cleveland, OH 44106, USA

E-mail addresses:
richard.watkins@akrongeneral.org (R.R. Watkins)
robert.bonomo@va.gov (R.A. Bonomo)

Overview: Global and Local Impact of Antibiotic Resistance

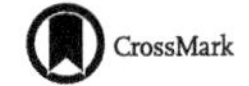

Richard R. Watkins, MD, MS[a,b], Robert A. Bonomo, MD[c,d,e,f,*]

KEYWORDS

- Antibiotic resistance • Infections • Agriculture • Public health

KEY POINTS

- The development and spread of antibiotic resistance (AR) in bacteria is a public health crisis.
- Antibiotic overuse in agriculture has created a large and diverse reservoir of resistant bacteria and resistance genes.
- Unless significant action is taken to turn the tide of AR, the daunting possibility that infections will no longer be treatable with antibiotics may be faced.

INTRODUCTION

The discovery and clinical implementation of antibiotics is one of the greatest achievements in the history of medicine. These miracle drugs treat infections ranging from minor to life threatening, enable surgeons to perform complex procedures in challenging anatomic locations, allow organ transplantation to be feasible, and empower oncologists to give higher doses of chemotherapy for cancer, thereby increasing the chance for cure. The global dissemination of AR bacteria, however, is threatening to undo all these advances and cause a return to the preantibiotic era.

Disclosures: R.R. Watkins has received grant support from the Akron General Foundation and Forest Laboratories. R.A. Bonomo has received grant support from AstraZeneca, Melinda, and Steris. R.A. Bonomo is also supported by grants from the National Institutes of Health, the Merit Review Program of the Veterans Health Administration, and the Harrington Foundation.
[a] Division of Infectious Diseases, Cleveland Clinic Akron General Medical Center, 224 West Exchange Street, Suite 290, Akron, OH 44302, USA; [b] Department of Internal Medicine, Northeast Ohio Medical University, Rootstown, OH, USA; [c] Medicine and Research Services, Louis Stokes Cleveland, Department of Veterans Affairs Medical Center, 10701 East Boulevard, Cleveland, OH 44106, USA; [d] Department of Medicine, Case Western Reserve University School of Medicine, Cleveland, OH, USA; [e] Department of Pharmacology, Case Western Reserve University School of Medicine, Cleveland, OH, USA; [f] Department of Molecular Biology and Microbiology, Case Western Reserve University School of Medicine, Cleveland, OH, USA
* Corresponding author. Department of Medicine, Case Western Reserve University School of Medicine, Cleveland, OH.
E-mail address: robert.bonomo@va.gov

http://dx.doi.org/10.1016/j.idc.2016.02.001

Approximately 2 million infections from AR bacteria occur annually in the United States, resulting in 23,000 deaths.[1] Moreover, these infections cause an increased risk of hospitalization and complications.[2] AR is an inevitable evolutionary outcome because all organisms develop genetic mutations to avoid lethal selective pressure (**Fig. 1**). As long as antibiotics are used against them, bacteria will continue to develop and use resistance mechanisms.[3] More than 70% of pathogenic bacteria are resistant to at least 1 antibiotic.[4] Notably, a recent survey of infectious diseases physicians in the United States found that 60% had encountered a bacterial infection resistant to available drugs in the previous year.[5]

AR is a complicated process that is driven by multiple factors (**Box 1**). Despite the global spread of AR, regulatory approval of new antibiotics has declined 90% during the past 30 years in the United States.[6] In addition to the high cost of antibiotic research and development, the rapid evolution of AR has meant diminished market returns for the pharmaceutical industry.[7] After many years out of the mainstream, the serious threat posed by AR has been increasingly recognized by the media and governmental organizations. For example, in September 2014, the White House proposed the National Strategy for Combating Antibiotic-Resistant Bacteria.[8] Herein, President Obama charged Congress with designing a research agenda to combat AR on multiple fronts.

The Centers for Disease Control and Prevention has prepared a list of AR bacteria in the United States that are of most concern (**Box 2**). Of these threats, the spread of AR gram-negative bacilli (GNB) is arguably the most worrisome. This is because of limited treatment options, the ease of plasmid-mediated transfer of resistance genes among GNB, the widespread distribution of Enterobacteriaceae as part of the human microbiome, the asymptomatic colonization present in certain individuals, and higher mortality associated with carbapenem-resistant Enterobacteriaceae compared with susceptible strains.[9] Moreover, risk factors have been identified for acquiring AR-GNB and include recent antibiotic usage, residence in extended care facilities, admission to an ICU, having an indwelling device or wounds, poor functional status, organ or stem cell transplantation, and travel to an endemic area.[10]

Of the drug classes to which AR can emerge, the most problematic is against the β-lactams. These are among the safest and most potent of antibiotics. β-lactam resistance in GNB is primarily acquired through plasmids that contain β-lactamases; β-lactamases are classified into 4 main groups based on their amino acid sequences (classes A, B, C, and D).[11] Class A includes extended-spectrum β-lactamases (ESBLs) and *Klebsiella pneumoniae* carbapenemase enzymes, class B enzymes are the metallo-β-lactamases, class C enzymes are the cephalosporinases, and class D enzymes are oxacillinases. Recently it was recognized that *Acinetobacter baumannii*, although often considered a less virulent pathogen compared with *K pneumoniae* and *Pseudomonas aeruginosa*, plays a significant role in spreading broad-spectrum resistance genes to other gram-negative organisms.[12]

EVOLUTION OF ANTIBIOTIC RESISTANCE

The first effective antimicrobial agent, sulfonamide, was introduced in 1937. Within 2 years, sulfonamide resistance was reported and the same AR mechanisms are still clinically present more than 70 years later.[13] One useful way of understanding the basic mechanisms of AR is through the bullet and target concept, whereby the sites of drug activity (the target) can be changed by enzymatic modification, transformed by genomic mutations, and bypassed metabolically (eg, sulfonamide resistance);

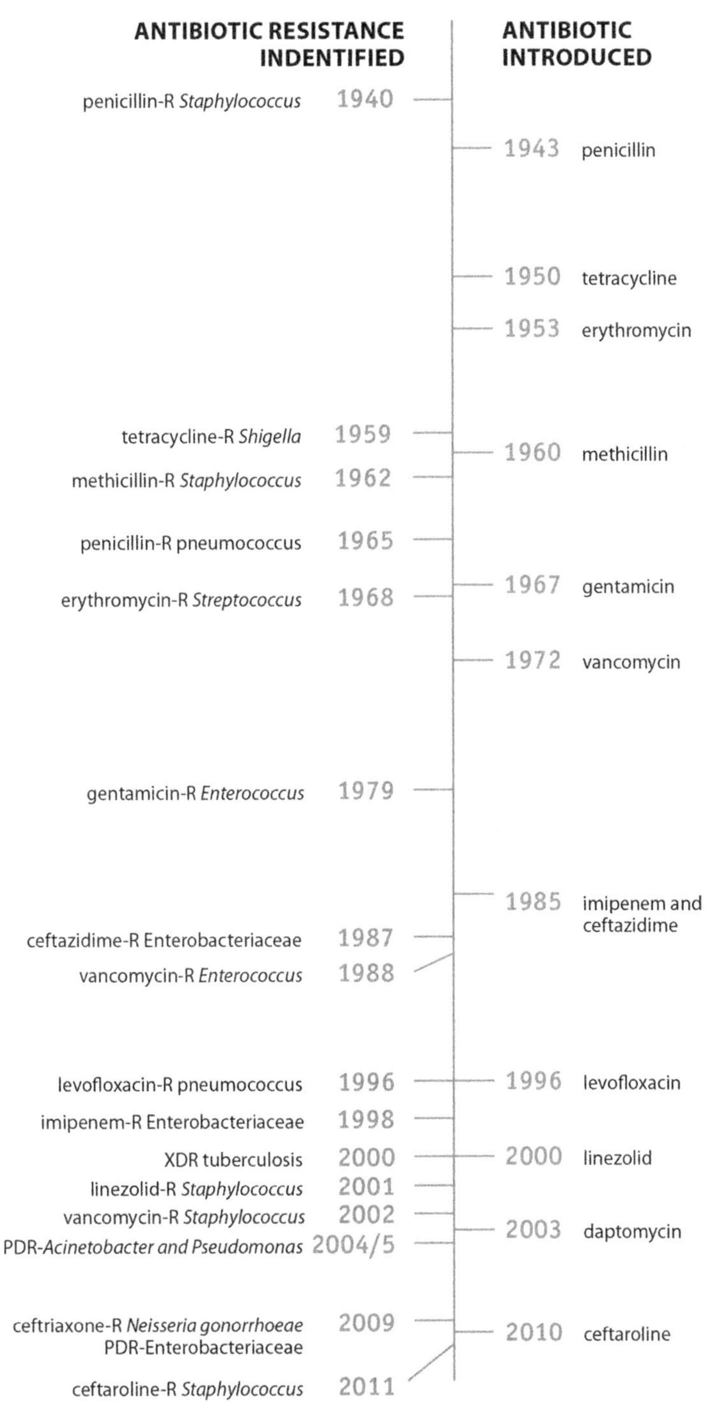

Fig. 1. Antibiotic timeline. PDR, penicillin drug resistant; R, resistant; XDR, extremely drug resistant. (*From* Centers for Disease Control and Prevention. Antibiotic/antimicrobial resistance. Available at: http://www.cdc.gov/drugresistance/about.html. Accessed March 3, 2016.)

Box 1
Factors that promote antibiotic resistance

- Bacterial population density in health care facilities; allows transfer of bacteria within a community and enables resistance to emerge
- Inadequate adherence to best infection control practices
- Increase of high risk patient populations (eg, chemotherapy, dialysis, and transplant patients and patients residing in long-term care facilities)
- Antibiotic overuse in agriculture
- Global travel and tourism (including medical tourism)
- Poor sanitation and contaminated water systems; can lead to the spread of resistant bacteria in sewage
- Improper antibiotic prescribing in human medicine (eg, for viral infections or for inappropriately long courses of therapy)
- Overprescription of broad-spectrum antibiotics; can exert selective pressure on commensal bacteria
- Paucity of rapid diagnostic tests to guide proper antibiotic prescribing
- Lack of approved vaccines for drug-resistant pathogens

Adapted from National Institute of Allergy and Infectious Diseases. NIAID's antibacterial resistance program: current status and future directions. 2014. Available at: http://www.niaid.nih.gov/topics/antimicrobialResistance/documents/arstrategicplan2014.pdf. Accessed March 3, 2016.

the antibiotic (the bullet) can undergo enzymatic inactivation and degradation (eg, β-lactamases), reduced access into the cell (eg, porin loss), and increased removal from the cell (eg, efflux pumps).[14,15]

There is emerging evidence that resistance mechanisms in *Mycobacterium tuberculosis* (MTb), one of the oldest and most widespread human pathogens, are induced by mutations caused by subinhibitory concentrations of antibiotics.[16] Patients with MTb who previously received quinolone antibiotics developed resistance to both this antibiotic class as well as to first-line anti-MTb drugs.[17] These data show a strong and direct correlation between the use of antibiotics and resistance.

One example of contemporary evolution in resistance mechanisms is *Salmonella* Typhi. Before the antimicrobial era, typhoid fever exacted a 20% mortality rate, which was significantly reduced with the introduction of effective therapy. Fluoroquinolones became the agents of choice in the 1990s, but 1 lineage of *Salmonella* with reduced susceptibility has widely disseminated.[18] Unfortunately efforts to develop novel therapies against *Salmonella* Typhi are minimal.[19] Thus, we are on the verge of widespread resistance with few effective alternatives for typhoid fever, raising the possibility of a return to the preantibiotic era for this disease.[20]

Although AR has traditionally been identified as a nosocomial problem, the impact of the environment is increasingly recognized. Certain environmental compartments (municipal wastewater systems, pharmaceutical manufacturing effluents, and agricultural waste products) are characterized by extremely high concentrations of bacteria coupled with subtherapeutic concentrations of antibiotics, leading to the discharge of AR bacteria and AR genes into the wider environment.[21] For example, river sediment downstream from a waste water treatment plant had 10 novel combinations of cephalosporin-resistance genes as well as an imipenem-resistant *Escherichia coli*.[22] Uncertainty exists as to whether AR genes that are acquired by both clinically relevant

Box 2
Antibiotic-resistant bacteria of concern in the United States

Urgent threat level

Clostridium difficile

Carbapenem-resistant Enterobacteriaceae

Drug-resistant *Neisseria gonorrhoeae*

Serious threat level

Multidrug-resistant *Acinetobacter*

Drug-resistant *Campylobacter*

ESBL-producing Enterobacteriaceae

Vancomycin-resistant *Enterococcus*

Multidrug-resistant *Pseudomonas*

Drug-resistant *Salmonella*

Drug-resistant *Shigella*

MRSA

Drug-resistant *Streptococcus pneumoniae*

Drug-resistant tuberculosis

Concerning threat level

Vancomycin-resistant *S aureus*

Erythromycin-resistant group A *Streptococcus*

Clindamycin-resistant group B *Streptococcus*

Adapted from Centers for Disease Control and Prevention. Antibiotic resistance threats in the United States. 2013. Available at: http://www.cdc.gov/drugresistance/threat-report-2013/pdf/ar-threats-2013-508.pdf. Accessed March 3, 2016.

bacteria and nonpathogenic ones in the environment originate from the same sources. Furthermore, the role of environmental bacterial in spreading AR genes to nosocomial pathogens is unknown. Finding answers to these questions should be paramount due to the global scale of AR.

ANTIBIOTICS AND AGRICULTURE

Recently, the use of antibiotics in agriculture has come under increasing scrutiny. More than 13 million kilograms of antibiotics are used annually in agriculture, approximately 80% of the antibiotics consumed in the United States.[23] Most of this usage is not for treating disease in animals (livestock) but for growth promotion and disease prevention, usually at subtherapeutic concentrations. Chang and colleagues[24] have suggested 3 mechanisms by which AR in agriculture could threaten human health: (1) a human is infected by a resistant pathogen through contact with livestock or through ingestion of bacteria from contaminated food or water; (2) a human becomes colonized by resistant bacteria through one of these means, then spreads it to another person who subsequently becomes ill; (3) resistance genes arising in agriculture are spread to humans through horizontal gene transfer and the resulting resistant strains are selected by antibiotic use in people. Evidence suggests several strains of pathogens that infect humans have originated from animals, including stains of AR *Campylobacter* spp,[25] *Salmonella* spp,[26] methicillin-resistant *Staphylococcus aureus* (MRSA),[27] vancomycin-resistant *Enterococcus*,[28] ESBL-producing Enterobacteriaceae,[29] and carbapenem-resistant Enterobacteriaceae.[30] The transfer of resistance determinants from animals to humans, however, is difficult to trace and the role of these animal reservoirs in clinical AR has not been adequately elucidated.

Given the link between AR and antibiotic use in farm animals, a possible solution is to ban antibiotics. The European Union banned all nontherapeutic antibiotics in animals in 2006 and the Food and Drug Administration issued a policy in 2012 asking farmers to voluntarily decrease their use of antibiotics. Theoretically, antibiotic selection pressure should be reduced by a ban leading to less resistant organisms in the environment, although evidence for this is lacking. For example, a clinical decline in ciprofloxacin resistance was observed after the 2005 ban of fluoroquinolones in poultry.[31] Despite the paucity of definitive data, a better argument for restricting antibiotics in agriculture may be to reduce the prevalence of resistant pathogens and, thereby, lower the chances for horizontal transfer of resistance genes.

Significant challenges exist for banning antibiotics in agriculture in the United States. Given the wide geographic distribution of farms, regulatory oversight would likely be difficult to enforce. Also, it could be problematic to clearly know what the antibiotics were being used for, such as treating sick animals versus prophylaxis against infections. Conceivably, some farmers might try to game the system and continue their old antibiotic practices. The additional costs to farmers in terms of lost productivity would be passed on to consumers in the form of higher food prices. Thus, strategies other than a ban are needed to reduce antibiotic usage. One proposed alternative is to impose a user fee. According to Hollis and Ahmed,[23] a user fee would be easier to administer because it could be collected at the manufacturing stage, would discourage low-value uses of antibiotics, would generate revenues that could help pay for new antibiotic development by the pharmaceutical industry or support antimicrobial stewardship efforts, and could encourage governments to collaborate, such as signing treaties to collect revenue generated by the user fees.[23] Further consideration of antibiotic user fees by US governmental agencies seems warranted.

SOCIETAL BURDEN OF ANTIBIOTIC RESISTANCE

The economic impact of AR is enormous. Overall, AR is estimated to cost $55 billion in the United States annually.[32] Moreover, an infection by an ESBL-producing *E coli* or *Klebsiella* spp was shown to increase hospitalization costs by $16,450 and add an additional 9.7 days to the length of stay.[33] The high costs of AR are not limited to industrialized countries. Novel AR genes disproportionately originate in lower-income countries, with downstream impact on both the originating country and in those outside the region.[18] For example, the New Delhi metallo-β-lactamase-1 was first identified in a strain of *K pneumoniae* from a Swedish patient who had returned from India.[34] Regarding the health impact of AR, the World Health Organization (WHO) reported a significant increase in all-cause mortality and 30-day mortality from infections caused by third-generation cephalosporin-resistant (including ESBL) and fluoroquinolone-resistant *E coli* as well as third-generation cephalosporin-resistant and carbapenem-resistant *K pneumoniae*.[35] MRSA infections lead to significant increases in all-cause mortality, bacterium-attributable mortality, ICU mortality, septic shock, length of stay and a 2-fold risk increase for discharge to long-term care compared with methicillin-sensitive *S aureus*.[36] Thus, the management of MRSA imposes important economic costs to health care organizations, although there is a scarcity of definitive evidence available to allow for a comprehensive evaluation of the economic burden. Also lacking are studies on the economic implications of changes in MRSA epidemiology, such as infections in patients who acquire MRSA from farm animals.[36]

WHAT CAN BE DONE TO AVERT A POSTANTIBIOTIC ERA?

Although identifying and developing new drugs is a potential solution to the AR problem, this is a costly and complicated endeavor. Therefore, alternative strategies are necessary, particularly in low-income countries. An important and effective way to limit the spread of AR is to reduce the consumption of antibiotics. In 2004, Bergman and colleagues[37] showed that regional macrolide use was closely associated with erythromycin resistance in *Streptococcus pyogenes*. Reducing antibiotics is one of the central tenets of antibiotic stewardship, now universally recognized as beneficial.[38] For example, a stewardship program from a Swedish university hospital decreased antibiotic usage by 27% without any negative impact on patient outcomes, primarily by limiting broad-spectrum agents.[39] However, reducing antibiotic consumption alone is not a panacea for stopping AR, which requires a multifaceted approach.

Recently, the World Alliance Against Antibiotic Resistance put forward a declaration that included 10 proposals for tackling AR.[40] Several of them (eg, more rapid diagnostic tests, antibiotic stewardship, and surveillance networks) were not new ideas but nonetheless are widely recognized as beneficial. Therefore, the value of the declaration is that it convincingly and authoritatively conveys the recommendations through a global perspective. One important concept in the document that deserves emphasis is the pressing need for a national surveillance mechanism in the United States. Currently there are several public databases and global surveillance projects, including *Antimicrobial Resistance: Global Report on Surveillance*, from the WHO; the European Antimicrobial Resistance Interactive Database; the Surveillance Network database in the United States and Australia; and the global Study for Monitoring Antimicrobial Resistance Trends. In 2002, this last study began to monitor in vitro resistance of GNB in intra-abdominal infections and more recently has focused on resistance to carbapenems and ESBLs.[41] What remains lacking is an integrated database that links data on resistance in environmental bacteria to existing databases on AR bacteria and AR genes in clinical, veterinary, and food-associated products.[21]

Despite increasing media attention, the general public largely remains unaware of the threat posed by AR. Of concern, a recent global survey conducted by the WHO found that even in countries where national antibiotic awareness programs had been conducted, there was still widespread belief that antibiotics were effective against viral illnesses.[42] Certainly better educational efforts are needed. Another disconcerting finding from the report was the widespread practice of antibiotics available without a prescription.[42] This undoubtedly leads to overconsumption, especially among commonly used drugs in low-income settings (eg, fluoroquinolones to treat viral illnesses where typhoid fever is endemic). Changing antibiotics to prescription status will require strong government action, which is also necessary to make improvements in infrastructure and to provide better access to health care providers and laboratory facilities.

SUMMARY

AR can only be tackled through a comprehensive approach that includes drug discovery and development, sustainable antibiotic usage policies, and disease prevention strategies, like improving sanitation in low-income countries, infection control practices in hospitals, and better diagnostic testing. The majority of the political will and necessary resources must come from high-income countries. AR is a complicated global threat that requires cooperation across a multitude of organizations and political boundaries. To quote Henry Ford, "coming together is a beginning, keeping together is progress, and working together is success."

REFERENCES

1. Centers for Disease Control and Prevention. Antibiotic resistance threats in the United States. 2013. Available at: http://www.cdc.gov/drugresistance/threat-report-2013/pdf/ar-threats-2013-508.pdf. Accessed March 3, 2016.
2. Livermore D. Current epidemiology and growing resistance of gram-negative pathogens. Korean J Intern Med 2012;27:128–42.
3. National Institute of Allergy and Infectious Diseases. NIAID's Antibacterial resistance program: current status and future directions. 2014. Available at: http://www.niaid.nih.gov/topics/antimicrobialResistance/documents/arstrategicplan2014.pdf. Accessed March 3, 2016.
4. Katz ML, Mueller LV, Polyakov M, et al. Where have all the antibiotic patents gone? Nat Biotechnol 2006;24:1529–31.
5. Hersh AL, Newland JG, Beekmann SE, et al. Unmet medical need in infectious diseases. Clin Infect Dis 2012;54:1677–8.
6. Shlaes DM, Sahm D, Opiela C, et al. The FDA reboot of antibiotic development. Antimicrobial Agents Chemother 2013;57:4605–7.
7. Payne DJ, Gwynn MD, Holmes DJ, et al. Drugs for bad bugs: confronting the challenges of antibiotic discovery. Nat Rev Drug Discov 2007;6:29–40.
8. Obama B. National strategy for combating antibiotic-resistant bacteria. Washington, DC: White House; 2014. p. 1–33.
9. Vasoo S, Barreto JN, Tosh PK. Emerging issues in gram-negative bacterial resistance: an update for the practicing clinician. Mayo Clin Proc 2015;90:395–403.
10. Tzouvelekis LS, Markogiannakis A, Psichogiou M, et al. Carbapenemases in Klebsiella pneumoniae and other Enterobacteriaceae: an evolving crisis of global dimensions. Clin Microbiol Rev 2012;25:682–707.
11. Hall BG, Barlow M. Revised Ambler classification of beta-lactamases. J Antimicrob Chemother 2005;55:1050–1.
12. Potron A, Poirel L, Nordmann P. Emerging broad-spectrum resistance to Pseudomonas aeruginosa and Acinetobacter baumannii: mechanisms and epidemiology. Int J Antimicrob Agents 2015;45(6):568–85.
13. Davies J, Davies D. Origins and evolution of antibiotic resistance. Microbiol Mol Biol Rev 2010;77:417–33.
14. Aminov RI. A brief history of the antibiotic era: lessons learned and challenges for the future. Front Microbiol 2010;1:134.
15. Tang SS, Apisarnthanarak A, Hsu LY. Mechanisms of β-lactam antimicrobial resistance and epidemiology of major community- and healthcare-associated multidrug-resistant bacteria. Adv Drug Deliv Rev 2014;78:3–13.
16. Fonseca JD, Knight GM, McHugh TD. The complex evolution of antibiotic resistance in Mycobacterium tuberculosis. Int J Infect Dis 2015;32:94–100.
17. Deutschendorf C, Goldani LZ, Santos RP. Previous use of quinolones: a surrogate marker for first line anti-tuberculosis drugs resistance in HIV-infected patients? Braz J Infect Dis 2012;16:142–5.

18. Kariuki S, Revathi G, Kiiru J, et al. Typhoid in Kenya is associated with a dominant multidrug-resistant Salmonella enterica serovar Typhi haplotype that is also widespread in Southeast Asia. J Clin Microbiol 2010;48:2171–6.
19. Baker S. A return to the pre-antimicrobial era? Science 2015;347:1064–6.
20. Koirala KD, Thanh DP, Thapa SD, et al. Highly resistant Salmonella enterica serovar Typhi with a novel gyrA mutation raises questions about the long-term efficacy of older fluoroquinolones for treating typhoid fever. Antimicrob Agents Chemother 2012;56:2761–2.
21. Berendonk TU, Manaia CM, Merlin C, et al. Tackling antibiotic resistance: the environmental framework. Nat Rev Microbiol 2015;13:310–7.
22. Amos GCA, Hawkey PM, Gaze WH, et al. Waste water effluent contributes to the dissemination of CTX-M-15 in the natural environment. J Antimicrob Chemother 2014;69:1785–91.
23. Hollis A, Ahmed Z. Preserving antibiotics, rationally. N Engl J Med 2013;369:2474–6.
24. Chang Q, Wang W, Regev-Yochay G, et al. Antibiotics in agriculture and the risk to human health: how worried should we be? Evol Appl 2015;8:240–7.
25. Travers K, Barza M. Morbidity of infections caused by antimicrobial-resistant bacteria. Clin Infect Dis 2002;34(Suppl 3):S131–4.
26. Brunelle BW, Bearson BL, Bearson SM. Chloramphenicol and tetracycline decrease motility and increase invasion and attachment gene expression in specific isolates of multi-drug resistant Salomella enterica serovar Typhimurium. Front Microbiol 2015;5:801.
27. Van der Mee-Marquet N, Francois P, Domelier-Valentin AS, et al. Emergence of unusual bloodstream infections associated with pig-borne-like Staphylococcus aureus ST398 in France. Clin Infect Dis 2011;52:152–3.
28. Lebreton F, van Schaik W, McGuire AM, et al. Emergence of epidemic multi-drug-resistant Enterococcus faecium from animal and commensal strains. MBio 2013;4 [pii:e00534-13].
29. Reich F, Atanassova V, Klein G. Extended-spectrum β-lactamase- and AmpC-producing enterobacteria in healthy broiler chickens, Germany. Emerg Infect Dis 2013;19:1253–9.
30. Wang Y, Wu C, Zhang Q, et al. Identification of New Delhi metallo-β-lactamase 1 in Acinetobacter lwoffii of food animal origin. PLoS One 2012;7:e37152.
31. Nannapaneni R, Hanning I, Wiggins KC, et al. Ciprofloxacin-resistant Campylobacter persists in raw retail chicken after the fluoroquinolone ban. Food Addit Contam Part A Chem Anal Control Expo Risk Assess 2009;26:1348–53.
32. Smith R, Coast J. The true cost of antimicrobial resistance. BMJ 2013;346:f1493.
33. Lee SY, Kotapati S, Kuti JL, et al. Impact of extended-spectrum beta-lactamase-producing Escherichia coli and Klebsiella species on clinical outcomes and hospital costs: a matched cohort study. Infect Control Hosp Epidemiol 2006;27:1226–32.
34. Walsh TR, Weeks J, Livermore DM, et al. Dissemination of NDM-1 positive bacteria in the New Delhi environment and its implications for human health: an environmental point prevalence study. Lancet Infect Dis 2011;11:355–62.
35. World Health Organization. Antimicrobial resistance: global report on surveillance. Geneva (Switzerland): WHO; 2014.
36. Antonanzas F, Lozano C, Torres C. Economic features of antibiotic resistance: the case of methicillin-resistant Staphylococcus aureus. Pharmacoeconomics 2015; 33:285–325.
37. Bergman M, Huikko S, Pihlajamäki M, et al. Effect of macrolide consumption on erythromycin resistance in Streptococcus pyogenes in Finland in 1997-2001. Clin Infect Dis 2004;38:1251–6.

38. Livermore DM. Of stewardship, motherhood and apple pie. Int J Antimicrob Agents 2014;43:319–22.
39. Nilholm H, Holmstrand L, Ahl J, et al. An audit-based, infectious disease specialist-guided antimicrobial stewardship program profoundly reduced antibiotic use without negatively affecting patient outcomes. Open Forum Infect Dis 2015;2(2):ofv042.
40. Claret J. The world alliance against antibiotic resistance: consensus for a declaration. Clin Infect Dis 2015;60(12):1837–41.
41. Morrissey I, Hackel M, Badal R, et al. A review of ten years of study for monitoring antimicrobial resistance trends (SMART) from 2002 to 2011. Pharmaceuticals (Basel) 2013;6:1335–46.
42. World Health Organization. Worldwide country situation analysis: response to antimicrobial resistance. Geneva (Switzerland): WHO; 2015.

The Changing Role of the Clinical Microbiology Laboratory in Defining Resistance in Gram-negatives

Andrea Endimiani, MD, PhD[a,*], Michael R. Jacobs, MD, PhD[b]

KEYWORDS

- AST • PCR • Real time • LAMP • Microarray • MALDI-TOF • Sequencing • Rapid

KEY POINTS

- Antimicrobial resistance in Gram-negatives is a major challenge.
- Multidrug-resistant strains, including carbapenem-resistant strains, are increasing.
- More rapid methods are needed.
- Considerable advances have been made with rapid genotypic methods.
- Advances have also been made with rapid phenotypic methods.

INTRODUCTION

The role of the clinical microbiology laboratory in defining resistance in Gram-negatives has been challenged by the evolution of resistance to antimicrobial agents because we are no longer able to rely on the efficacy of the empiric use of "broad-spectrum" agents. In particular, development and spread of extended-spectrum β-lactamases (ESBLs; eg, CTX-Ms) and carbapenemases have presented major challenges. The mutation of narrow-spectrum β-lactamases (which degrade penicillins) into ESBLs (which add cephalosporins and monobactams to their spectrum) has limited the activity of advanced generation cephalosporins. Acquisition of carbapenemases such as KPC, NDM, IMP, and VIM results in resistance to virtually all available β-lactams in common use. Moreover, these strains are frequently resistant to many other drug classes, rendering them resistant to typical empiric therapy combinations.[1–3]

Disclosure Statement: The authors do not have any commercial or financial conflicts of interest. A. Endimiani is supported by the Swiss National Science Foundation (project No.: 32003B_153377) and SwissTransMed (project: Rapid Diagnosis of Antibiotic Resistance in Gonorrhea, Radar-Go).
[a] Institute for Infectious Diseases, Faculty of Medicine, University of Bern, Friedbühlstrasse 51, Bern CH-3010, Switzerland; [b] Department of Pathology, University Hospitals Case Medical Center, Case Western Reserve University, 11100 Euclid Avenue, Cleveland, OH 44106, USA
* Corresponding author.
E-mail addresses: andrea.endimiani@ifik.unibe.ch; aendimiani@gmail.com

Infect Dis Clin N Am 30 (2016) 323–345
http://dx.doi.org/10.1016/j.idc.2016.02.002
id.theclinics.com

These challenges have led to the realization of the need for more rapid diagnosis, particularly of bloodstream infections, and for more rapid antimicrobial susceptibility testing (AST). A mean decrease in survival of 7.6% for each hour after onset of infection until effective antibiotics are administered has been reported, as well as a 5-fold increase in mortality when inappropriate antimicrobials were administered within 6 hours after recognition of septic shock.[4] Recent studies have also documented the value of more rapid diagnosis, which allows earlier appropriate, targeted antimicrobial use.[5] This has been shown to improve patient outcomes, lower mortality, decrease hospital length of stay, lower superinfection and adverse drug reaction rates, and decrease costs.

Although the rapid detection of bacteria and their resistance mechanisms directly from blood specimens is still an elusive target, this has been achieved on growing blood cultures, which typically become positive after 18 to 24 hours of incubation. Many systems for rapid bacterial identification from growing blood cultures have been developed, such as fluorescence in situ hybridization (FISH) tests, mass spectroscopy (MS), and automated polymerase chain reaction (PCR) systems.[6] Many of these systems can also detect antimicrobial resistance genes. For instance, a recent study of an automated molecular system documented the value of one such system, the Verigene Gram-negative blood culture nucleic acid test (BC-GN; Nanosphere), a multiplex, automated test for the identification of 8 Gram-negative organisms and 6 resistance markers from blood cultures with a turnaround time (TAT) of approximately 2 hours. The test correctly identified 95.6% of isolates and detected CTX-M and OXA resistance determinants, with an intervention group having a significantly shorter duration to both effective (3.3 vs 7.0 h; *P*<.01) and optimal (23.5 vs 41.8 h; *P*<.01) antibiotic therapy.[7]

AVAILABLE METHODS

Standard Antimicrobial Susceptibility Test Methods

Conventional AST procedures have been in use for many decades and follow methods and interpretations of various organizations such as European Committee on Antimicrobial Susceptibility Testing and Clinical and Laboratory Standards Institute,[8,9] as well as regulatory agencies such as US Food and Drug Administration and European Agency for the Evaluation of Medicinal Products. These organizations and agencies have established "reference" AST methods based on minimum inhibitory concentration (MIC) determination by microdilution and agar dilution, with incubation times ranging from 18 to 48 hours. Disk diffusion methods have also been standardized by these groups.

Many commercial methods for AST are available and are based on using these reference methods directly, or by methods correlated to reference methods and providing comparable results. Commercial methods using reference microdilution methods include MicroScan WalkAway (Siemens Healthcare Diagnostics, Erlangen, Germany) and Sensititre (Trek Diagnostic Systems, Independence, OH). Methods providing results comparable with reference testing include gradient diffusion MIC determination (Etest), Vitek (bioMérieux, Marcy l'Etoile, France), Phoenix (BD Diagnostic Systems, Franklin Lake, NJ), as well as rapid versions of MicroScan and Sensititre. Several of the methods have faster TAT than reference methods, and many are automated with machine-generated results. Instruments that record and interpret disk diffusion zone are also available (eg, BIOMIC V3, Giles Scientific, Santa Barbara, CA; ADAGIO, Bio-Rad, Hercules, CA; Scan 1200, Interscience, Boston MA; SirSCAN, i2a Diagnostics, Montpellier Cedex 2, France).

These reference AST methods also include methods for determination of resistance mechanisms, such as the presence of ESBLs in some *Enterobacteriaceae* using cefotaxime and ceftazidime alone and combined with clavulanate, and the presence of carbapenemases in *Enterobacteriaceae* using lowered carbapenem breakpoints and the modified Hodge test.[8] Many commercial AST systems incorporate these methods and many other tests for detection of these resistance mechanisms are available commercially and are discussed.

Rapid Biochemical Tests to Detect Extended-spectrum β-Lactamase and Carbapenemase Producers

The ESBL NDP test is a rapid (from 15 min to 1 h) and cost-effective biochemical test used to detect ESBL producers. It is based on the recognition of cefotaxime hydrolysis that is inhibited by tazobactam. ESBL production is evidenced by a color change (red to yellow) of the pH indicator phenol red owing to acid formation resulting from cefotaxime hydrolysis that is reversed by adding tazobactam. Its sensitivity and specificity for detecting ESBL-producing *Enterobacteriaceae* are 93% and 100%, respectively.[10] The test has been evaluated on blood culture and urine samples, showing excellent sensitivity and specificity (>98% and >99%, respectively).[10–12]

The Carba NP test was specifically designed to detect carbapenemase producers. It detects a change in pH owing to the hydrolysis of imipenem in presence of carbapenemase enzymes in less than 2 hours. Without the need for any particular equipment, β-lactamases are rapidly extracted from bacterial cells and then incubated with imipenem and phenol red.[10,13,14] This test demonstrated an excellent ability to detect different classes of carbapenemases (eg, KPC, GES, NDM, VIM, IMP, and OXA-48) in *Enterobacteriaceae*, *Pseudomonas* spp., and *Acinetobacter* spp.,[10,13–16] although some concerns regarding the low sensitivity for OXA-48–like carbapenemase producers have arisen.[17–20] The test has also been directly implemented on positive blood cultures with carbapenemase-producing *Enterobacteriaceae* and *Pseudomonas* spp., demonstrating a sensitivity and specificity of greater than 98% and 100%, respectively.[21,22] Notably, the Carba NP test is recommended for the confirmation of carbapenemase production in Gram-negatives by the Clinical and Laboratory Standards Institute.[8] Recently, this test became available commercially in an easy-to-use rapid kit (RAPIDEC Carba NP test; bioMérieux).[23]

The Blue-Carba test is another biochemical assay for carbapenemase production, using a different indicator (bromothymol blue) and a simplified protocol compared with the Carba NP test. The main advantage of this test is its faster TAT, because there is no need to extract the β-lactamase from colonies.[24] Overall, the Blue-Carba test shows comparable performance to the Carba NP test, but it seems to have better sensitivity, especially for OXA-type carbapenemases.[24] A commercially available version (Rapid CARB Screen; Rosco Diagnostics, Stamford, CT) has shown similar sensitivity (97% vs 98%), but superior specificity (100% vs 83%) compared with the Carba NP test during an evaluation with *Enterobacteriaceae* producing different classes of carbapenemases.[25] In contrast, in another comparison the Carba NP test had sensitivities of 91% for *Enterobacteriaceae* and 100% *Pseudomonas aeruginosa*, whereas those for the Rapid CARB Screen kit were 73% and 67%, respectively; the specificity of both tests was 100%. The cost of reagents for performing Carba NP test was 0.31 Euro and for CARB Screen was 1.25 Euro.[26]

Single and Multiplex Endpoint Polymerase Chain Reactions

The single PCR is advantageous if the detection of a single gene, such as KPC, is sufficient.[27] However, for specific gene characterization, DNA sequencing is frequently necessary (eg, distinguishing SHV mutations with ESBL spectrum from those with non-ESBL activity). PCR also requires a high copy number of the target gene to produce a detectable amplification product.[28] Results can be obtained in less than 3 to 4 hours for simple amplification to 24 hours or longer (for determination of DNA sequences). Examples of single PCRs designed to detect antibiotic resistance genes include detection of CTX-M,[29,30] TEM, SHV,[31] KPC,[32] IMP, VIM,[33] NDM,[34] Qnr,[35] aminoglycoside modifying enzymes,[36] and outer membrane porin genes.[37]

The multiplex endpoint PCRs use multiple primer sets allowing the simultaneous amplification of different targets in the same reaction.[38] Numerous multiplex PCRs able to detect resistance genes have been proposed. One paradigmatic example is the multiplex reaction designed by Perez-Perez and Hanson to detect the plasmid-mediated AmpC (pAmpC) genes with a total time from primary incubation to test results of about 3 hours.[39] Voets and colleagues[40] presented a design to simultaneously detect different families of ESBLs (SHV, TEM, CTX-M, GES, PER, VEB). Doyle and colleagues[41] designed a multiplex reaction for the concurrent detection of KPC, NDM, VIM, IMP, and OXA-48–like carbapenemase genes. Cattoir and colleagues[42] designed a multiplex reaction for the detection of different *qnr* genes. Berçot and colleagues[43] developed a protocol for the detection of 16S rRNA methylase genes.

Recently, Amplex Diagnostics (Giessen, Germany) has designed 3 commercial kits combining PCR and enzyme-linked immunosorbent assay reactions to rapidly detect (2.5–4 h) *bla* genes. In particular, hyplex ESBL ID, hyplex SuperBug ID, and hyplex CarbOXA ID detect, respectively: (i) TEM, SHV, CTX-M, and OXA; (ii) KPC, IMP, VIM, NDM, and OXA-48–like; and (iii) OXA-23, OXA-24/40, OXA-51–like genes. Hyplex SuperBug ID showed a 97% agreement with the standard PCR/sequencing.[44,45] In another study, the combination of hyplex ESBL ID and hyplex SuperBug ID was able to detect all class A and B enzymes among *Enterobacteriaceae* with high sensitivity (100%) and specificity (98%).[46] Curetis AG has industrialized the Unyvero pneumonia assay, a fully automated multiplex PCR platform to identify 18 species and 22 resistance genes, including SHV, TEM, CTX-M, and OXA, in approximately 4 hours directly from respiratory samples.[47] However, comparison with conventional microbiological diagnostics showed poor performance of the assay.[48,49]

Single and Multiplex Real-time Polymerase Chain Reactions

The real-time PCR consists of an amplification reaction of the target gene coupled with the detection of the exponentially amplified DNA by monitoring fluorescence emission (eg, with SYBR Green or TaqMan probes).[50,51] The real-time apparatus can also analyze the denaturing temperature (high-resolution melting analysis) of synthesized DNA products, giving information on small variations (single nucleotide polymorphisms) in the sequence. The real-time PCR avoids time consuming steps such as running gels, and is more sensitive, reliable, and cost effective, and usually does not require DNA sequencing.[52,53]

Many in-house real-time PCRs for detecting ESBL and carbapenemase genes in Gram-negatives have been designed in the past.[54–58] Platforms to detect pAmpCs and plasmid-mediated quinolone resistance genes, or even perform multilocus sequencing typing–like analysis, have also been developed.[59–61] These in-house platforms have also been used extensively to test clinical samples. For instance, Oxacelay and colleagues[62] engineered an HYB probe for detecting CTX-M genes in urine. Naas and colleagues[63,64] engineered TaqMan probes for detecting NDM and OXA-48 producers in fecal specimens with detection limits of 10 colony-forming units (CFU)/100 mg and 10 to 50 CFU/100 mg, respectively. Two different TaqMan designs enabled detection of KPC genes directly from rectal swabs, showing superior sensitivity compared with selective cultures.[65,66] One of these protocols was also adapted for detecting KPC genes within 4 hours in blood culture bottles.[67]

BioMérieux has developed a very rapid (<2 h), highly sensitive and specific commercial real-time PCR kit (New NucliSENS EasyQ KPC) for the detection of KPC genes.[68] Check-Points Health BV (Wageningen, Netherlands) provides a rapid (3.5 h) multiplex real-time PCR kit (Check-MDR ESBL) to detect SHV/TEM (distinguishing ESBLs from non-ESBLs) and CTX-M genes.[69] Similarly, the Check-MDR Carba kit rapidly identifies KPC, IMP, VIM, NDM, and OXA-48 genes.[70] The Check-Direct CPE assay is another commercial multiplex test that targets carbapenemases, and it has been recently evaluated directly from rectal swabs: when compared with the selective culture approach, the sensitivity and specificity of the assay were 100% and 94%, respectively.[71] BD Diagnostics has developed a multiplex SYBR green real-time PCR coupled with high-resolution melting analysis for the detection of important carbapenemases in cultured isolates, showing both sensitivity and specificity of 100%.[72] Panagene designed a peptide nucleic acid probe-based multiplex real-time PCR kits to detect carbapenemase genes, including KPC, OXA-48, GES, IMP, VIM, NDM, OXA-23, and OXA-58. For a collection of 318 Gram-negatives, the sensitivity and specificity of the assay were greater than 99%; the detection limit was of 100 copies/25 μL reaction and the genes were all detected in less than 3 hours.[73] GeneXpert (Cepheid, Sunnyvale, CA) has developed the Xpert multiple drug-resistant organisms cartridge kit for detecting KPC, NDM, and VIM genes, requiring 2 minutes of hands-on time and 47 minutes to achieve results. High sensitivity and specificity (100% and ≥99%, respectively) have been recorded for fecal samples containing KPC or VIM producers.[74] Recently, an updated version (Xpert Carba-R test), designed for the detection of KPC, NDM, VIM, IMP, and OXA-48–like genes, has become available.[75]

Loop-mediated Isothermal Amplification

By engineering the primers to form continuous loops rather than single bands, the loop-mediated isothermal amplification (LAMP) method allows amplification and fluorescent detection at a constant temperature (no need for a thermocycler) of the target DNA.[76] This rapid and inexpensive method represents a promising alternative to PCRs and real-time PCRs. With in-house designs, Anjum and colleagues[77] correctly amplified CTX-M and OXA-10–like genes from food samples, and Liu and associates[78] detected the NDM-1 gene in pure cultures as well as in sputum, urine, and fecal samples with a very rapid protocol (1 h) and with a detection limit of 10.7 pg/mL (which correspond with 10^3 vs 10^5 CFU/mL for the endpoint PCR used as comparator).[78] With a platform designed to detect KPC and NDM-1 genes, Solanki and colleagues[79] showed that LAMP had greater sensitivity and specificity than endpoint PCRs. Nakano and coworkers[80] recognized homologous regions of all KPC genes at 68°C in 25 minutes; the detection limit was 10 CFU/tube (10-fold more sensitive than PCR) both for pure DNA extracts and clinical samples (sputum, urine, feces, and blood). Cheng and colleagues[81] developed a LAMP to detect KPC, NDM, IMP, and VIM carbapenemase genes. The lower detection limit was 10 CFU/reaction for real-time detection and 100 CFU/reaction for visual inspection.

The commercially available Eazyplex LAMP system (Amplex Diagnostics) is a qualitative genotypic diagnostic test consisting of a freeze-dried, ready-to-use kit. It was initially evaluated for the detection of carbapenemase enzymes (KPC, NDM, OXA-48, VIM, OXA-23, OXA-24/40, and OXA-58) in a collection of 82 well-characterized and non–clonally related *Acinetobacter* spp. strains. Using 1 colony, all isolates were correctly characterized in less than 30 minutes.[82] More recently, the Eazyplex SuperBug CRE kit has been evaluated to detect carbapenemases (KPC, VIM, NDM, and OXA-48-like) and CTX-M-1/-9–like genes in previously characterized *Enterobacteriaceae* recovered in Spain. In this study, all carbapenemase and/or CTX-M producers were correctly identified in 15 minutes.[83] Extended kit versions able to further detect OXA-23-, OXA-24/40-, OXA-58-, and OXA-181–like genes are also available. The possible implementation of Eazyplex directly from clinical swab and without DNA extraction is promising but not yet validated.

Next-generation Sequencing

The Sanger methodology is still the most frequently used method for the sequencing of resistance genes. However, because this method is laborious, recent efforts have been made to overcome these limitations giving rise to the so-called "Next-Generation Sequencing (NGS)" methodologies. These methods are based on the "real-time" fluorescence detection occurring during the sequencing process. Their commercialization promises to be revolutionary for the improvement of antimicrobial resistance determination because they are fast, reasonably cheap, and easy to interpret owing to the development of bioinformatics tools.[84–87]

An example of an NGS system is the bench-top 454 pyrosequencing system (GS Junior+, Roche, Basel, Switzerland).[88] It has been used to discriminate the 5 CTX-M groups after real-time PCR by 13-bp DNA region analysis,[89] characterize carbapenemase GES variants,[90] and distinguish chromosomal broad-spectrum SHVs from the acquired SHV ESBLs.[91] Moreover, the technology can also efficiently applied for the discernment of *aac(6)-Ib* from variant *aac(6)-Ib-cr*,[92] and for the detection of *gyrA/parC* mutations conferring quinolone resistance.[93]

Other promising NGS methods are also available. The sequencing by synthesis, commercially referred to as "Illumina," consists of the neosynthesis of DNA, which is detected in real time.[86] The sequencing by ligation, implemented by Life Technology (Norwalk, CT) with the commercial name "SOLiD," is based on the action of a DNA ligase, which adds fluorescent-labeled dNTPs to an anchor probe hybridizing a single strand DNA.[86] The Ion torrent sequencing method (Life Technologies) is another powerful NGS approach based on the detection of the hydrogen ions released at each addition of a nucleic base.[86] Oxford Nanopore Technologies (Oxford, UK) introduced 2 nanopore sequencing platforms capable of delivering high-throughput and ultralong sequence reads at low cost[94]: the GridION (for genome-scale sequencing) and the MinION (a disposable memory-key device that can be plugged into a laptop providing a gigabase of DNA sequence) use nanopores embedded within a synthetic membrane; as a DNA strand passes through the pore, each nucleotide induces changes in an electric current that can be translated into a DNA sequence.[95]

Whole-genome Sequencing

In many studies, the whole-genome sequencing (WGS) of single or relatively small numbers of interesting clinical isolates has been obtained. Genomic data are usually used to determine overall antibiotic resistance and virulence backgrounds,[96,97] evolution/adaptation under antibiotic selective conditions or diverse environments,[98,99] and clonal relationship of bacteria in different settings or geographic regions.[87,100]

For instance, Wright and colleagues,[101] characterizing 49 *Acinetobacter baumannii* isolates from 1 US integrated hospital system with the Illumina method, observed wide variations in gene content, even among strains that were almost identical phylogenetically. Transfer of mobile genetic elements, mobilization of insertion sequences, and genome-wide homologous recombination contributed to this diversity. Performing WGS with Illumina for a collection of 103 *Acinetobacter* spp., Périchon and colleagues[102] were able to detect 50 new OXA β-lactamases and 65 new *Acinetobacter*-derived cephalosporinases. Snitkin and associates[98] performed WGS with Roche 454 on longitudinal *A baumannii* isolates from patients undergoing colistin treatment. Colistin resistance evolved via mutations at the *pmr* locus, but after colistin withdrawal susceptible strains were found, indicating a fitness cost preventing evolution to stable colistin resistance.[98] Holt and colleagues[96] presented a detailed WGS analysis with Illumina HiSeq of 300 human and animal *Klebsiella pneumoniae* isolates (including KPC and NDM producers) found on 4 continents. Strains could be split into 3 distinct species: *K pneumoniae*, *K quasipneumoniae*, and *K variicola*. Human *K pneumoniae* isolates had a large accessory genome, including virulence functions associated with community-acquired invasive disease. In contrast, antimicrobial resistance genes were common in isolates colonizing patients or causing hospital-acquired infections.[96]

Notably, the NGS methodologies can also be implemented to perform whole sequence analysis of plasmids carrying antibiotic resistance genes.[103] Thanks to the design and developed of supportive, easy-to-use web tools (PlasmidFinder), this information has become of great importance to study the epidemiology, evolution, and clinical impact of plasmids.[104] The importance of these novel methodologies in redefining the classes of epidemic plasmids has also been demonstrated.[105]

Microarrays

Microarrays possess great diagnostic capacity because they can simultaneously detect and analyze a very large number of target genes.[106,107] In the past, numerous in-house assays have been designed to characterize virulence, surface antigens, insertion sequences, plasmids, and resistance genes. However, their implementation in a clinical laboratory is difficult because of problems related to the standardization of the procedures.[108–112] Recently, commercially available microarrays have solved this problem. These platforms are easy to perform and be updated, but the TAT is moderately high (6–8 h) and commercial kits are quite expensive.[113,114]

Check-Points has developed several automated DNA microarrays to detect *bla* genes.[107,115–118] One of these platforms (Check KPC/ESBL) was used to detect ESBL and KPC genes directly in positive blood cultures, reducing the reporting time of ESBL and/or KPC production by 18 to 20 hours.[119,120] Check-MDR CT101 assay, which detects ESBL, KPC, pAmpCs, and NDM genes, showed 100% agreement with standard PCR/DNA sequencing.[114] Check-MDR CT102, which detects ESBLs and the most important carbapenemase (VIM, IMP, OXA-48–like, KPC, and NDM) genes, showed an agreement with PCR/DNA sequencing of 99%.[121] Check-MDR CT103 merged the characteristics of CT101 and CT102, showing the same overall performances.[106] More recently, more clinically significant targets (ie, OXA-23, OXA-24/40, OXA-58, GES, GIM, SPM, BEL, and PER enzymes) have been added to the CT103XL assay to obtain an advanced platform useful for the characterization of *Enterobacteriaceae, Acinetobacter* spp., and *Pseudomonas* spp.

Alere Inc (Upper Saddle River, NJ) prepared a large microarray assay containing probes to detect the virulence factors of *Escherichia coli* and further important resistance alleles (including CTX-M, KPC, NDM, GIM, OXA-23, OXA-48, VIM, IMP, and Qnr).[113,122–124] This platform was evaluated against a panel of 117 Gram-negative isolates, showing an overall 100% concordance rate with the PCR method.[125] Nanosphere Technology (Northbrook, IL) has developed a promising automated microarray (Verigene Nucleic Acid Test) for detecting bacterial species and resistance genes within 2 hours.[126,127] In particular, the Verigene Gram-negative Blood Culture Nucleic Acid Test is able to identify the most frequent Gram-negative species along with CTX-M, KPC, NDM, VIM, IMP, and OXA enzymes. Several authors evaluated its performance for positive blood cultures, obtaining sensitivities and specificities of 87% to 90% and 100%, respectively.[7,126,127]

Matrix-Assisted Laser Desorption Ionization-Time of Flight Mass Spectroscopy

The matrix-assisted laser desorption ionization-time of flight mass spectroscopy (MALDI-TOF MS) is nowadays often used routinely by clinical microbiologists to discriminate unique protein signatures (ie, 16S ribosomal proteins) to identify bacterial species.[128] Overall, the main advantages of MALDI-TOF MS are its rapidity, very low costs, and consistency.[129–132] Recently, this system has also been applied to (i) recognize antibiotic degradation owing to resistance proteins[133–142]; (ii) discover mutations within resistance genes through DNA minisequencing[142]; and (iii) study clonality of Gram-negative pathogens (eg, detection of ST131 or ST405 *E coli*).[143,144]

Numerous studies have assessed specifically the usefulness of MALDI-TOF MS for the identification of β-lactam degradation products in the presence of hydrolyzing β-lactamases,[137–141,145,146] including directly from positive blood cultures.[147–150] In particular, many studies have evaluated the identification of carbapenemase producers.[132,137,138,140,146,151] Antibiotics (imipenem or meropenem) are incubated with the enzyme extract and then analyzed for degradation products with the MS; the time required to do this assay is about 1 to 4 hours. However, we should note that this method can only detect the presence of β-lactam hydrolysis as a resistance mechanism and not the specific enzyme (eg, distinguishing NDM from KPC) that can be determined with PCR- or microarray-based methodology. Therefore, the implementation of the MALDI-TOF MS for this aspect may be of limited value and this information can be easily obtained by implementing the rapid and cost-effective Carba NP and Blue-Carba tests.[10,16,24] On the other hand, MALDI-TOF MS possess higher sensitivity than the Carba-NP assay owing to its ability to better identify OXA or GES carbapenemase producers.[152,153]

PROMISING TECHNOLOGIES IN DEVELOPMENT

Rapid Antimicrobial Susceptibility Testing

Inhibition zone diameters around antibiotic disk can be continuously read using instruments consisting of a real-time high-resolution video imager in dedicated incubators. For instance, with the Advencis (Mutzig, France) Bio-System instrument, susceptibility to imipenem and production of ESBLs in Gram-negative bacteria can be detected in approximately 4 hours.[154] This approach is also extended for use with microcolonies under selective pressure or absence of antibiotics. A good example is the BACcel Digital Microscopy System (Accelerate Diagnostics, Tucson, AZ).[5,155]

The ATP-bioluminescence method provides a fast and reliable AST in 2 to 3 hours. Testing both Gram-positive and Gram-negative strains, the sensitivity of this method compared with commercial systems (Microscan, Vitek) was 100%.[156] The method was also implemented to directly perform AST in urine samples, showing an overall accuracy of 91%.[157]

The cell lysis method can be implemented to evaluate the activity of β-lactams against peptidoglycan. Cells incubated with the antibiotic are embedded in an agarose microgel on a slide, incubated in a lysis buffer, stained with a DNA fluorochrome, and observed under fluorescence microscopy. When the bacterium is susceptible to the antibiotic, the debilitated cell wall is affected by the lysing solution, the DNA is released, and hybridized with a specific probes.[158] Similarly, the effect of quinolones on the chromosomal DNA can be evaluated.[159] Bou and coworkers[160] combined these 2 techniques to test a collection of *A baumannii* strains for meropenem and ciprofloxacin susceptibility. All strains were correctly categorized in 100 minutes according to the MIC results interpreted with Clinical and Laboratory Standards Institute criteria.[160]

Flow cytometric analysis can be used to detect ESBL producers. Cells are incubated with ceftazidime or cefotaxime for 1 to 2 hours in the presence or absence of clavulanate and then stained with a fluorescent dye able to diffuse across depolarized membranes. After incubation, non-ESBL isolates display increased fluorescence, whereas those producing ESBLs show this phenomenon only when incubated with clavulanate. The assay is rapid (approximately 3 h) and correlated well with standard methods, but it cannot be performed with bacteria in stationary growth phase.[161] This principle was also implemented to perform a rapid AST (3 h) on positive blood culture bottles using the Sysmex (Kobe, Japan) UF-1000i flow cytometer. The essential agreement of the test with the commercial methods was 99%.[162]

Numerous further potential AST configurations are under development. These near or more distant future technologies have been reviewed by other authors.[5,6,163] Among them, we should note that microfluidic methods are the most promising tools for obtaining rapid AST results (see discussion below).

Microfluidics and Nanotechnology

The rapidly evolving development of microfluidic and nanotechnology devices represents a basis for future applications in the laboratory diagnosis of antibiotic resistance. These lab-on-chip miniaturized and automated diagnostics will become the point-of-care tests in the future, significantly affecting the outcome of patients.[164–166] These devices (i) use very small amounts of sample (from nano- to picoliters) and reagents, (ii) incorporate multitasking functions in a disposable single cartridge performing different steps (eg, cell lysis, hybridization, amplification), (iii) do not need expensive equipment, and (iv) ensure high sensitivity, rapid results, and less work load for the operators owing to innovative detection methods (eg, optical, magnetic, electrochemical).[167–169]

Several authors have used microfluidic technologies to perform rapid AST for Gram-negatives. By observing the growth of *E coli* in gas permeable polymeric microchannels, Chen and colleagues[170] demonstrated that the large surface-to-volume ratio of microfluidic systems facilitates rapid growth of bacteria and analysis of antibiotic resistance profiles in 2 hours. Mach and colleagues[171] implemented a biosensor-based AST device for urine samples. Growth of Gram-negative pathogens was determined in the presence of antibiotics in 2.5 hours by electrochemical measurement of 16S rRNA, showing 94% accuracy compared with standard microbiological analyses. Tang and colleagues[172] used a microfluidic pH sensor to perform real-time rapid MIC determination. Confinement of bacterial cells in a nanoliter-size channel eliminates the need for long incubation (16–24 h), thus reducing the detection time to less than 2 hours. Choi and colleagues[173] designed a microfluidic agarose channel chip that reduces the AST time to 3-4 hours. The system immobilizes single bacterial cells by using agarose in a microfluidic culture chamber so that growth can be followed by microscopy time lapse imaging under different antibiotic conditions.[173] Kim and colleagues[174] implemented a microfluidic device where continuous concentration gradients of antibiotics were generated to measure the minimal biofilm eradication concentration of *P aeruginosa*. Mohan and colleagues[175] used a small volume (<6 μL) microfluidic multiplexed platform that relies on fluorescence detection of bacteria for highly sensitive (1 cell) and rapid ASTs (2–4 h) against *E coli*. Recently, Hou and colleagues[176] described a method to isolate low abundance pathogens (approximately 100/mL) from whole blood using inertial microfluidics and directly determine species identification and resistance patterns in approximately 8 hours with hybridization-based RNA detection.

Fluorescence In Situ Hybridization

The FISH is a cheap, rapid, and easy to standardize methodology traditionally used to identify bacterial pathogens. In this context, it is based on the hybridization of short and specific (approximately 18–25 bp) fluorescent-labelled, single-stranded probes to the rRNA target with subsequent analysis using fluorescent microscopes. The main advantage of FISH is its potential use directly from clinical specimens. This method has also been implemented to detect resistance genes, as confirmed for several commercial tests implemented for detecting clarithromycin resistance in *Helicobacter pylori* or *Campylobacter* spp. and the presence of *mecA* gene in *Staphylococcus aureus*.[6] Palasubramaniam and colleagues[177] applied this approach to detect SHV variants with ESBL spectrum in positive blood cultures in approximately 1 hour and with a limit of detection of 1.5×10^5 CFU/mL.

FilmArray

Idaho Technology (now BioFire Diagnostics, Salt Lake City, UT) developed the FilmArray technique, a closed, very rapid (1 h) and fully automated system that combines DNA extraction from clinical samples, nested multiplex PCRs, after PCR amplicon melt curve analysis, and automated interpretation of results.[178] So far, this method has been applied to the detection of respiratory pathogens.[179] Recently, the FilmArray Blood Culture ID was evaluated in blood cultures to rapidly identify the causative pathogens and to detect several antibiotic resistance genes, including KPCs. However, data regarding the ability to detect KPC producers were not provided.[180–182]

Rapid Whole-genome Sequencing

In the past, it was stated commonly that the use of WGS for routine susceptibility testing was not practical owing to its long TAT and the elevated costs compared with standard techniques.[183] Nowadays, the latest generation benchtop platforms (eg, Illumina MiSeq and nanopore MinION) have almost eliminated these problems, making pathogen WGS data available to the diagnostic microbiology laboratory in less than a day for about US$100.[184–186] The challenge for the next few years will be the development of rapid and fully automated sequence interpretation software able to provide information (eg, AST- and multilocus sequencing typing–like results) understandable by laboratory workers and clinicians with no experience with WGS.[187]

Polymerase Chain Reaction/Electrospray Ionization Mass Spectrometry

The polymerase chain reaction/electrospray ionization mass spectrometry (PCR/ESI MS) is a very promising technology that performs mini-sequencing–like of small PCR products (from 100 to 450 bp) by measuring their exact molecular mass and interpreting such data as a DNA sequence. This system has demonstrated success in the identification of pathogens and has been developed into a fully automated system (PLEX-ID; Abbott Biosciences, Carlsbad, CA) with results available within 4 to 6 hours starting from clinical samples.[129–131,188,189] The rapid and fully automated ability to detect multiple genes (not only those conferring antibiotic resistance but also certain pathogens and virulence factors) in one reaction may represent a revolution for the diagnosis of infectious diseases.[190] Moreover, this platform offers the ability to detect pathogens at very low copy numbers and to determine genetic relatedness based on a multilocus sequencing typing–like approach,[191–194] thus providing "real-time" data essential to detect outbreaks and limit spread of Gram-negative multidrug-resistant clones. Notably, the detection of DNA from organisms that are noncultured (eg, during antibiotic treatment) is a major step forward in the diagnosis of "culture-negative infections."[195–198] Unfortunately, PCR/ESI MS is still under development and currently only available for research applications and at a high cost.

The application of PCR/ESI MS for the detection of resistance mechanisms and single nucleotide polymorphisms within resistance genes in Gram-negative pathogens has been studied.[188,199] Its usefulness for detecting KPC genes, evaluated using 110 well-characterized *Enterobacteriaceae*, indicated that the system correctly detected 100% of the KPC producers.[200] In another study, PCR ESI-MS quickly and accurately identified quinolone resistance mediated by mutations in the *gyrA* and *parC* genes of *Acinetobacter* spp. Single point mutations detected by PCR ESI-MS correctly correlated with susceptibility testing and DNA sequencing.[201]

DISCUSSION

The development of resistance in Gram-negatives has challenged the clinical microbiology laboratory to recognize the presence of these resistance mechanisms, appreciate their clinical significance, and develop methods to rapidly detect their presence. These challenges have been significant and in many instances difficult to address when conventional AST fails to recognize the presence of weak, but clinically significant, resistance mechanisms such as carbapenemases and ESBLs. A further challenge has been to rapidly detect these resistance mechanisms in established cultures as well as directly from specimens. Review of methods to address these issues show the advances that have been made in rapid detection of resistance in cultures, but limited progress in direct detection from specimens.

There is also the inherent conflict between choosing between phenotypic and genotypic methods. Genotypic methods are rapid, can be used to test specimens as well as cultures, but are limited by the complexity of some targets and the evolution of new resistance mechanisms. Phenotypic methods are slow and best suited for use on cultures, but speed has been improved using microfluidics and progress is being made on direct specimen testing. It is likely that these challenges will continue as new resistance mechanisms emerge, and that both phenotypic and genotypic methods will continue to be needed and used.

REFERENCES

1. Nordmann P, Poirel L. The difficult-to-control spread of carbapenemase producers among enterobacteriaceae worldwide. Clin Microbiol Infect 2014;20(9):821–30.
2. Nordmann P. Carbapenemase-producing enterobacteriaceae: overview of a major public health challenge. Med Mal Infect 2014;44(2):51–6.
3. Perez F, Endimiani A, Hujer KM, et al. The continuing challenge of ESBLs. Curr Opin Pharmacol 2007;7(5):459–69.
4. Kothari A, Morgan M, Haake DA. Emerging technologies for rapid identification of bloodstream pathogens. Clin Infect Dis 2014;59(2):272–8.
5. van Belkum A, Durand G, Peyret M, et al. Rapid clinical bacteriology and its future impact. Ann Lab Med 2013;33(1):14–27.
6. Frickmann H, Masanta WO, Zautner AE. Emerging rapid resistance testing methods for clinical microbiology laboratories and their potential impact on patient management. Biomed Res Int 2014;2014:375681.
7. Bork JT, Leekha S, Heil EL, et al. Rapid testing using the Verigene gram-negative blood culture nucleic acid test in combination with antimicrobial stewardship intervention against gram-negative bacteremia. Antimicrob Agents Chemother 2015;59(3):1588–95.

8. Clinical and Laboratory Standards Institute (CLSI). Performance standards for antimicrobial susceptibility testing: 25th informational supplement. Wayne (PA): Clinical and Laboratory Standard Institute; 2015. CLSI document m100-s25.
9. EUCAST. European Committee on Antimicrobial Susceptibility Testing Breakpoint Tables for interpretation of MICs and zone diameters. Version 5.0, valid from 2015-01-01.
10. Nordmann P, Dortet L, Poirel L. Rapid detection of extended-spectrum-β-lactamase-producing *Enterobacteriaceae*. J Clin Microbiol 2012;50(9):3016–22.
11. Dortet L, Poirel L, Nordmann P. Rapid detection of extended-spectrum-β-lactamase-producing *Enterobacteriaceae* from urine samples by use of the ESBL NDP test. J Clin Microbiol 2014;52(10):3701–6.
12. Dortet L, Poirel L, Nordmann P. Rapid detection of ESBL-producing *Enterobacteriaceae* in blood cultures. Emerg Infect Dis 2015;21(3):504–7.
13. Dortet L, Brechard L, Poirel L, et al. Impact of the isolation medium for detection of carbapenemase-producing *Enterobacteriaceae* using an updated version of the carba NP test. J Med Microbiol 2014;63(Pt 5):772–6.
14. Dortet L, Poirel L, Errera C, et al. Carbacineto NP test for rapid detection of carbapenemase-producing *Acinetobacter* spp. J Clin Microbiol 2014;52(7):2359–64.
15. Dortet L, Poirel L, Nordmann P. Rapid detection of carbapenemase-producing *Pseudomonas* spp. J Clin Microbiol 2012;50(11):3773–6.
16. Nordmann P, Poirel L, Dortet L. Rapid detection of carbapenemase-producing *Enterobacteriaceae*. Emerg Infect Dis 2012;18(9):1503–7.
17. Tijet N, Boyd D, Patel SN, et al. Evaluation of the carba NP test for rapid detection of carbapenemase-producing *Enterobacteriaceae* and *Pseudomonas aeruginosa*. Antimicrob Agents Chemother 2013;57(9):4578–80.
18. Osterblad M, Hakanen AJ, Jalava J. Evaluation of the carba NP test for carbapenemase detection. Antimicrob Agents Chemother 2014;58(12):7553–6.
19. Tijet N, Boyd D, Patel SN, et al. Reply to "further proofs of concept for the carba NP test". Antimicrob Agents Chemother 2014;58(2):1270.
20. Dortet L, Poirel L, Nordmann P. Further proofs of concept for the carba NP test. Antimicrob Agents Chemother 2014;58(2):1269.
21. Dortet L, Brechard L, Poirel L, et al. Rapid detection of carbapenemase-producing *Enterobacteriaceae* from blood cultures. Clin Microbiol Infect 2014; 20(4):340–4.
22. Dortet L, Boulanger A, Poirel L, et al. Bloodstream infections caused by *Pseudomonas* spp.: How to detect carbapenemase producers directly from blood cultures. J Clin Microbiol 2014;52(4):1269–73.
23. Poirel L, Nordmann P. Rapidec carba NP test for rapid detection of carbapenemase producers. J Clin Microbiol 2015;53(9):3003–8.
24. Pires J, Novais A, Peixe L. Blue-carba, an easy biochemical test for detection of diverse carbapenemase producers directly from bacterial cultures. J Clin Microbiol 2013;51(12):4281–3.
25. Huang TD, Berhin C, Bogaerts P, et al. Comparative evaluation of two chromogenic tests for rapid detection of carbapenemase in *Enterobacteriaceae* and in *Pseudomonas aeruginosa* isolates. J Clin Microbiol 2014;52(8):3060–3.
26. Yusuf E, Van Der Meeren S, Schallier A, et al. Comparison of the carba NP test with the rapid carb screen kit for the detection of carbapenemase-producing *Enterobacteriaceae* and *Pseudomonas aeruginosa*. Eur J Clin Microbiol Infect Dis 2014;33(12):2237–40.

27. Mullis KB, Faloona FA. Specific synthesis of DNA in vitro via a polymerase-catalyzed chain reaction. Methods Enzymol 1987;155:335–50.
28. Schrader C, Schielke A, Ellerbroek L, et al. PCR inhibitors - occurrence, properties and removal. J Appl Microbiol 2012;113(5):1014–26.
29. Pitout JD, Hossain A, Hanson ND. Phenotypic and molecular detection of CTX-M-β-lactamases produced by *Escherichia coli* and *Klebsiella* spp. J Clin Microbiol 2004;42(12):5715–21.
30. Boyd DA, Tyler S, Christianson S, et al. Complete nucleotide sequence of a 92-kilobase plasmid harboring the CTX-M-15 extended-spectrum β-lactamase involved in an outbreak in long-term-care facilities in Toronto, Canada. Antimicrob Agents Chemother 2004;48(10):3758–64.
31. De Champs C, Chanal C, Sirot D, et al. Frequency and diversity of class A extended-spectrum β-lactamases in hospitals of the Auvergne, France: a 2 year prospective study. J Antimicrob Chemother 2004;54(3):634–9.
32. Bradford PA, Bratu S, Urban C, et al. Emergence of carbapenem-resistant *Klebsiella* species possessing the class a carbapenem-hydrolyzing KPC-2 and inhibitor-resistant TEM-30 β-lactamases in New York City. Clin Infect Dis 2004; 39(1):55–60.
33. Pitout JD, Gregson DB, Poirel L, et al. Detection of *Pseudomonas aeruginosa* producing metallo-β-lactamases in a large centralized laboratory. J Clin Microbiol 2005;43(7):3129–35.
34. Nordmann P, Poirel L, Carrer A, et al. How to detect NDM-1 producers. J Clin Microbiol 2011;49(2):718–21.
35. Robicsek A, Strahilevitz J, Sahm DF, et al. Qnr prevalence in ceftazidime-resistant *Enterobacteriaceae* isolates from the United States. Antimicrob Agents Chemother 2006;50(8):2872–4.
36. Miro F, Grunbaum F, Gomez L, et al. Characterization of aminoglycoside-modifying enzymes in *Enterobacteriaceae* clinical strains and characterization of the plasmids implicated in their diffusion. Microb Drug Resist 2012;19(2): 94–9.
37. Lee CH, Chu C, Liu JW, et al. Collateral damage of flomoxef therapy: In vivo development of porin deficiency and acquisition of $bla_{dha\text{-}1}$ leading to ertapenem resistance in a clinical isolate of *Klebsiella pneumoniae* producing CTX-M-3 and SHV-5 β-lactamases. J Antimicrob Chemother 2007;60(2):410–3.
38. Markoulatos P, Siafakas N, Moncany M. Multiplex polymerase chain reaction: a practical approach. J Clin Lab Anal 2002;16(1):47–51.
39. Perez-Perez FJ, Hanson ND. Detection of plasmid-mediated AmpC β-lactamase genes in clinical isolates by using multiplex PCR. J Clin Microbiol 2002;40(6): 2153–62.
40. Voets GM, Fluit AC, Scharringa J, et al. A set of multiplex PCRs for genotypic detection of extended-spectrum β-lactamases, carbapenemases, plasmid-mediated AmpC β-lactamases and OXA β-lactamases. Int J Antimicrob Agents 2011;37(4):356–9.
41. Doyle D, Peirano G, Lascols C, et al. Laboratory detection of *Enterobacteriaceae* that produce carbapenemases. J Clin Microbiol 2012;50(12):3877–80.
42. Cattoir V, Poirel L, Rotimi V, et al. Multiplex PCR for detection of plasmid-mediated quinolone resistance QNR genes in ESBL-producing enterobacterial isolates. J Antimicrob Chemother 2007;60(2):394–7.
43. Berçot B, Poirel L, Nordmann P. Updated multiplex polymerase chain reaction for detection of 16s RRNA methylases: High prevalence among NDM-1 producers. Diagn Microbiol Infect Dis 2011;71(4):442–5.

44. Kaase M, Szabados F, Wassill L, et al. Detection of carbapenemases in *Enterobacteriaceae* by a commercial multiplex PCR. J Clin Microbiol 2012;50(9): 3115–8.
45. Avlami A, Bekris S, Ganteris G, et al. Detection of metallo-β-lactamase genes in clinical specimens by a commercial multiplex PCR system. J Microbiol Methods 2010;83(2):185–7.
46. Ambretti S, Gaibani P, Berlingeri A, et al. Evaluation of phenotypic and genotypic approaches for the detection of class a and class b carbapenemases in enterobacteriaceae. Microb Drug Resist 2013;19(3):212–5.
47. Jamal W, Al Roomi E, AbdulAziz LR, et al. Evaluation of Curetis Unyvero, a multiplex PCR-based testing system, for rapid detection of bacteria and antibiotic resistance and impact of the assay on management of severe nosocomial pneumonia. J Clin Microbiol 2014;52(7):2487–92.
48. Kunze N, Moerer O, Steinmetz N, et al. Point-of-care multiplex PCR promises short turnaround times for microbial testing in hospital-acquired pneumonia - an observational pilot study in critical ill patients. Ann Clin Microbiol Antimicrob 2015;14:33.
49. Schulte B, Eickmeyer H, Heininger A, et al. Detection of pneumonia associated pathogens using a prototype multiplexed pneumonia test in hospitalized patients with severe pneumonia. PLoS One 2014;9(11):e110566.
50. Higuchi R, Fockler C, Dollinger G, et al. Kinetic PCR analysis: real-time monitoring of DNA amplification reactions. Biotechnology (N Y) 1993;11(9):1026–30.
51. Heid CA, Stevens J, Livak KJ, et al. Real time quantitative PCR. Genome Res 1996;6(10):986–94.
52. Tong SY, Giffard PM. Microbiological applications of high-resolution melting analysis. J Clin Microbiol 2012;50(11):3418–21.
53. Erali M, Voelkerding KV, Wittwer CT. High resolution melting applications for clinical laboratory medicine. Exp Mol Pathol 2008;85(1):50–8.
54. Hammond DS, Schooneveldt JM, Nimmo GR, et al. Bla(SHV) genes in *Klebsiella pneumoniae*: Different allele distributions are associated with different promoters within individual isolates. Antimicrob Agents Chemother 2005;49(1): 256–63.
55. Birkett CI, Ludlam HA, Woodford N, et al. Real-time TaqMan PCR for rapid detection and typing of genes encoding CTX-M extended-spectrum β-lactamases. J Med Microbiol 2007;56(Pt 1):52–5.
56. Raghunathan A, Samuel L, Tibbetts RJ. Evaluation of a real-time PCR assay for the detection of the *Klebsiella pneumoniae* carbapenemase genes in microbiological samples in comparison with the modified Hodge test. Am J Clin Pathol 2011;135(4):566–71.
57. Kruttgen A, Razavi S, Imohl M, et al. Real-time PCR assay and a synthetic positive control for the rapid and sensitive detection of the emerging resistance gene New Delhi metallo-β-lactamase-1 ($bla_{\text{ndm-1}}$). Med Microbiol Immunol 2011;200(2):137–41.
58. Bisiklis A, Papageorgiou F, Frantzidou F, et al. Specific detection of bla_{vim} and bla_{imp} metallo-β-lactamase genes in a single real-time PCR. Clin Microbiol Infect 2007;13(12):1201–3.
59. Geyer CN, Reisbig MD, Hanson ND. Development of a TaqMan multiplex PCR assay for detection of plasmid-mediated AmpC β-lactamase genes. J Clin Microbiol 2012;50(11):3722–5.

60. Guillard T, Moret H, Brasme L, et al. Rapid detection of qnr and *qepa* plasmid-mediated quinolone resistance genes using real-time PCR. Diagn Microbiol Infect Dis 2011;70(2):253–9.
61. Chen L, Chavda KD, Mediavilla JR, et al. Multiplex real-time PCR for detection of an epidemic KPC-producing *Klebsiella pneumoniae* st258 clone. Antimicrob Agents Chemother 2012;56(6):3444–7.
62. Oxacelay C, Ergani A, Naas T, et al. Rapid detection of CTX-M-producing *Enterobacteriaceae* in urine samples. J Antimicrob Chemother 2009;64(5):986–9.
63. Naas T, Ergani A, Carrer A, et al. Real-time PCR for detection of NDM-1 carbapenemase genes from spiked stool samples. Antimicrob Agents Chemother 2011;55(9):4038–43.
64. Naas T, Cotellon G, Ergani A, et al. Real-time PCR for detection of $bla_{oxa\text{-}48}$ genes from stools. J Antimicrob Chemother 2013;68(1):101–4.
65. Hindiyeh M, Smollen G, Grossman Z, et al. Rapid detection of bla_{kpc} carbapenemase genes by real-time PCR. J Clin Microbiol 2008;46(9):2879–83.
66. Singh K, Mangold KA, Wyant K, et al. Rectal screening for *Klebsiella pneumoniae* carbapenemases: Comparison of real-time PCR and culture using two selective screening agar plates. J Clin Microbiol 2012;50(8):2596–600.
67. Hindiyeh M, Smollan G, Grossman Z, et al. Rapid detection of bla_{kpc} carbapenemase genes by internally controlled real-time PCR assay using bactec blood culture bottles. J Clin Microbiol 2011;49(7):2480–4.
68. Spanu T, Fiori B, D'Inzeo T, et al. Evaluation of the new Nuclisens EasyQ KPC test for rapid detection of *Klebsiella pneumoniae* carbapenemase genes (bla_{kpc}). J Clin Microbiol 2012;50(8):2783–5.
69. Nijhuis R, van Zwet A, Stuart JC, et al. Rapid molecular detection of extended-spectrum β-lactamase gene variants with a novel ligation-mediated real-time PCR. J Med Microbiol 2012;61(Pt 11):1563–7.
70. Cuzon G, Naas T, Bogaerts P, et al. Probe ligation and real-time detection of KPC, OXA-48, VIM, IMP, and NDM carbapenemase genes. Diagn Microbiol Infect Dis 2013;76(4):502–5.
71. Huang TD, Bogaerts P, Ghilani E, et al. Multicentre evaluation of the check-direct CPE(r) assay for direct screening of carbapenemase-producing *Enterobacteriaceae* from rectal swabs. J Antimicrob Chemother 2015;70(6):1669–73.
72. Hofko M, Mischnik A, Kaase M, et al. Detection of carbapenemases by real-time PCR and melt curve analysis on the BD max system. J Clin Microbiol 2014;52(5):1701–4.
73. Jeong S, Kim JO, Jeong SH, et al. Evaluation of peptide nucleic acid-mediated multiplex real-time PCR kits for rapid detection of carbapenemase genes in gram-negative clinical isolates. J Microbiol Methods 2015;113:4–9.
74. Tenover FC, Canton R, Kop J, et al. Detection of colonization by carbapenemase-producing gram-negative bacilli in patients by use of the Xpert MDRO assay. J Clin Microbiol 2013;51(11):3780–7.
75. Lafeuille E, Laouira S, Sougakoff W, et al. Detection of OXA-48-like carbapenemase genes by the xpert(r) carba-r test: Room for improvement. Int J Antimicrob Agents 2015;45(4):441–2.
76. Notomi T, Okayama H, Masubuchi H, et al. Loop-mediated isothermal amplification of DNA. Nucleic Acids Res 2000;28(12):E63.
77. Anjum MF, Lemma F, Cork DJ, et al. Isolation and detection of extended spectrum β-lactamase (ESBL)-producing *Enterobacteriaceae* from meat using chromogenic agars and isothermal loop-mediated amplification (LAMP) assays. J Food Sci 2013;78(12):M1892–8.

78. Liu W, Zou D, Li Y, et al. Sensitive and rapid detection of the New Delhi metallo-β-lactamase gene by loop-mediated isothermal amplification. J Clin Microbiol 2012;50(5):1580–5.
79. Solanki R, Vanjari L, Ede N, et al. Evaluation of LAMP assay using phenotypic tests and conventional PCR for detection of blandm-1 and bla_{kpc} genes among carbapenem-resistant clinical gram-negative isolates. J Med Microbiol 2013; 62(Pt 10):1540–4.
80. Nakano R, Nakano A, Ishii Y, et al. Rapid detection of the Klebsiella pneumoniae carbapenemase (KPC) gene by loop-mediated isothermal amplification (LAMP). J Infect Chemother 2015;21(3):202–6.
81. Cheng C, Zheng F, Rui Y. Rapid detection of bla_{ndm}, bla_{kpc}, bla_{imp}, and bla_{vim} carbapenemase genes in bacteria by loop-mediated isothermal amplification. Microb Drug Resist 2014;20(6):533–8.
82. Vergara A, Zboromyrska Y, Mosqueda N, et al. Evaluation of a loop-mediated isothermal amplification-based methodology to detect carbapenemase carriage in *Acinetobacter* clinical isolates. Antimicrob Agents Chemother 2014;58(12): 7538–40.
83. Garcia-Fernandez S, Morosini MI, Marco F, et al. Evaluation of the Eazyplex(r) Superbug CRE system for rapid detection of carbapenemases and ESBLs in clinical *Enterobacteriaceae* isolates recovered at two Spanish hospitals. J Antimicrob Chemother 2015;70(4):1047–50.
84. Maxam AM, Gilbert W. A new method for sequencing DNA. Proc Natl Acad Sci U S A 1977;74(2):560–4.
85. Sanger F, Nicklen S, Coulson AR. DNA sequencing with chain-terminating inhibitors. Proc Natl Acad Sci U S A 1977;74(12):5463–7.
86. Liu L, Li Y, Li S, et al. Comparison of next-generation sequencing systems. J Biomed Biotechnol 2012;2012:251364.
87. Gilchrist CA, Turner SD, Riley MF, et al. Whole-genome sequencing in outbreak analysis. Clin Microbiol Rev 2015;28(3):541–63.
88. Ronaghi M, Karamohamed S, Pettersson B, et al. Real-time DNA sequencing using detection of pyrophosphate release. Anal Biochem 1996;242(1):84–9.
89. Naas T, Oxacelay C, Nordmann P. Identification of CTX-M-type extended-spectrum-β-lactamase genes using real-time PCR and pyrosequencing. Antimicrob Agents Chemother 2007;51(1):223–30.
90. Poirel L, Naas T, Nordmann P. Pyrosequencing as a rapid tool for identification of ges-type extended-spectrum β-lactamases. J Clin Microbiol 2006;44(8): 3008–11.
91. Haanpera M, Forssten SD, Huovinen P, et al. Typing of SHV extended-spectrum β-lactamases by pyrosequencing in *Klebsiella pneumoniae* strains with chromosomal SHV β-lactamase. Antimicrob Agents Chemother 2008;52(7):2632–5.
92. Guillard T, Duval V, Moret H, et al. Rapid detection of *aac(6')-ib-cr* quinolone resistance gene by pyrosequencing. J Clin Microbiol 2010;48(1):286–9.
93. Hopkins KL, Arnold C, Threlfall EJ. Rapid detection of *GyrA* and *ParC* mutations in quinolone-resistant *Salmonella enterica* using pyrosequencing technology. J Microbiol Methods 2007;68(1):163–71.
94. Branton D, Deamer DW, Marziali A, et al. The potential and challenges of nanopore sequencing. Nat Biotechnol 2008;26(10):1146–53.
95. Maitra RD, Kim J, Dunbar WB. Recent advances in nanopore sequencing. Electrophoresis 2012;33(23):3418–28.

96. Holt KE, Wertheim H, Zadoks RN, et al. Genomic analysis of diversity, population structure, virulence, and antimicrobial resistance in *Klebsiella pneumoniae*, an urgent threat to public health. Proc Natl Acad Sci U S A 2015;112(27):E3574–81.
97. Fournier PE, Vallenet D, Barbe V, et al. Comparative genomics of multidrug resistance in *Acinetobacter baumannii*. PLoS Genet 2006;2(1):e7.
98. Snitkin ES, Zelazny AM, Gupta J, et al. Genomic insights into the fate of colistin resistance and *Acinetobacter baumannii* during patient treatment. Genome Res 2013;23(7):1155–62.
99. Nielsen LE, Snesrud EC, Onmus-Leone F, et al. IS5 element integration, a novel mechanism for rapid in vivo emergence of tigecycline nonsusceptibility in *Klebsiella pneumoniae*. Antimicrob Agents Chemother 2014;58(10):6151–6.
100. Onori R, Gaiarsa S, Comandatore F, et al. Tracking nosocomial *Klebsiella pneumoniae* infections and outbreaks by whole genome analysis: small-scale Italian scenario within a single hospital. J Clin Microbiol 2015;53(9):2861–8.
101. Wright MS, Haft DH, Harkins DM, et al. New insights into dissemination and variation of the health care-associated pathogen *Acinetobacter baumannii* from genomic analysis. MBio 2014;5(1):e00963–1013.
102. Périchon B, Goussard S, Walewski V, et al. Identification of 50 class d β-lactamases and 65 Acinetobacter-derived cephalosporinases in *Acinetobacter* spp. Antimicrob Agents Chemother 2014;58(2):936–49.
103. Carattoli A. Plasmids and the spread of resistance. Int J Med Microbiol 2013; 303(6–7):298–304.
104. Carattoli A, Zankari E, Garcia-Fernandez A, et al. In silico detection and typing of plasmids using Plasmidfinder and plasmid multilocus sequence typing. Antimicrob Agents Chemother 2014;58(7):3895–903.
105. Carattoli A, Seiffert SN, Schwendener S, et al. Differentiation of IncL and IncM plasmids associated with the spread of clinically relevant antimicrobial resistance. PLoS One 2015;10(5):e0123063.
106. Cuzon G, Naas T, Bogaerts P, et al. Evaluation of a DNA microarray for the rapid detection of extended-spectrum β-lactamases (TEM, SHV and CTX-M), plasmid-mediated cephalosporinases (CMY-2-like, DHA, FOX, ACC-1, ACT/MIR and CMY-1-like/MOX) and carbapenemases (KPC, OXA-48, VIM, IMP and NDM). J Antimicrob Chemother 2012;67(8):1865–9.
107. Endimiani A, Hujer AM, Hujer KM, et al. Evaluation of a commercial microarray system for detection of SHV-, TEM-, CTX-M-, and KPC-type β-lactamase genes in gram-negative isolates. J Clin Microbiol 2010;48(7):2618–22.
108. Glenn LM, Lindsey RL, Folster JP, et al. Antimicrobial resistance genes in multidrug-resistant *Salmonella enterica* isolated from animals, retail meats, and humans in the United States and Canada. Microb Drug Resist 2013; 19(3):175–84.
109. Huehn S, Bunge C, Junker E, et al. Poultry-associated *Salmonella enterica* subsp. Enterica serovar 4,12:D:- reveals high clonality and a distinct pathogenicity gene repertoire. Appl Environ Microbiol 2009;75(4):1011–20.
110. Hauser E, Hebner F, Tietze E, et al. Diversity of *Salmonella enterica* serovar derby isolated from pig, pork and humans in Germany. Int J Food Microbiol 2011;151(2):141–9.
111. Hauser E, Tietze E, Helmuth R, et al. Pork contaminated with *Salmonella enterica* serovar 4,[5],12:I:-, an emerging health risk for humans. Appl Environ Microbiol 2010;76(14):4601–10.

112. van Hoek AH, Scholtens IM, Cloeckaert A, et al. Detection of antibiotic resistance genes in different *Salmonella* serovars by oligonucleotide microarray analysis. J Microbiol Methods 2005;62(1):13–23.
113. Batchelor M, Hopkins KL, Liebana E, et al. Development of a miniaturised microarray-based assay for the rapid identification of antimicrobial resistance genes in gram-negative bacteria. Int J Antimicrob Agents 2008;31(5):440–51.
114. Bogaerts P, Hujer AM, Naas T, et al. Multicenter evaluation of a new DNA microarray for rapid detection of clinically relevant *bla* genes from β-lactam-resistant gram-negative bacteria. Antimicrob Agents Chemother 2011;55(9):4457–60.
115. Cohen Stuart J, Dierikx C, Al Naiemi N, et al. Rapid detection of TEM, SHV and CTX-M extended-spectrum β-lactamases in *Enterobacteriaceae* using ligation-mediated amplification with microarray analysis. J Antimicrob Chemother 2010;65(7):1377–81.
116. Platteel TN, Stuart JW, Voets GM, et al. Evaluation of a commercial microarray as a confirmation test for the presence of extended-spectrum β-lactamases in isolates from the routine clinical setting. Clin Microbiol Infect 2011;17(9):1435–8.
117. Naas T, Cuzon G, Truong H, et al. Evaluation of a DNA microarray, the check-points ESBL/KPC array, for rapid detection of TEM, SHV, and CTX-M extended-spectrum β-lactamases and KPC carbapenemases. Antimicrob Agents Chemother 2010;54(8):3086–92.
118. Lascols C, Hackel M, Hujer AM, et al. Using nucleic acid microarrays to perform molecular epidemiology and detect novel β-lactamases: a snapshot of extended-spectrum β-lactamases throughout the world. J Clin Microbiol 2012; 50(5):1632–9.
119. Fishbain JT, Sinyavskiy O, Riederer K, et al. Detection of extended-spectrum β-lactamase and *Klebsiella pneumoniae* carbapenemase genes directly from blood cultures by use of a nucleic acid microarray. J Clin Microbiol 2012; 50(9):2901–4.
120. Wintermans BB, Reuland EA, Wintermans RG, et al. The cost-effectiveness of ESBL detection: towards molecular detection methods? Clin Microbiol Infect 2013;19(7):662–5.
121. Naas T, Cuzon G, Bogaerts P, et al. Evaluation of a DNA microarray (check-MDR CT102) for rapid detection of TEM, SHV, and CTX-M extended-spectrum β-lactamases and of KPC, OXA-48, VIM, IMP, and NDM-1 carbapenemases. J Clin Microbiol 2011;49(4):1608–13.
122. Vogt D, Overesch G, Endimiani A, et al. Occurrence and genetic characteristics of third-generation cephalosporin-resistant *Escherichia coli* in Swiss retail meat. Microb Drug Resist 2014;20(5):485–94.
123. Szmolka A, Anjum MF, La Ragione RM, et al. Microarray based comparative genotyping of gentamicin resistant *Escherichia coli* strains from food animals and humans. Vet Microbiol 2012;156(1–2):110–8.
124. Geue L, Stieber B, Monecke S, et al. Development of a rapid microarray-based DNA subtyping assay for the alleles of *Shiga* toxins 1 and 2 of *Escherichia coli*. J Clin Microbiol 2014;52(8):2898–904.
125. Braun SD, Monecke S, Thurmer A, et al. Rapid identification of carbapenemase genes in gram-negative bacteria with an oligonucleotide microarray-based assay. PLoS One 2014;9(7):e102232.
126. Mancini N, Infurnari L, Ghidoli N, et al. Potential impact of a microarray-based nucleic acid assay for rapid detection of gram-negative bacteria and resistance markers in positive blood cultures. J Clin Microbiol 2014;52(4):1242–5.

127. Sullivan KV, Deburger B, Roundtree SS, et al. Rapid detection of inpatient gram-negative bacteremia; extended-spectrum beta-lactamases and carbapenemase resistance determinants with the Verigene BC-GN test: a multi-center evaluation. J Clin Microbiol 2014;52:2416–21.
128. Wieser A, Schneider L, Jung J, et al. MALDI-TOF MS in microbiological diagnostics-identification of microorganisms and beyond (mini review). Appl Microbiol Biotechnol 2012;93(3):965–74.
129. Emonet S, Shah HN, Cherkaoui A, et al. Application and use of various mass spectrometry methods in clinical microbiology. Clin Microbiol Infect 2010; 16(11):1604–13.
130. Ho YP, Reddy PM. Advances in mass spectrometry for the identification of pathogens. Mass Spectrom Rev 2011;30(6):1203–24.
131. Lavigne JP, Espinal P, Dunyach-Remy C, et al. Mass spectrometry: a revolution in clinical microbiology? Clin Chem Lab Med 2012;0(0):1–14.
132. Lasserre C, De Saint Martin L, Cuzon G, et al. Efficient detection of carbapenemase activity in enterobacteriaceae by matrix-assisted laser desorption ionization-time of flight mass spectrometry in less than 30 minutes. J Clin Microbiol 2015;53(7):2163–71.
133. Schaumann R, Knoop N, Genzel GH, et al. A step towards the discrimination of β-lactamase-producing clinical isolates of *Enterobacteriaceae* and *Pseudomonas aeruginosa* by MALDI-TOF mass spectrometry. Med Sci Monit 2012; 18(9):MT71–7.
134. Cai JC, Hu YY, Zhang R, et al. Detection of OmpK36 porin loss in *Klebsiella* spp. By matrix-assisted laser desorption ionization-time of flight mass spectrometry. J Clin Microbiol 2012;50(6):2179–82.
135. Camara JE, Hays FA. Discrimination between wild-type and ampicillin-resistant *Escherichia coli* by matrix-assisted laser desorption/ionization time-of-flight mass spectrometry. Anal Bioanal Chem 2007;389(5):1633–8.
136. Hrabak J, Chudackova E, Walkova R. Matrix-assisted laser desorption ionization-time of flight (MALDI-TOF) mass spectrometry for detection of antibiotic resistance mechanisms: From research to routine diagnosis. Clin Microbiol Rev 2013;26(1):103–14.
137. Hrabak J, Walkova R, Studentova V, et al. Carbapenemase activity detection by matrix-assisted laser desorption ionization-time of flight mass spectrometry. J Clin Microbiol 2011;49(9):3222–7.
138. Burckhardt I, Zimmermann S. Using matrix-assisted laser desorption ionization-time of flight mass spectrometry to detect carbapenem resistance within 1 to 2.5 hours. J Clin Microbiol 2011;49(9):3321–4.
139. Sparbier K, Schubert S, Weller U, et al. Matrix-assisted laser desorption ionization-time of flight mass spectrometry-based functional assay for rapid detection of resistance against β-lactam antibiotics. J Clin Microbiol 2012; 50(3):927–37.
140. Hrabak J, Studentova V, Walkova R, et al. Detection of NDM-1, VIM-1, KPC, OXA-48, and OXA-162 carbapenemases by matrix-assisted laser desorption ionization-time of flight mass spectrometry. J Clin Microbiol 2012;50(7):2441–3.
141. Hooff GP, van Kampen JJ, Meesters RJ, et al. Characterization of β-lactamase enzyme activity in bacterial lysates using MALDI-mass spectrometry. J Proteome Res 2012;11(1):79–84.
142. Ikryannikova LN, Shitikov EA, Zhivankova DG, et al. A MALDI Tof MS-based minisequencing method for rapid detection of TEM-type extended-spectrum

β-lactamases in clinical strains of *Enterobacteriaceae*. J Microbiol Methods 2008;75(3):385–91.

143. Lafolie J, Sauget M, Cabrolier N, et al. Detection of Escherichia coli sequence type 131 by matrix-assisted laser desorption ionization time-of-flight mass spectrometry: Implications for infection control policies? J Hosp Infect 2015;90(3): 208–12.
144. Matsumura Y, Yamamoto M, Nagao M, et al. Detection of extended-spectrum-β-lactamase-producing *Escherichia coli* ST131 and ST405 clonal groups by matrix-assisted laser desorption ionization-time of flight mass spectrometry. J Clin Microbiol 2014;52(4):1034–40.
145. Hoyos-Mallecot Y, Cabrera-Alvargonzalez JJ, Miranda-Casas C, et al. MALDI-TOF MS, a useful instrument for differentiating metallo-beta-lactamases in *Enterobacteriaceae* and *Pseudomonas* spp. Lett Appl Microbiol 2014;58(4):325–9.
146. Wang L, Han C, Sui W, et al. MALDI-TOF MS applied to indirect carbapenemase detection: A validated procedure to clearly distinguish between carbapenemase-positive and carbapenemase-negative bacterial strains. Anal Bioanal Chem 2013;405(15):5259–66.
147. Jung JS, Popp C, Sparbier K, et al. Evaluation of matrix-assisted laser desorption ionization-time of flight mass spectrometry for rapid detection of beta-lactam resistance in enterobacteriaceae derived from blood cultures. J Clin Microbiol 2014;52(3):924–30.
148. Oviano M, Fernandez B, Fernandez A, et al. Rapid detection of enterobacteriaceae producing extended spectrum beta-lactamases directly from positive blood cultures by matrix-assisted laser desorption ionization-time of flight mass spectrometry. Clin Microbiol Infect 2014;20(11):1146–57.
149. Hoyos-Mallecot Y, Riazzo C, Miranda-Casas C, et al. Rapid detection and identification of strains carrying carbapenemases directly from positive blood cultures using MALDI-TOF MS. J Microbiol Methods 2014;105:98–101.
150. Carvalhaes CG, Cayo R, Visconde MF, et al. Detection of carbapenemase activity directly from blood culture vials using MALDI-TOF MS: a quick answer for the right decision. J Antimicrob Chemother 2014;69(8):2132–6.
151. Papagiannitsis CC, Studentova V, Izdebski R, et al. Matrix-assisted laser desorption ionization-time of flight mass spectrometry meropenem hydrolysis assay with NH4HCO3, a reliable tool for direct detection of carbapenemase activity. J Clin Microbiol 2015;53(5):1731–5.
152. Chong PM, McCorrister SJ, Unger MS, et al. MALDI-TOF MS detection of carbapenemase activity in clinical isolates of *Enterobacteriaceae* spp., *Pseudomonas aeruginosa*, and *Acinetobacter baumannii* compared against the carba-NP assay. J Microbiol Methods 2015;111:21–3.
153. Knox J, Jadhav S, Sevior D, et al. Phenotypic detection of carbapenemase-producing *Enterobacteriaceae* by use of matrix-assisted laser desorption ionization-time of flight mass spectrometry and the carba NP test. J Clin Microbiol 2014;52(11):4075–7.
154. Le Page S, Raoult D, Rolain JM. Real-time video imaging as a new and rapid tool for antibiotic susceptibility testing by the disc diffusion method: a paradigm for evaluating resistance to imipenem and identifying extended-spectrum beta-lactamases. Int J Antimicrob Agents 2015;45(1):61–5.
155. Douglas IS, Price CS, Overdier KH, et al. Rapid automated microscopy for microbiological surveillance of ventilator-associated pneumonia. Am J Respir Crit Care Med 2015;191(5):566–73.

156. March Rossello GA, Garcia-Loygorri Jordan de Urries MC, Gutierrez Rodriguez MP, et al. A two-hour antibiotic susceptibility test by ATP-bioluminescence. Enferm Infecc Microbiol Clin 2015. [Epub ahead of print].
157. Ivancic V, Mastali M, Percy N, et al. Rapid antimicrobial susceptibility determination of uropathogens in clinical urine specimens by use of ATP bioluminescence. J Clin Microbiol 2008;46(4):1213–9.
158. Santiso R, Tamayo M, Gosalvez J, et al. A rapid in situ procedure for determination of bacterial susceptibility or resistance to antibiotics that inhibit peptidoglycan biosynthesis. BMC Microbiol 2011;11:191.
159. Tamayo M, Santiso R, Gosalvez J, et al. Rapid assessment of the effect of ciprofloxacin on chromosomal DNA from *Escherichia coli* using an in situ DNA fragmentation assay. BMC Microbiol 2009;9:69.
160. Bou G, Otero FM, Santiso R, et al. Fast assessment of resistance to carbapenems and ciprofloxacin of clinical strains of *Acinetobacter baumannii*. J Clin Microbiol 2012;50(11):3609–13.
161. Faria-Ramos I, Espinar MJ, Rocha R, et al. A novel flow cytometric assay for rapid detection of extended-spectrum β-lactamases. Clin Microbiol Infect 2013;19(1):E8–15.
162. March GA, Garcia-Loygorri MC, Simarro M, et al. A new approach to determine the susceptibility of bacteria to antibiotics directly from positive blood culture bottles in two hours. J Microbiol Methods 2015;109:49–55.
163. van Belkum A, Dunne WM Jr. Next-generation antimicrobial susceptibility testing. J Clin Microbiol 2013;51(7):2018–24.
164. Pulido MR, Garcia-Quintanilla M, Martin-Pena R, et al. Progress on the development of rapid methods for antimicrobial susceptibility testing. J Antimicrob Chemother 2013;68(12):2710–7.
165. Jayamohan H, Sant HJ, Gale BK. Applications of microfluidics for molecular diagnostics. Methods Mol Biol 2013;949:305–34.
166. Sin ML, Mach KE, Wong PK, et al. Advances and challenges in biosensor-based diagnosis of infectious diseases. Expert Rev Mol Diagn 2014;14(2):225–44.
167. Nuchtavorn N, Suntornsuk W, Lunte SM, et al. Recent applications of microchip electrophoresis to biomedical analysis. J Pharm Biomed Anal 2015;113:72–96.
168. Kokalj T, Perez-Ruiz E, Lammertyn J. Building bio-assays with magnetic particles on a digital microfluidic platform. N Biotechnol 2015;32(5):485–503.
169. Jubery TZ, Srivastava SK, Dutta P. Dielectrophoretic separation of bioparticles in microdevices: a review. Electrophoresis 2014;35(5):691–713.
170. Chen CH, Lu Y, Sin ML, et al. Antimicrobial susceptibility testing using high surface-to-volume ratio microchannels. Anal Chem 2010;82(3):1012–9.
171. Mach KE, Mohan R, Baron EJ, et al. A biosensor platform for rapid antimicrobial susceptibility testing directly from clinical samples. J Urol 2011;185(1):148–53.
172. Tang Y, Zhen L, Liu J, et al. Rapid antibiotic susceptibility testing in a microfluidic pH sensor. Anal Chem 2013;85(5):2787–94.
173. Choi J, Jung YG, Kim J, et al. Rapid antibiotic susceptibility testing by tracking single cell growth in a microfluidic agarose channel system. Lab Chip 2013; 13(2):280–7.
174. Kim KP, Kim YG, Choi CH, et al. In situ monitoring of antibiotic susceptibility of bacterial biofilms in a microfluidic device. Lab Chip 2010;10(23):3296–9.
175. Mohan R, Mukherjee A, Sevgen SE, et al. A multiplexed microfluidic platform for rapid antibiotic susceptibility testing. Biosens Bioelectron 2013;49:118–25.

176. Hou HW, Bhattacharyya RP, Hung DT, et al. Direct detection and drug-resistance profiling of bacteremias using inertial microfluidics. Lab Chip 2015; 15(10):2297–307.
177. Palasubramaniam S, Muniandy S, Navaratnam P. Rapid detection of ESBL-producing *Klebsiella pneumoniae* in blood cultures by fluorescent in-situ hybridization. J Microbiol Methods 2008;72(1):107–9.
178. Poritz MA, Blaschke AJ, Byington CL, et al. Filmarray, an automated nested multiplex PCR system for multi-pathogen detection: Development and application to respiratory tract infection. PLoS One 2011;6(10):e26047.
179. Babady NE. The FilmArray(r) respiratory panel: An automated, broadly multiplexed molecular test for the rapid and accurate detection of respiratory pathogens. Expert Rev Mol Diagn 2013;13(8):779–88.
180. Blaschke AJ, Heyrend C, Byington CL, et al. Rapid identification of pathogens from positive blood cultures by multiplex polymerase chain reaction using the FilmArray system. Diagn Microbiol Infect Dis 2012;74(4):349–55.
181. Vasoo S, Cunningham SA, Greenwood-Quaintance KE, et al. Evaluation of the FilmArray(R) blood culture (BCID) panel on biofilms dislodged from explanted arthroplasties for prosthetic joint infection diagnosis. J Clin Microbiol 2015; 53(8):2790–2.
182. Southern TR, VanSchooneveld TC, Bannister DL, et al. Implementation and performance of the biofire FilmArray(r) blood culture identification panel with antimicrobial treatment recommendations for bloodstream infections at a Midwestern academic tertiary hospital. Diagn Microbiol Infect Dis 2015;81(2):96–101.
183. Dunne WM Jr, Westblade LF, Ford B. Next-generation and whole-genome sequencing in the diagnostic clinical microbiology laboratory. Eur J Clin Microbiol Infect Dis 2012;31(8):1719–26.
184. Long SW, Williams D, Valson C, et al. A genomic day in the life of a clinical microbiology laboratory. J Clin Microbiol 2013;51(4):1272–7.
185. Wright MS, Stockwell TB, Beck E, et al. SISPA-Seq for rapid whole genome surveys of bacterial isolates. Infect Genet Evol 2015;32:191–8.
186. Quick J, Ashton P, Calus S, et al. Rapid draft sequencing and real-time nanopore sequencing in a hospital outbreak of *Salmonella*. Genome Biol 2015; 16(1):114.
187. Koser CU, Ellington MJ, Cartwright EJ, et al. Routine use of microbial whole genome sequencing in diagnostic and public health microbiology. PLoS Pathog 2012;8(8):e1002824.
188. Wolk DM, Kaleta EJ, Wysocki VH. PCR-electrospray ionization mass spectrometry: the potential to change infectious disease diagnostics in clinical and public health laboratories. J Mol Diagn 2012;14(4):295–304.
189. Kaleta EJ, Clark AE, Johnson DR, et al. Use of PCR coupled with electrospray ionization mass spectrometry for rapid identification of bacterial and yeast bloodstream pathogens from blood culture bottles. J Clin Microbiol 2011; 49(1):345–53.
190. Ecker DJ, Sampath R, Massire C, et al. Ibis T5000: a universal biosensor approach for microbiology. Nat Rev Microbiol 2008;6(7):553–8.
191. Ecker JA, Massire C, Hall TA, et al. Identification of *Acinetobacter* species and genotyping of *Acinetobacter baumannii* by multilocus PCR and mass spectrometry. J Clin Microbiol 2006;44(8):2921–32.
192. Sarovich DS, Colman RE, Price EP, et al. Molecular genotyping of *Acinetobacter* spp. Isolated in Arizona, USA, using multilocus PCR and mass spectrometry. J Med Microbiol 2013;62(Pt 9):1295–300.

193. Decker BK, Perez F, Hujer AM, et al. Longitudinal analysis of the temporal evolution of *Acinetobacter baumannii* strains in Ohio, USA, by using rapid automated typing methods. PLoS One 2012;7(4):e33443.
194. Perez F, Endimiani A, Ray AJ, et al. Carbapenem-resistant *Acinetobacter baumannii* and *Klebsiella pneumoniae* across a hospital system: Impact of post-acute care facilities on dissemination. J Antimicrob Chemother 2010;65(8): 1807–18.
195. Farrell JJ, Hujer AM, Sampath R, et al. Salvage microbiology: Opportunities and challenges in the detection of bacterial pathogens following initiation of antimicrobial treatment. Expert Rev Mol Diagn 2015;15(3):349–60.
196. Nagalingam S, Lisgaris M, Rodriguez B, et al. Identification of occult *Fusobacterium nucleatum* central nervous system infection by use of PCR-electrospray ionization mass spectrometry. J Clin Microbiol 2014;52(9):3462–4.
197. Farrell JJ, Larson JA, Akeson JW, et al. *Ureaplasma parvum* prosthetic joint infection detected by PCR. J Clin Microbiol 2014;52(6):2248–50.
198. Brinkman CL, Vergidis P, Uhl JR, et al. PCR-electrospray ionization mass spectrometry for direct detection of pathogens and antimicrobial resistance from heart valves in patients with infective endocarditis. J Clin Microbiol 2013; 51(7):2040–6.
199. Endimiani A, Hujer KM, Hujer AM, et al. Are we ready for novel detection methods to treat respiratory pathogens in hospital-acquired pneumonia? Clin Infect Dis 2011;52(Suppl 4):S373–83.
200. Endimiani A, Hujer KM, Hujer AM, et al. Rapid identification of bla_{KPC}-possessing *Enterobacteriaceae* by PCR/electrospray ionization-mass spectrometry. J Antimicrob Chemother 2010;65(8):1833–4.
201. Hujer KM, Hujer AM, Endimiani A, et al. Rapid determination of quinolone resistance in *Acinetobacter* spp. J Clin Microbiol 2009;47(5):1436–42.

The Continuing Plague of Extended-spectrum β-lactamase–producing Enterobacteriaceae Infections

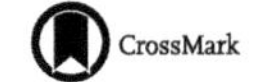

Amos Adler, MD[a,b], David E. Katz, MD, MPH[c],
Dror Marchaim, MD[b,d,*]

KEYWORDS

- Gram-negative • MDROs • *Escherichia coli* • *Klebsiella pneumoniae*
- *Proteus mirabilis*

KEY POINTS

- The continued spread of extended-spectrum β-lactamase (ESBL) infections is correlated with shifts in medical care.
- The overuse and misuse of prolonged 'prophylactic' courses of antimicrobials is a modifiable independent predictor for ESBL acquisition.
- Agriculture and food products might have an additional role in dissemination of ESBL-producing organisms in community settings.
- Emergence of a new class of ESBL enzymes, the CTX-Ms, might have resulted the epidemiologic evolution of human ESBL infections in community settings.
- Appropriate antimicrobial therapy is frequently delayed in patients with ESBL infections; rapid diagnostics and reliable clinical predicting tools could aid in reducing delays and might improve patient outcomes.

D. Marchaim had received in the past payments for lectures and a research grant from Merck (all not related to this paper).
Funding: This study was not supported financially by any external source.
Conflicts of Interest: No potential conflicts of interest.
[a] Clinical Microbiology Laboratory, Tel-Aviv Sourasky Medical Center, Tel-Aviv, Israel; [b] Sackler School of Medicine, Tel-Aviv University, Tel-Aviv, Israel; [c] Department of Internal Medicine D, Shaare Zedek Medical Center, Hebrew University School of Medicine, Jerusalem, Israel; [d] Division of Infectious Diseases, Assaf Harofeh Medical Center, Zerifin 70300, Israel
* Corresponding author. Division of Infectious Diseases, Assaf Harofeh Medical Center, Zerifin 70300, Israel.
E-mail address: drormarchaim@gmail.com

Infect Dis Clin N Am 30 (2016) 347–375
http://dx.doi.org/10.1016/j.idc.2016.02.003 id.theclinics.com
0891-5520/16/$ – see front matter

INTRODUCTION

The incidence of infections caused by multidrug-resistant (MDR) Gram-negative bacilli pathogens, affecting humans in hospitals, outpatient health care facilities, and community settings, is continually growing worldwide.[1–3] The Infectious Diseases Society of America defined the "ESKAPE" pathogens as the pathogens that currently cause the majority of hospital infections and can effectively "escape" the effects of available therapeutics.[1] Among the ESKAPE pathogens are common Enterobacteriaceae (eg, *Klebsiella pneumoniae*, *Enterobacter* species, *and Escherichia coli*).[1] *Proteus mirabilis* is another enteric pathogen in which the rate of resistance to multiple antimicrobials is rising, more commonly outside of the United States.[4,5] Emergence of resistance to a wide range of antibiotics among the most common human pathogens,[6] namely, the Enterobacteriaceae, is hazardous, and it poses a huge burden on individual patients and the general public.[1,7,8]

THE EMERGENCE OF EXTENDED-SPECTRUM β-LACTAMASES

The incremental growth in resistance to β-lactam agents (eg, penicillins and cephalosporins) among Enterobacteriaceae is a worrisome trend. β-Lactams are among the oldest and safest therapeutics.[9,10] Given susceptible isolates, they are potent bacteriocidic agents.[11] In addition, well-controlled data on their clinical efficacy against Enterobacteriaceae are readily available because of their extended years of usage.[1,12] Owing to their safety, tolerability, potency, and (usually) low price, β-lactams are the most commonly prescribed drugs worldwide.[13] β-Lactams are used universally as first-line agents for many infectious clinical syndromes resulting from Enterobacteriaceae infections.[14,15]

The first report of a naturally occurring β-lactam hydrolyzing enzyme in *Escherichia coli* was published even before penicillin was marketed for use.[16] In 1960, the plasmid-mediated β-lactamase TEM was first reported from Greece.[17] Later, additional transmissible types of β-lactamases were identified, for example, SHV-1.[12] These β-lactamases confer resistance to penicillins and narrow-spectrum cephalosporins, but not to extended-spectrum penicillins or cephalosporins of advanced generations.[12] Soon thereafter, new broader spectrum β-lactam agents became widely used (eg, cephalosporins with oxymino side chain, cephamycins, carbapenems, and monobactam). Subsequently, new families of β-lactamases soon started to emerge.[18,19] One of the most epidemiologically 'successful' groups of such enzymes are the extended-spectrum β-lactamases (ESBLs).

The ESBLs are serine β-lactamases, characterized according to their biochemically functional Ambler classification as class A, and are therefore hydrolyzed by β-lactamase inhibitors such as clavulanate or tazobactam.[10] This feature constitutes the basis for the phenotypic diagnosis of ESBL-producing bacteria in many laboratories; measuring the zone of inhibition of the isolates in the presence and absence of a β-lactamase inhibitor (ie, the "ESBL test").[10] According to the functional Bush–Jacoby–Medeiros classification, ESBLs are classified under group 2be.[20,21]

ESBLs confer resistance to most β-lactam antibiotics, including third- and fourth-generation cephalosporins and monobactams, but not to carbapenems and cephamycins.[15,17,22] Although ESBL-producing Enterobacteriaceae hydrolyze penicillins, cephalosporins (excluding cephamycins) and monobactam, their degree of hydrolytic activity can vary greatly. This results in both diagnostic challenges and controversies pertaining to treatment efficacy of agents for which isolates are supposedly "susceptible."[23] It took several years before clinicians realized that treatment with β-lactams for an ESBL-producing strain, even when the strain is supposedly 'susceptible' (per older criteria[24]), could fail in various infectious syndromes.[22,23,25,26] Moreover, ESBL-producing Enterobacteriaceae are often co-resistant to other classes of antibiotics such as fluoroquinolones, aminoglycosides, and trimethoprim/sulfamethoxazole (TMP/SMX).[27,28] This further limits available therapeutic options and increases the epidemiologic significance posed by these pathogens.[23,29,30]

ESBLs have been reported in Gram-negatives, most commonly in *K pneumoniae*, *E coli*, and *P mirabilis*, as well as in other enteric bacteria (eg, *Klebsiella oxytoca*, *Citrobacter*, *Enterobacter*, *Salmonella*, *Serratia*), and in nonfermenting nosocomial pathogens (eg, *Acinetobacter baumannii*, *Pseudomonas aeruginosa*).[19] Some Enterobacteriaceae (eg, *Enterobacter*, *Citrobacter*, *Providencia*, *Morganella*, *Serratia*) inherently possess chromosomal genes (bla_{AmpC}) that confer resistance to the same extended-spectrum cephalosporins and penicillins through an Ambler C hydrolyzing bla_{AmpC} β-lactamases.[19,21] This review focuses solely on Ambler A ESBL producing *K pneumoniae*, *E coli*, and *P mirabilis* infections, because this has proved to be a somewhat distinct epidemiologic clinical entity.

WORLDWIDE PREVALENCE OF EXTENDED-SPECTRUM β-LACTAMASES

Overall, the rates and types of ESBL-producing Enterobacteriaceae infections have increased dramatically in the past 30 years; however, distinct geographic patterns and institutional variation do exist.[17,31] Huge surveillance programs are periodically reporting the prevalence of ESBLs among offending pathogens from all over the world.[32,33] Database from 2004 to 2006 illustrated for example, that the rates of ESBL production in Latin America was 44% among *K pneumoniae* and 13.5% among *E coli* isolations.[32] In Europe, the rates reported during the same years were 13.3% of *K pneumoniae* and 7.6% of *E coli*, in Asia/Pacific Rim 22.4% of *K pneumoniae* and 12% of *E coli*, and in North America rates were 7.5% in *K pneumoniae* and 2.2% among *E coli*.[32,34–36] Presently, the rates reported from many facilities are much higher, that is, up to 45% among *K pneumoniae* and up to 35% among *E coli*.[37–39]

THE HISTORIC EVOLUTION OF TEM AND SHV-TYPES EXTENDED-SPECTRUM β-LACTAMASES–PRODUCING ENTEROBACTERIACEAE INFECTIONS

Third-generation (extended-spectrum) cephalosporins were introduced to clinical practice in the early 1980s.[40,41] In many institutions, they were prescribed in high volumes and with very little regulation.[42] These agents were safe, potent, accessible, relatively cheap, and extremely effective against a wide array of human pathogens.[43,44] In many facilities, they became the backbone of empiric regimens for various indications.[45] Frequently, administration of these broad-spectrum agents was continued, even after the isolation of a more susceptible causative pathogen.[42]

Soon thereafter, plasmid-encoded β-lactamases, which hydrolyze extended-spectrum cephalosporins, started to appear in western Europe (Germany, 1983), Asia, and the Americas.[17] The first ESBLs reported were developed via point mutations in the narrow-spectrum β-lactamases SHV-1, TEM-1, and TEM-2.[46] These substitutions resulted in amino acid substitutions that changed the active site of the β-lactamase and consequently resulted in resistance also to the extended-spectrum cephalosporins, to all penicillins, and to monobactams.[47] As new alleles of the SHV and TEM families of enzymes were discovered, they were named in chronologic order (ie, SHV-2, SHV-3, etc; and TEM-3, TEM-4, etc, respectively)[19,21,47] but not necessarily according to their antimicrobial spectrum. For instance, the SHV-9 is categorized as a type 2be (ie, ESBL) enzyme whereas the SHV-11 is a type 2b (narrow spectrum) enzyme (available: http://www.lahey.org/Studies/).

Initially, ESBL-producing pathogens were isolated primarily in acute care tertiary care facilities, particularly from very sick patients hospitalized in intensive care units.[17,48–50] These patients were heavily exposed to broad spectrum antibiotics and had multiple invasive devices and exposure to instrumentation.[51,52] After establishing endemicity in certain facilities, reports of nosocomial outbreaks of Enterobacteriaceae producing bla_{SHV} or bla_{TEM} ESBLs were starting to emerge, consisting mostly of ESBL-producing *K pneumoniae*.[51,53–55] In the mid to late 1990s, case reports and case series suggested that ESBL-producing Enterobacteriaceae had started to spread to outpatient settings as well.[56–63] This phenomenon was extremely worrisome at that time, and was defined by experts as a global sentinel event that should be closely monitored and controlled.[51,64]

One hypothesis explaining this spread of ESBL producers to community settings stems from the dramatic change related to the continuum of medical care that gradually took place during those years. Medically complex patients, who previously were exclusively managed in acute care settings (eg, the severely ill, patients with chronic invasive foreign devices, central lines, urinary catheter, and even ventilated patients), were now being managed for prolonged periods in long-term care facilities (LTCF).[65] The motivation for this gradual change was primarily fiscal.[65] These LTCFs are in many instances 'for-profit' facilities, and were initially reluctant to invest in infection control and antimicrobial stewardship measures.[65,66] Therefore, LTCFs soon became an important pathway between the hospital and the community settings, contributing to the exponential rise in the prevalence of multidrug-resistant organisms (MDROs),[67] including ESBL-producing Enterobacteriaceae.[68,69] These patients with complicated medical conditions were continually transmitted back and forth between health care facilities, serving as "Trojan horses" for MDROs.[68,70] Multiple case-control analyses conducted in various locations worldwide showed that an LTCF stay was an independent predictor for acquisition of various MDROs, including ESBLs.[30,71–74] Misuse of antimicrobials, which facilitate the predominance of resistance strains and emergence of resistance among susceptible strains, coupled with nonimplementation of infection control measures, which facilitate patient-to-patient transmission of MDROs within the institution, accompanied by patients' basic deteriorated characteristics, were all common in certain LTCFs.[7,65,68,69] This evolution of the continuum of medical care probably aided the spread of formerly pure nosocomial ESBLs, for example, bla_{SHV} and bla_{TEM}, into nonhospital settings.[74]

The epidemiology of ESBL-producing strains further evolved soon thereafter. Approximately a decade ago, ESBL-producing Enterobacteriaceae began to appear in the community among patients with no prior documented contact with LTCFs, no recent antibiotic exposure, and no other known risk factors for ESBL acquisition and carriage.[30,71,72,75,76] This created an additional clinical challenge; apart from being resistant to extended-spectrum β-lactam agents, resistances to commonly prescribed oral agents, frequently prescribed in community settings, became prevalent as well.[27,71] The plasmid harboring the ESBL gene (ie, the "resistome"[77]) was carrying additional genes conferring resistance to commonly prescribed oral antimicrobials such as fluoroquinolones and TMP/SMX.[71,72,74,78–80] This resulted in delays in instituting appropriate therapy in the community setting, and worse outcomes for relatively "simple" infections among previously healthy and young individuals.[22,30,79,81]

THE CTX-M–PRODUCING *E COLI* OUTBREAK IN NONHOSPITAL SETTINGS

After the reports of increased incidence of ESBL infections in nonhospital settings among patients with none of the known "traditional" risk factors (ie, associated with health care exposures), molecular investigations revealed that a change in ESBL types might be related to this epidemiologic shift.[28,48,69,71,73,75,76,82–90] As mentioned, *K pneumoniae* was the main isolate harboring ESBL genes (most often bla_{TEM} and bla_{SHV} types) during the 1990s.[10] However, a decade later, *E coli*–producing ESBLs became prevalent in various regions, producing a different class of ESBLs, that is, the CTX-Ms.[75,76,90] The CTX-Ms were discovered over a decade earlier, but were not prevalent initially among ESBL pathogens associated with human infections (with the exception of few alleles, ie, CTX-M-93[91]).[12,20,92]

In recent years, the CTX-M families have seen a tremendous diversification. They can be divided into 5 main groups,[93] with different enzymes prevalent in different locations worldwide.[94,95] In comparison with the "old epidemiology," where *K pneumoniae* ESBL infections (ie, mainly SHVs and TEMs) were associated with various infectious clinical syndromes (eg, pneumonia, intra-abdominal infections, urinary tract infections [UTI], and skin and soft tissue infections), the majority of $bla_{CTX\text{-}M}$–producing *E coli* infections from the community were UTIs.[27,76,78]

The risk factors for $bla_{CTX\text{-}M}$–producing *E coli* infections were assessed in multiple analyses.[71,96–100] One of the unique features of this endemic strain is the tight statistical correlation to prior use of fluoroquinolones and recent invasive urologic procedures.[27,71,76] The common practice of many urologists is to prescribe "prophylactic" regimens of antimicrobials, mostly consisting of fluoroquinolones, for several days before and after an invasive urologic procedure. This practice is not supported by professional guidelines[101,102] or based on solid scientific clinical data.[103–105] Regardless, this practice is still common with urologists and primary practitioners worldwide.[101,102] The increase in the number of such ambulatory urologic procedures in the modern era might have also contributed to the spread of $bla_{CTX\text{-}M}$–producing *E coli* infections in some community settings.[71] Some risk factor analyses even pointed to the fact that being a middle-aged male became an independent risk factor for $bla_{CTX\text{-}M}$–producing *E coli* infection, although UTIs are usually much more common among women in this age group. Sex might have served as a possible confounder for urologic invasive procedures in some of these studies.[27,72]

Additional contributing factors to the epidemic of ESBL infections in the community in general, and of $bla_{CTX\text{-}M}$–producing *E coli* infections in particular, may be related to the agriculture and food industries.[106–109] Unfortunately, misuse of antibiotics in these industries is common and not tightly regulated.[110–112] Many community outbreaks of $bla_{CTX\text{-}M}$–producing *E coli* infections, originating from the agriculture and food industries, were reported in the past decade.[85,106–109,113–121] One of the largest ever reported was an outbreak in 2011 of a $bla_{CTX\text{-}M}$–producing *E coli* strain that was associated with hemolytic uremic syndrome and several deaths among previously healthy and young individuals, mainly from Germany and France.[122,123] It was suggested that the outbreak resulted from contaminated food products that were distributed in various European countries.[121] CTX-Ms have also been isolated from wild birds, poultry, urban rats, companion animals, and retail meat from supermarkets in various states in the United States.[85,89,115,124–132] These findings led several investigators to suggest that CTX-M enzymes could potentially spread from the community to the health care environment, and not universally vice versa.[27,54] Despite the appeal of this concept, the importance of this connection beyond isolated outbreaks (as mentioned) is questionable. Although ESBLs are certainly not uncommon in livestock, there are important differences in the prevalence of specific genes and clones in animals versus humans.[132] This is in contrast with other organisms, for example, *Staphylococcus aureus*, where specific clones have been shown to be transferred from livestock to human.[133] More important, considering the production process of food products from livestock, the transmission mechanism of living organisms from food to human is not clear.

International travel to certain locations (eg, India, the Middle East, and Africa) used to be an additional factor that had facilitated the spread of *bla*$_{CTX-M}$–producing strains in the community, specifically in certain countries (particularly in North America).[134] A detailed Canadian risk factor analysis found that the distribution of CTX-M enzymes among travelers was highly correlated with the predominant CTX-Ms that were reported from the respective travel destinations.[134] However, these enzymes had already established endemicity in most regions. As of 2013, CTX-Ms are considered the most common ESBLs in Latin America, Canada, South America, and in many parts of Europe and the United States.[54,75,94,135,136] Thus, unlike carbapenemases that are still rare in the community of many parts of the world, ESBLs endemicity is much wider and thus the contribution of international travel to current spread is probably minor.

THE CLONAL EXPANSION OF A SPECIFIC *bla*$_{CTX-M}$–PRODUCING *E COLI* STRAIN IN THE COMMUNITY

After the recognition that CTX-Ms might be related in part to the epidemiologic shift in ESBL human infections and its dissemination into community settings, advanced investigational molecular techniques soon revealed the predominance of a specific *E coli* clone producing mainly *bla*$_{CTX-M15}$ enzymes on at least 3 continents.[137,138] This successful clone was classified as (1) sequence type (ST) 131 per multilocus sequence typing[71,75,137,139–143]; (2) phylogenetic group B2 (classified according to major *E coli* phylogenetic groups [A, B1, B2, D])[144]; and (3) serotype O25:H4.[145] This clone, referred to as ST-131 for the rest of this review, is a pandemic clone that has disseminated exponentially since 2003.[146] Although other lineages such as the ST-405 or ST-38 have also played an important role in the dissemination of CTX-M–producing *E coli*,[138] they have been less predominant compared with the ST-131 clone. This clone is primarily associated with community-associated ESBL UTIs, which are frequently accompanied by bloodstream infections (BSI).[147] The vast majority of ST-131 isolates are resistant to fluoroquinolones.[148]

Until recently, the reasons that made this specific clone so successful were obscure. It was isolated from companion animals, seagulls, rats, poultry, and even retail chicken, with all of these sources suggested as possible reservoirs.[147] In a recent trial conducted in Seville, Spain, a case-control and cohort investigation of the risk factors and clinical outcomes, respectively, were compared between 110 patients with ST-131 *E coli* ESBL infections versus 288 patients with non–ST-131 ESBL *E coli* infections.[149] Previous use of antibiotics was the main modifiable risk factor for infections caused by ST-131 strains. The severity of sepsis, rates of bacteremia and mortality were similar among ST-131 and non–ST-131 groups.[149] These same findings were later reported from a US site[76] and from Nepal as well.[150] These analyses suggest that misuse of antimicrobials, particularly in the community, plays an important role in the acquisition and spread of this clone. Other common mode of MDRO acquisition, that is, patient-to-patient transmission, probably plays a lesser role in the dissemination of this clone in the community.[7] This understanding led to the initiation of extensive systematic efforts to reduce the misuse of antibiotics in the "community": that is, in ambulatory clinical settings and in the agriculture and the food industries.[151] This also contributes to the ongoing debate over whether patients with ESBL carriage should be subjected to contact isolation precautions while they are admitted to the hospital.[152]

WHAT ARE THE PREDICTORS FOR EXTENDED-SPECTRUM β-LACTAMASES–PRODUCING ENTEROBACTERIACEAE INFECTIONS ACQUIRED OUTSIDE OF THE HOSPITAL SETTINGS?

Many risk factor analyses pertaining to ESBLs acquired outside the hospital settings have been published from diverse geographic settings using various definitions.[62,63,134,153–159] The debate on how best to define "community-onset infections" is beyond the scope of this paper and is reviewed in detail elsewhere.[8] The risk factors analyses that were published up until 2008 were nicely summarized by Pitout and Laupland.[28] However, this was before the magnitude of the $bla_{CTX\text{-}Ms}$–producing ST-131 *E coli* pandemia was fully acknowledged.[72] Their review highlighted the different predictors of hospital-onset and community-onset infections. In the hospital setting, ESBL infections were significantly linked to intensive care unit stay, prolonged "time at risk" (ie, time from admission to culture), presence of foreign medical devices (eg, central line, nasogastric tube, urinary catheter, endotracheal tube), recent prior invasive procedures, and recent prior administration of antimicrobials (especially third-generation cephalosporins).[10,17,160–162] In community-onset infections, or infections upon admission to hospitals, admission from an LTCF was the major risk factor for ESBL infection.[10,27,71] Other risk factors for community-onset ESBL infections were recurrent UTIs coupled with underlying renal pathology, recent exposure to fluoroquinolones, previous hospitalization, advanced age, diabetes mellitus, and underlying liver disease.[28] Later in 2008, Rodriguez-Bano and associates[72] published a detailed prospective analysis of risk factors for 'community-acquired' ESBL-producing *E coli* infections in 11 Spanish hospitals. The independent predictors based on this multivariable model were age older than 60 years, female sex, diabetes mellitus, recurrent UTIs, previous urologic invasive procedures, follow-up visits to outpatient clinics, and previous recent receipt of antibiotics (in particular β-lactams or fluoroquinolones).[72] Many of these independent predictors simply reflected health care–associated exposures, as set in the past by Friedman and colleagues.[163] The misuse of antibiotics before and after minimally invasive urologic procedures (by urologists and primary care physicians), frequently with no established indication,[164] may have contributed to the emergence and spread of ESBLs in nonhospital settings of this region.[72]

This former epidemiologic era of community-onset ESBL infections is also well-summarized by a multinational metasynthesis investigation conducted by Ben-Ami and coworkers.[71] This study included a synthesis of data collected from 6 centers in Europe, Asia, and North America. A total of 983 patient-specific isolates were reviewed (91% were *E coli*, 7% were *Klebsiella* species, and 2% were *P mirabilis*). CTX-M types were already the most frequent ESBLs in this united cohort (65%). Independent significant predictors for community-onset ESBL infections included recent antibiotic use, residence in an LTCF, recent hospitalization, age greater than 65 years, and male sex (in contrast with the female predominance reported from Seville[72]). This comprehensive analysis illustrates again the resemblance of independent predictors for ESBL infections acquired outside of a hospital, and the definition of health care-associated infections as set in the past by Friedman and colleagues,[163] that is, ESBL infections upon admission to acute care hospitals should be suspected when health care exposure is documented.[39,165]

A multicenter prospective case-control study conducted in 10 Israeli hospitals (2007–2009) was published in 2010.[30] This was already after $bla_{CTX\text{-}M}$–producing strains had established endemicity in most of Israel.[6,27] Overall, 447 patients with bacteremia owing to Enterobacteriaceae were enrolled: 205 cases with ESBLs and 242 controls with susceptible strains. Independent predictors of ESBL were advanced age, multiple comorbid conditions, poor functional status, recent contact with health care settings, invasive procedures, and prior receipt of antimicrobial therapy. An interesting, and previously unreported, finding of this prospective study was that patients presenting with septic shock and/or multiorgan failure were more likely to have an ESBL infections (ie, as opposed to infection resulting from susceptible Enterobacteriaceae). This may be related indirectly to the increased virulence properties of these ESBL producing strains. It is very common in MDRO epidemiologic analyses that patients affected by the resistant strain suffer worse outcomes compared with its susceptible counterpart strain.[166–170] However, when controlling for various confounders, particularly for delays in initiation of appropriate antimicrobial therapy (DAAT), antimicrobial resistance alone has not always been shown to be independently associated with worse clinical outcomes[171]; many times, the opposite was actually evident.[171,172] With ESBL strains, however, this might be different, and it is postulated by some that virulence properties are coupled with resistance genes on some of the transmissible "resistomes" in some of the circulating ESBL strains.[173,174] This aspect, however, is beyond the scope of this review. An additional finding of this multicenter Israeli study, was that patients infected with ESBL strains, suffered more frequently from DAAT (odds ratio, 4.7). This again highlights the importance of early pathogen detection and identification (ie, by rapid diagnostics), and the standardization of appropriate empirical regimens, and the development of reliable prediction tools. These measures could shorten the time to initiation of appropriate therapy, thereby improving patient outcomes,[81] while adhering to stewardship guidelines and recommendations.[30,39]

The spread of human ESBL infections caused by $bla_{CTX\text{-}M}$–producing *E coli* strains was introduced to the United States a few years after earlier reports from other locations.[76,83,175–177] A prospective observational study to examine the epidemiology of community-associated (both community-acquired and health care–associated) infections owing specifically to ESBL-producing *E coli* at 5 centers in the United States was published in 2013.[75] Of the 291 patients infected or colonized with ESBL-producing *E coli* who were enrolled either as outpatients or within 48 hours of hospitalization, 107 (36.8%) had community-acquired infections (with none of the health care–associated exposures set by Friedman and colleagues[163]) and in 81.5% of them, the infectious syndrome was UTI.[75] Independent risk factors for health care associated infection (with ≥1 health care exposures per Friedman criteria[163]) were the presence of cardiovascular disease, chronic renal failure, dementia, solid organ malignancy, and hospitalization within the previous 12 months. Of the community-acquired infections (ie, no health care exposures[163]), 54.2% were caused by the globally epidemic ST131 strain, and 91.3% of the isolates produced CTX-M–type ESBL.[75]

A case–case-control study of risk factors for CTX-M–producing *E coli* was conducted later on in Detroit.[76] Overall 575 patients with community-onset ESBL-producing *E coli* were enrolled, and 491 (85.4%) of the isolates contained a CTX-M ESBL gene. Independent risk factors for CTX-M *E coli* isolation compared with non–CTX-M *E coli* included male gender, impaired consciousness, H2 blocker use, immunosuppression, and exposure to penicillins and/or TMP/SMX. Compared with uninfected controls, independent risk factors for isolation of CTX-M *E coli* included the presence of a urinary catheter, previous UTI, exposure to oxyimino-cephalosporins, dependent functional status, nonhome residence, and multiple comorbid conditions. In addition, CTX-M strains were more resistant to multiple antibiotics than non–CTX-M ESBL strains.[76]

To summarize this section, independent predictors for ESBL infections acquired in the community resemble some of the criteria set by Friedman and colleagues[163] for defining health care–associated exposures. These include LTCF stay, recent hospitalization in acute care facilities, exposure to antibiotics, recent invasive procedures (specifically urologic), presence of foreign devices, and certain complex comorbidities.

WHAT IS THE ISOLATED IMPACT OF EXTENDED-SPECTRUM β-LACTAMASE ACQUISITION ON PATIENTS' CLINICAL OUTCOMES?

In a matched case–case-control analysis (ie, the preferred methodology to study the epidemiology of MDROs[178,179]), patients with ESBL infections have been shown to experience worse clinical outcomes compared with patients with susceptible Enterobacteriaceae, and compared with uninfected controls.[72,79,81,180–182] In a metaanalysis looking at the impact of ESBL-production on mortality, comprising 16 studies conducted from 1996 to 2003, there was a significant rise in mortality among patients with ESBL-associated BSIs (relative risk, 1.85; $P<.001$). Moreover, patients with ESBL infections had significant DAAT (relative risk, 5.56; $P<.001$).[81] Because DAAT is the strongest independent modifiable predictor for mortality in sepsis,[183] and because every hour of DAAT in septic shock reduces survival rates by approximately 7.6%,[184] this might be one of the main reasons for worse outcomes among these patients.[81]

There are various methods for reducing DAAT, including implementation of rapid diagnostic techniques and developing genuine prediction tools for early identification of ESBL infections, all to aid in reducing DAAT and avoiding the inappropriate administration of wide spectrum antibiotics.[185] In an attempt to reduce DAAT, several approaches to hasten the diagnosis of ESBLs have been explored including the detection of bla_{ESBL} genes by microarray[186] or by using MALDI-ToF to detect cefotaxime-hydrolyzing Gram negatives from positive blood cultures.[187] Unfortunately, these methods are both expensive and require significant amount of work and expertise. In addition, unlike other important resistance traits, such as methicillin resistance in *S aureus* that are conferred by a single molecular mechanism, cephalosporin resistance may be caused by a multitude of genetic mechanisms that are difficult to detect by a single test. Thus, such methods are unlikely to be implemented on a routine basis in the majority of clinical microbiology laboratories. There were also attempts to develop prediction tools for ESBL infection upon admission to hospitals, with the aim of reducing DAAT, and avoiding misuse of broad spectrum antimicrobials in patients without ESBL infection.[185] However, these tools have not yet been validated or implemented in many centers.[188] Difficulty in developing these tools arises from the fact that MDRO infections upon admission are not limited only to Enterobacteriaceae.[39,165,189]

TREATMENT OPTIONS FOR EXTENDED-SPECTRUM β-LACTAMASES–PRODUCING ENTEROBACTERIACEAE INFECTIONS IN HOSPITAL SETTINGS

Despite being prevalent pathogens, both in hospital and community settings, no prospective randomized controlled trials have ever been conducted addressing the most efficacious therapy for ESBL-producing Enterobacteriaceae infections. The efficacy of some of the antimicrobial classes are reviewed in these sections.[8]

Carbapenems

This class is considered by many as first-line agents, particularly for serious invasive ESBL infections.[14] Carbapenems have favorable pharmacokinetic/pharmacodynamic (PK/PD) properties, are relatively safe, and have the most established clinical track record in this field.[14,15,190] A multicenter prospective observational trial, which was published more than a decade ago, demonstrated a significant association between carbapenems and lower mortality rates in *K pneumoniae* BSIs, compared with other supposedly appropriate agents.[190] Notably, this was at a time when the prevalent ESBLs were TEM and SHV, not like the current epidemiology. Other relative older trials, summarized in a review in 2008,[28] consisted of relatively small retrospective trials, with multiple methodological flaws.[28] More recently, a metaanalysis comparing carbapenems with alternative antibiotics demonstrated superiority of carbapenems over other therapeutic regimens.[191]

Group 1 (eg, ertapenem) and group 2 (eg, imipenem, meropenem, and doripenem) carbapenems cannot be hydrolyzed by ESBLs. Group 1 has a potential advantage in terms of reducing selective pressure among non–glucose-fermenting Gram-negative bacilli pathogens (eg, *A baumannii*, *P aeruginosa*).[192] However, group 1 carbapenems were not thoroughly trialed against serious invasive ESBL infections (eg, BSIs); therefore, initial expert reviews recommended group 2 carbepenems for serious ESBL infections.[14] A retrospective analysis of 261 patients with ESBL BSIs from Detroit showed that the outcomes of infections were equivalent between patients treated with ertapenem versus those treated with group 2 carbapenems.[15] The authors stratified the analysis based on the systemic inflammatory response syndrome[193] level, and group 1 was equivalent to group 2 even in patients with severe sepsis, septic shock, or multiorgan failure.[15] A recent published paper confirms this finding, though it stresses the fact that further studies are needed specifically for patients with severe sepsis/septic shock.[194]

Despite being the agents of choice for microbiologically confirmed ESBL infections, the empiric use of carbapenems should be limited, owing to the emergence and spread of carbapenem-resistant Enterobacteriaceae (CRE).[7,195,196] Although a direct correlation between carbapenem usage and CRE acquisition on an ecological level (not patient level) is still a matter of debate,[7,192] the strongest independent predictor for CRE acquisition, on a patient level, is exposure to antimicrobials in general.[166]

Cephalosporins

Although most cephalosporins are effectively inhibited by ESBLs, certain cephalosporins may retain in vitro activity (per older higher Clinical and Laboratory Standards Institute [CLSI] breakpoints[24]) against specific ESBL-producing isolates (eg, ceftazidime for $bla_{\text{CTX-M}}$–producing strains).[197] However, studies (usually small retrospective observational case series analyses) have shown that clinical outcomes are often unsatisfactory even when the drug is administered to a seemingly susceptible isolate.[22,198,199] This also pertains to cefepime, for which CLSI breakpoints were not yet reduced.[22] Other more conclusive studies found significant correlations between cephalosporin use and increased mortality among patients with ESBL infection.[200] As of 2010, the American CLSI has joined the European Committee on Antimicrobial Susceptibility Testing in recommending that ESBL testing should not be used for breakpoints determination (it might still be done for epidemiologic purposes). This was combined with recommendation to lower the minimum inhibitory concentration (MIC) breakpoints for cephalosporins.[201] These recommendations are still debated, because some experts are advocating that resistance mechanisms, including ESBL, are of importance to clinical decision making.[202] The implications of these changes in diagnostic policies on both the epidemiology and diagnosis of ESBL-producing bacteria has yet to be determined.[23]

Fluoroquinolones

Some older data suggested that fluoroquinolones could be as effective as carbapenems for treatment of infections caused by ESBLs.[203] Kang and colleagues (2004)[200] found similar 30-day mortality rates with ciprofloxacin and carbapenem therapy for patients with BSIs caused by ESBL-producing *E coli* and *K pneumoniae*. However, owing to exponential increases in resistance to fluoroquinolones (in both community and health care settings), and mainly the spread of certain CTX-Ms, this therapeutic option became nearly irrelevant in certain locations, with more than 90% of offending ESBL isolates becoming resistant to all fluoroquinolones.[80,204] Moreover, few reports have identified fluoroquinolone exposure as a strong independent predictor for ESBL acquisition.[204,205]

Cephamycins

By definition this group of β-lactams (eg, cefoxitin, cefotetan, and cefmetazole) is stable to hydrolysis by ESBL-producing Enterobacteriaceae.[10] A small retrospective study from Taiwan found flomoxef is as effective at treating ESBL-producing *K pneumoniae* infections as carbapenems[206]; however, these compounds have unfavorable PK/PD properties and are no longer distributed and marketed in many countries. Additionally, there are reports of emerging coresistances to these molecules as a result of either decreased expression of external membrane porins or cocarriage of AmpC enzyme conveying cephamycin resistance in some ESBL-producing strains.[48]

β-Lactam–β-lactamase Inhibitors Combinations

Although ESBLs (as Ambler A enzymes) are inhibited by β-lactamase inhibitors such as clavulonic acid and tazobactam, data and expert opinions pertaining to the efficacy of β-lactam–β-lactamase inhibitors (BLBLI) for treating ESBL infections are conflicting.[10,11,15] The efficacy of BLBLI is doubtful because of the mostly theoretic "inoculum effect" phenomenon, hypothesizing that at certain hypoperfused infected tissues (eg, lungs), the bacteria inoculum is high compared with the concentration of the β-lactamase inhibitor concentration that reaches that tissue.[207,208] The clinical impact of this phenomenon is not supported by strong scientific data, although worse outcomes were consistently reported, mainly in high inoculum infectious syndromes, such as in endovascular infections and endocarditis.[209] Owing to these reports, the common practice among most experts in the field was to consider BLBLI as an inappropriate alternative for ESBL infections.[14] Many microbiologic laboratories converted the susceptibility results to BLBLI of ESBL-producing strains to "resistant" so that prescribers would not consider BLBLI for ESBL infections.[23]

In 2012, a post hoc analysis of 6 prospective studies from Spain was published comparing the efficacy of BLBLI to carbapenems in BSIs caused by ESBL-producing *E coli*.[210] A total of 192 patients were included in the final analysis consisting of 2 distinct cohorts—one for empiric therapy and the other for definitive therapy. The authors did not find significant correlations between any of the regimens to any of the measured outcomes. However, outcomes in general were better among the group of patients who received BLBLI, and in the definitive treatment arm this difference nearly reached statistical significance for some of the outcomes.[210] The authors concluded that BLBLIs should be perceived as legitimate alternatives to carbapenems for *E coli* ESBL BSIs.[210] However, as displayed in the editorial that accompanied this publication,[211] it is problematic to extrapolate these results to all ESBL-producing Enterobacteriaceae (not solely to *E coli*) and to all clinical infectious syndromes, for the following reasons. First, nearly 70% of BSIs originated from the urinary (or biliary) tract. β-Lactamase inhibitors, the only 'active' ingredient in the BLBLI combination, are excreted almost exclusively unchanged in urine (or bile).[212] Because UTIs are relatively "low inoculum infections,"[213] a somewhat reverse inoculum effect might be expected in ESBL UTIs. Second, nearly 90% of ESBL *E coli* BSIs were owing to $bla_{\text{CTX-M}}$–producing pathogens, and these enzymes are known to be hydrolyzed more efficiently by tazobactam compared with other ESBLs (eg, bla_{TEM}, bla_{SHV}), which are more prevalent among other Enterobacteriaceae (eg, *K pneumoniae* and *P mirabilis*). Third, the investigators found an obvious and significant correlation between the piperacillin–tazobactam MIC and the clinical outcome: that is, mortality increased when the MIC was greater than 4 mg/L.[210,214] Many ESBL isolates in multiple locations worldwide, particularly non *E coli* and non-$bla_{CTX\text{-}M}$–producing strains, exhibit much higher MICs to piperacillin–tazobactam.[23] Fourth, bla_{CMY}-producing *E coli* strains, which are not inhibited by tazobactam, are as common as ESBL-producing strains in certain areas.[211] Fifth, the recent spread of the ST-131 *E coli* clone, which is the prevalent strain in this Spanish region,[45] is known to have lower MICs to BLBLIs.[215] Despite all these issues, this was a meticulously executed analysis, which questioned a concept that was already well-accepted in many regions worldwide, although it was based on poor scientific clinical data. Interestingly, the authors pointed out that the sickest patients of their cohort were treated with carbapenems,[210] perhaps implying that carbapenems are still more trusted. To test whether BLBLI are equal to carbapenems in treating ESBL-producing BSIs (all ESBL-producing Enterobacteriaceae), a study focusing on BSIs arising from a nonurinary, high inoculum source (eg, pneumonia), is warranted. Such studies were conducted concurrently at a US and Israeli center.[216] Although both centers were endemic for ESBLs, only 10 patients were enrolled to the piperacillin–tazobactam arm (ie, in the majority of patients, the treatment with BLBLI was discontinued after obtaining results of a confirmed ESBL isolate from blood). Nonetheless, despite the very low sample size, the mortality risk with piperacillin–tazobactam was significantly and independently greater compared with carbapenems (adjusted odds ratio, 7.9; *P* = .03).[216] Because it is difficult to enroll patients with ESBL BSIs to a BLBLI consolidative regimen for a well-designed controlled trial, a group from Johns Hopkins University School of Medicine had studied the isolated impact of the empiric regimen (only), on the clinical outcomes of patients with ESBL BSI.[217] The adjusted 14-day mortality risk was 1.92 times higher for 103 patients who received empiric piperacillin–tazobactam, compared with 110 patients who received empiric carbapenems (95% CI, 1.07–3.45).[217]

In a metaanalysis published in 2012, carbapenems were associated with lower mortality rates than other regimens.[191] However, rates of resistance among ESBL-producing Enterobacteriaceae were higher for BLBLIs than for carbapenems. This might suggest that carbapenems should be perceived as superior in terms of empiric regimen, to reduce DAAT for ESBL BSIs.[191]

To summarize, current data are inconclusive as to the use of BLBLIs as definitive treatment for ESBL infections. Further research is needed to better understand the role that BLBLI may play in the treatment of severe infections originating from various infectious syndromes and caused by various ESBL-producing bacteria.

Aminoglycosides

The susceptibility rates of certain aminoglycosides (eg, gentamicin, amikacin, and tobramycin) to common ESBL-producing offending Enterobacteriaceae isolates might still be relatively high in some locales.[218–220] Despite its well-known elevated toxicity rates and unfavorable PK/PD properties,[221] aminoglycosides might still have a role for treatment of ESBL infections in hospital settings, particularly in mild to moderate (but not severe or life-threatening) UTIs, in patients without underlying renal or auditory compromise.[222] Aminoglycoside use may be advantageous in terms of antimicrobial stewardship efforts on a population level, particularly as a substitute for carbapenems.[223] However, there is a lack of well-controlled clinical data pertaining to aminoglycosides efficacy for the treatment of mild to moderate UTIs.[222] For non–UTI infectious syndromes, aminoglycosides should serve only as adjuncts, and should not be trusted as the single effective agent.[221,224]

Tigecycline and Polymyxins

ESBL-producing *E coli* and, to a lesser extent, *K pneumoniae*, have shown high susceptibility rates to these compounds.[48,225] Tigecycline is a drug with unfavorable pharmacodynamic properties for BSI, and there was a warning from the US Food and Drug Administration pertaining to its use.[226] Colistin, the polymyxin used most often, is toxic, and its PK/PD properties have not been determined thoroughly after its revived usage over the past decade.[227] However, the main reason to avoid these agents for treating ESBL infections is that these are frequently the only remaining therapeutic options for CRE and other extensively drug resistant Gram-negative MDROs (eg, *A baumannii* and *P aeruginosa*).[8] Therefore, it is of paramount importance to avoid these therapeutics while additional options are available.[14,228]

TREATING EXTENDED-SPECTRUM β-LACTAMASE INFECTIONS IN AMBULATORY SETTINGS

ESBLs have become prevalent in "the community" of many regions worldwide, particularly since the spread of the ESBL-producing *E coli* ST131 strain.[139,149,176] In ambulatory settings, DAAT is probably even more common than in acute care hospitals,[8] and it probably impact patients' outcomes, although controlled data on this issue are lacking.[8] Some mild to moderate ESBL infections could probably be managed outside the hospital settings[29,222]; however, oral therapeutics that possess potential activity against ESBLs are lacking, and controlled data of their efficacy are lacking as well.[8]

Fluoroquinolones and TMP-SMX can be used as definitive therapy against susceptible isolates.[25,203,229–232] Susceptibility rates from recent years, however, have been shown to be consistently low.[10,60,232–234] In a prospective multicenter observational study of community-associated infections caused by ESBL-producing *E coli* from the United States, only 11% and 32% of the isolates were susceptible to fluoroquinolones and TMP-SMX, respectively, and 64% were resistant to both agents.[75]

Nitrofurantoin and fosfomycin are 2 additional oral therapeutic options in ambulatory settings for mild to moderate ESBL UTIs. In vitro susceptibility to nitrofurantoin was shown to be 71.3% in a microbiological survey from Spain, conducted in 2006,[235] and 90% in 2013 in 1 US center.[75] Susceptibility rates to fosfomycin among Enterobacteriaceae (mostly CRE) recovered from a single US center was more than 90%.[29] Fosfomycin is approved in many countries for mild ESBL UTI.[236] In a retrospective study from Spain, the cure rate of patients with cystitis was 93% with fosfomycin therapy and all ESBL-producing offending strains were susceptible to fosfomycin.

Another potential option to manage ESBL infections in the community are oral BLBLI (eg, amoxicillin–clavulanate). A large Spanish multicenter publication demonstrated the significant association between BLBLI MIC and clinical outcome. Cure rates were up to 93% for susceptible isolates (MIC $\leq$8 μg/mL) but only 56% for intermediate or resistant isolates (MIC $\geq$16 μg/mL).[72] Susceptibility rates to oral BLBLI vary greatly, with some areas reporting more than 70% resistance rates.[237] For UTIs, the inherent broad spectrum activity of BLBLI (covering many prevalent Gram-positives, Gram-negatives, and anaerobes) might pose an additional disadvantage, in terms of antimicrobial stewardship, when additional oral alternatives are available.

FUTURE PERSPECTIVE

Antimicrobial resistance is a worldwide prevalent iatrogenic complication of modern medical care. ESBL-producing Enterobacteriaceaeare are one of the most common features of this complication. These infections are prevalent both in health care settings and in the community. Appropriate therapy is frequently delayed in these patients, who experience worse clinical outcomes as a result. Moreover, no prospective randomized controlled trials have ever been conducted in this field and there are still several debates and controversies pertaining to the most efficacious management of these common infections. There are few investigational efforts, which we think could significantly aid on this research front in the future:

1. Studies that propose, develop, and validate a reliable bedside score that predict ESBL infections upon admission to acute care hospitals, to reduce DAAT among patients with severe invasive ESBL infections.
2. Improve the availability and applicability of rapid diagnostics tools, both for invasive ESBL infections (from blood cultures) and for ESBL asymptomatic carriage (from rectal samplings).
3. Invest efforts and conduct more studies, which will aid in the control and regulation of ESBL carriage, and of antimicrobial usage in general, in the food and agriculture industries.
4. Invest efforts and conduct more studies of innovations in the field of antimicrobial stewardship in ambulatory settings and its impact on "emergence" and spread of ESBLs in the community settings.
5. Study the role of oral agents (eg, fluoroquinolones, TMP/SMX, fosfomycin, nitrofurantoin, amoxicillin–clavulonate) for treating mild to moderate ESBL infections that are managed in ambulatory settings.
6. Conduct prospective randomized control trial of ertapenem versus BLBLI for ESBL BSIs.
7. The implications of the changes in breakpoint reporting according to the current CLSI and EUCAST recommendations on both the epidemiology and diagnosis of ESBL-producing bacteria has to be monitored and studied.

REFERENCES

1. Boucher HW, Talbot GH, Bradley JS, et al. Bad bugs, no drugs: no ESKAPE! An update from the Infectious Diseases Society of America. Clin Infect Dis 2009; 48(1):1–12.
2. Livermore DM. Has the era of untreatable infections arrived? J Antimicrob Chemother 2009;64(Suppl 1):i29–36.
3. Marchaim D, Perez F, Lee J, et al. "Swimming in resistance": co-colonization with carbapenem-resistant enterobacteriaceae and Acinetobacter baumannii or pseudomonas aeruginosa. Am J Infect Control 2012;40(9):830–5.
4. Cohen-Nahum K, Saidel-Odes L, Riesenberg K, et al. Urinary tract infections caused by multi-drug resistant Proteus mirabilis: risk factors and clinical outcomes. Infection 2010;38(1):41–6.
5. Endimiani A, Luzzaro F, Brigante G, et al. Proteus mirabilis bloodstream infections: risk factors and treatment outcome related to the expression of extended-spectrum beta-lactamases. Antimicrob Agents Chemother 2005;49(7):2598–605.
6. Marchaim D, Zaidenstein R, Lazarovitch T, et al. Epidemiology of bacteremia episodes in a single center: increase in gram-negative isolates, antibiotics resistance, and patient age. Eur J Clin Microbiol Infect Dis 2008;27(11):1045–51.

7. Bogan C, Marchaim D. The role of antimicrobial stewardship in curbing carbapenem resistance. Future Microbiol 2013;8(8):979–91.
8. Tal Jasper R, Coyle JR, Katz DE, et al. The complex epidemiology of extended-spectrum beta-lactamase-producing enterobacteriaceae. Future Microbiol 2015;10:819–39.
9. Bonomo RA, Rossolini GM. Importance of antibiotic resistance and resistance mechanisms. Foreword. Expert Rev Anti Infect Ther 2008;6(5):549–50.
10. Paterson DL, Bonomo RA. Extended-spectrum beta-lactamases: a clinical update. Clin Microbiol Rev 2005;18(4):657–86.
11. Peterson LR. Antibiotic policy and prescribing strategies for therapy of extended-spectrum beta-lactamase-producing enterobacteriaceae: the role of piperacillin-tazobactam. Clin Microbiol Infect 2008;14(Suppl 1):181–4.
12. Bush K, Fisher JF. Epidemiological expansion, structural studies, and clinical challenges of new beta-lactamases from gram-negative bacteria. Annu Rev Microbiol 2011;65:455–78.
13. Gerber JS, Kronman MP, Ross RK, et al. Identifying targets for antimicrobial stewardship in children's hospitals. Infect Control Hosp Epidemiol 2013; 34(12):1252–8.
14. Peleg AY, Hooper DC. Hospital-acquired infections due to gram-negative bacteria. N Engl J Med 2010;362(19):1804–13.
15. Collins VL, Marchaim D, Pogue JM, et al. Efficacy of ertapenem for treatment of bloodstream infections caused by extended-spectrum-beta-lactamase-producing enterobacteriaceae. Antimicrob Agents Chemother 2012;56(4): 2173–7.
16. Abraham EP, Chain E. An enzyme from bacteria able to destroy penicillin. 1940. Rev Infect Dis 1988;10(4):677–8.
17. Bradford PA. Extended-spectrum beta-lactamases in the 21st century: characterization, epidemiology, and detection of this important resistance threat. Clin Microbiol Rev 2001;14(4):933–51, table of contents.
18. Medeiros AA. Evolution and dissemination of beta-lactamases accelerated by generations of beta-lactam antibiotics. Clin Infect Dis 1997;24(Suppl 1):S19–45.
19. Jacoby GA, Munoz-Price LS. The new beta-lactamases. N Engl J Med 2005; 352(4):380–91.
20. Bush K, Jacoby GA, Medeiros AA. A functional classification scheme for beta-lactamases and its correlation with molecular structure. Antimicrob Agents Chemother 1995;39(6):1211–33.
21. Jacoby GA, Bush K. Beta-lactamase nomenclature. J Clin Microbiol 2005; 43(12):6220.
22. Chopra T, Marchaim D, Veltman J, et al. Impact of cefepime therapy on mortality among patients with bloodstream infections caused by extended-spectrum-beta-lactamase-producing Klebsiella pneumoniae and Escherichia coli. Antimicrob Agents Chemother 2012;56(7):3936–42.
23. Marchaim D, Sunkara B, Lephart PR, et al. Extended-spectrum beta-lactamase producers reported as susceptible to piperacillin-tazobactam, cefepime, and cefuroxime in the era of lowered breakpoints and no confirmatory tests. Infect Control Hosp Epidemiol 2012;33(8):853–5.
24. Clinical and Laboratory Standards Institute (CLSI). Performance standards for antimicrobial susceptibility testing. In: Clinical and Laboratory Standards Institute, editor. Nineteenth informational supplement. Approved standard m100–s19. Wayne (PA): Clinical and Laboratory Standards Institute; 2009.

25. Endimiani A, Paterson DL. Optimizing therapy for infections caused by enterobacteriaceae producing extended-spectrum beta-lactamases. Semin Respir Crit Care Med 2007;28(6):646–55.
26. Marchaim D, Lazarovitch Z, Efrati S, et al. Serious consequences to the use of cephalosporins as the first line of antimicrobial therapy administered in hemodialysis units. Nephron Clin Pract 2005;101(2):c58–64.
27. Ben-Ami R, Schwaber MJ, Navon-Venezia S, et al. Influx of extended-spectrum beta-lactamase-producing enterobacteriaceae into the hospital. Clin Infect Dis 2006;42(7):925–34.
28. Pitout JD, Laupland KB. Extended-spectrum beta-lactamase-producing enterobacteriaceae: an emerging public-health concern. Lancet Infect Dis 2008;8(3): 159–66.
29. Pogue JM, Marchaim D, Abreu-Lanfranco O, et al. Fosfomycin activity versus carbapenem-resistant enterobacteriaceae and vancomycin-resistant enterococcus, Detroit, 2008-10. J Antibiot (Tokyo) 2013;66(10):625–7.
30. Marchaim D, Gottesman T, Schwartz O, et al. National multicenter study of predictors and outcomes of bacteremia upon hospital admission caused by enterobacteriaceae producing extended-spectrum beta-lactamases. Antimicrob Agents Chemother 2010;54(12):5099–104.
31. Reinert RR, Low DE, Rossi F, et al. Antimicrobial susceptibility among organisms from the Asia/Pacific rim, Europe and Latin and North America collected as part of test and the in vitro activity of tigecycline. J Antimicrob Chemother 2007; 60(5):1018–29.
32. Nagy E, Dowzicky MJ. In vitro activity of tigecycline and comparators against a European compilation of anaerobes collected as part of the tigecycline evaluation and surveillance trial (test). Scand J Infect Dis 2010;42(1):33–8.
33. Jones RN, Biedenbach DJ, Gales AC. Sustained activity and spectrum of selected extended-spectrum beta-lactams (carbapenems and cefepime) against Enterobacter spp. And ESBL-producing Klebsiella spp.: report from the sentry antimicrobial surveillance program (USA, 1997-2000). Int J Antimicrob Agents 2003;21(1):1–7.
34. Bouchillon SK, Iredell JR, Barkham T, et al. Comparative in vitro activity of tigecycline and other antimicrobials against gram-negative and gram-positive organisms collected from the asia-pacific rim as part of the tigecycline evaluation and surveillance trial (test). Int J Antimicrob Agents 2009;33(2): 130–6.
35. Rodloff AC, Leclercq R, Debbia EA, et al. Comparative analysis of antimicrobial susceptibility among organisms from France, Germany, Italy, Spain and the UK as part of the tigecycline evaluation and surveillance trial. Clin Microbiol Infect 2008;14(4):307–14.
36. Hoban DJ, Bouchillon SK, Johnson BM, et al. In vitro activity of tigecycline against 6792 gram-negative and gram-positive clinical isolates from the global tigecycline evaluation and surveillance trial (test program, 2004). Diagn Microbiol Infect Dis 2005;52(3):215–27.
37. Badura A, Feierl G, Pregartner G, et al. Antibiotic resistance patterns of more than 120 000 clinical Escherichia coli isolates in southeast Austria, 1998-2013. Clin Microbiol Infect 2015;21(6):569.e1–7.
38. Calbo E, Garau J. The changing epidemiology of hospital outbreaks due to ESBL-producing Klebsiella pneumoniae: the ctx-m-15 type consolidation. Future Microbiol 2015;10:1063–75.

39. Leibman V, Martin ET, Tal-Jasper R, et al. Simple bedside score to optimize the time and the decision to initiate appropriate therapy for carbapenem-resistant enterobacteriaceae. Ann Clin Microbiol Antimicrob 2015;14:31.
40. Livermore DM. Current epidemiology and growing resistance of gram-negative pathogens. Korean J Intern Med 2012;27(2):128–42.
41. Livermore DM. Defining an extended-spectrum beta-lactamase. Clin Microbiol Infect 2008;14(Suppl 1):3–10.
42. Dellit TH, Owens RC, McGowan JE Jr, et al. Infectious Diseases Society of America and the Society for Healthcare Epidemiology of America guidelines for developing an institutional program to enhance antimicrobial stewardship. Clin Infect Dis 2007;44(2):159–77.
43. del Rio MA, Chrane D, Shelton S, et al. Ceftriaxone versus ampicillin and chloramphenicol for treatment of bacterial meningitis in children. Lancet 1983; 1(8336):1241–4.
44. Bernstein Hahn L, Barclay CA, Iribarren MA, et al. Ceftriaxone, a new parenteral cephalosporin, in the treatment of urinary tract infections. Chemotherapy 1981; 27(Suppl 1):75–9.
45. Efficacy and toxicity of single daily doses of amikacin and ceftriaxone versus multiple daily doses of amikacin and ceftazidime for infection in patients with cancer and granulocytopenia. The international antimicrobial therapy cooperative group of the European Organization for Research and Treatment of Cancer. Ann Intern Med 1993;119(7 Pt 1):584–93.
46. Kliebe C, Nies BA, Meyer JF, et al. Evolution of plasmid-coded resistance to broad-spectrum cephalosporins. Antimicrob Agents Chemother 1985;28(2): 302–7.
47. Bush K. Extended-spectrum beta-lactamases in North America, 1987-2006. Clin Microbiol Infect 2008;14(Suppl 1):134–43.
48. Falagas ME, Karageorgopoulos DE. Extended-spectrum beta-lactamase-producing organisms. J Hosp Infect 2009;73(4):345–54.
49. Brun-Buisson C, Legrand P, Philippon A, et al. Transferable enzymatic resistance to third-generation cephalosporins during nosocomial outbreak of multiresistant Klebsiella pneumoniae. Lancet 1987;2(8554):302–6.
50. Babini GS, Livermore DM. Antimicrobial resistance amongst Klebsiella spp. Collected from intensive care units in southern and western Europe in 1997-1998. J Antimicrob Chemother 2000;45(2):183–9.
51. Livermore DM, Yuan M. Antibiotic resistance and production of extended-spectrum beta-lactamases amongst Klebsiella spp. From intensive care units in Europe. J Antimicrob Chemother 1996;38(3):409–24.
52. Decre D, Gachot B, Lucet JC, et al. Clinical and bacteriologic epidemiology of extended-spectrum beta-lactamase-producing strains of Klebsiella pneumoniae in a medical intensive care unit. Clin Infect Dis 1998;27(4):834–44.
53. Pitout JD, Nordmann P, Laupland KB, et al. Emergence of enterobacteriaceae producing extended-spectrum beta-lactamases (ESBLs) in the community. J Antimicrob Chemother 2005;56(1):52–9.
54. Canton R, Coque TM. The ctx-m beta-lactamase pandemic. Curr Opin Microbiol 2006;9(5):466–75.
55. Hobson RP, MacKenzie FM, Gould IM. An outbreak of multiply-resistant Klebsiella pneumoniae in the Grampian region of Scotland. J Hosp Infect 1996;33(4): 249–62.

56. Borer A, Gilad J, Menashe G, et al. Extended-spectrum beta-lactamase-producing enterobacteriaceae strains in community-acquired bacteremia in southern Israel. Med Sci Monit 2002;8(1):CR44–7.
57. Goldstein FW, Pean Y, Gertner J. Resistance to ceftriaxone and other beta-lactams in bacteria isolated in the community. The vigil'roc study group. Antimicrob Agents Chemother 1995;39(11):2516–9.
58. Blomberg B, Jureen R, Manji KP, et al. High rate of fatal cases of pediatric septicemia caused by gram-negative bacteria with extended-spectrum beta-lactamases in Dar es Salaam, Tanzania. J Clin Microbiol 2005;43(2):745–9.
59. Mirelis B, Navarro F, Miro E, et al. Community transmission of extended-spectrum beta-lactamase. Emerg Infect Dis 2003;9(8):1024–5.
60. Pitout JD, Hanson ND, Church DL, et al. Population-based laboratory surveillance for Escherichia coli-producing extended-spectrum beta-lactamases: importance of community isolates with blactx-m genes. Clin Infect Dis 2004; 38(12):1736–41.
61. Woodford N, Kaufmann ME, Karisik E, et al. Molecular epidemiology of multiresistant Escherichia coli isolates from community-onset urinary tract infections in Cornwall, England. J Antimicrob Chemother 2007;59(1):106–9.
62. Cormican M, Morris D, Corbett-Feeeney G, et al. Extended spectrum beta-lactamase production and fluorquinolone resistance in pathogens associated with community acquired urinary tract infection. Diagn Microbiol Infect Dis 1998;32(4):317–9.
63. Goldstein FW. Antibiotic susceptibility of bacterial strains isolated from patients with community-acquired urinary tract infections in France. Multicentre study group. Eur J Clin Microbiol Infect Dis 2000;19(2):112–7.
64. Centers for Disease Control and Prevention (CDC). Laboratory capacity to detect antimicrobial resistance, 1998. MMWR Morb Mortal Wkly Rep 2000; 48(51–52):1167–71.
65. Munoz-Price LS. Long-term acute care hospitals. Clin Infect Dis 2009;49(3): 438–43.
66. Denman SJ, Burton JR. Fluid intake and urinary tract infection in the elderly. JAMA 1992;267(16):2245–9.
67. de Medina T, Carmeli Y. The pivotal role of long-term care facilities in the epidemiology of Acinetobacter baumannii: another brick in the wall. Clin Infect Dis 2010;50(12):1617–8.
68. Marchaim D, Chopra T, Bogan C, et al. The burden of multidrug-resistant organisms on tertiary hospitals posed by patients with recent stays in long-term acute care facilities. Am J Infect Control 2012;40(8):760–5.
69. Adler A, Gniadkowski M, Baraniak A, et al. Transmission dynamics of ESBL-producing Escherichia coli clones in rehabilitation wards at a tertiary care centre. Clin Microbiol Infect 2012;18(12):E497–505.
70. Sengstock DM, Thyagarajan R, Apalara J, et al. Multidrug-resistant Acinetobacter baumannii: an emerging pathogen among older adults in community hospitals and nursing homes. Clin Infect Dis 2010;50(12):1611–6.
71. Ben-Ami R, Rodriguez-Bano J, Arslan H, et al. A multinational survey of risk factors for infection with extended-spectrum beta-lactamase-producing enterobacteriaceae in nonhospitalized patients. Clin Infect Dis 2009;49(5):682–90.
72. Rodriguez-Bano J, Alcala JC, Cisneros JM, et al. Community infections caused by extended-spectrum beta-lactamase-producing Escherichia coli. Arch Intern Med 2008;168(17):1897–902.

73. Rodriguez-Bano J, Lopez-Cerero L, Navarro MD, et al. Faecal carriage of extended-spectrum beta-lactamase-producing Escherichia coli: prevalence, risk factors and molecular epidemiology. J Antimicrob Chemother 2008;62(5): 1142–9.
74. Rodriguez-Bano J, Paterson DL. A change in the epidemiology of infections due to extended-spectrum beta-lactamase-producing organisms. Clin Infect Dis 2006;42(7):935–7.
75. Doi Y, Park YS, Rivera JI, et al. Community-associated extended-spectrum beta-lactamase-producing Escherichia coli infection in the united states. Clin Infect Dis 2013;56(5):641–8.
76. Hayakawa K, Gattu S, Marchaim D, et al. Epidemiology and risk factors for isolation of Escherichia coli producing ctx-m-type extended-spectrum beta-lactamase in a large U.S. Medical center. Antimicrob Agents Chemother 2013;57(8):4010–8.
77. Wright GD. The antibiotic resistome: the nexus of chemical and genetic diversity. Nat Rev Microbiol 2007;5(3):175–86.
78. Rodriguez-Bano J, Navarro MD, Romero L, et al. Risk-factors for emerging bloodstream infections caused by extended-spectrum beta-lactamase-producing Escherichia coli. Clin Microbiol Infect 2008;14(2):180–3.
79. Schwaber MJ, Navon-Venezia S, Kaye KS, et al. Clinical and economic impact of bacteremia with extended- spectrum-beta-lactamase-producing enterobacteriaceae. Antimicrob Agents Chemother 2006;50(4):1257–62.
80. Schwaber MJ, Navon-Venezia S, Schwartz D, et al. High levels of antimicrobial coresistance among extended-spectrum-beta-lactamase-producing enterobacteriaceae. Antimicrob Agents Chemother 2005;49(5):2137–9.
81. Schwaber MJ, Carmeli Y. Mortality and delay in effective therapy associated with extended-spectrum beta-lactamase production in enterobacteriaceae bacteraemia: a systematic review and meta-analysis. J Antimicrob Chemother 2007; 60(5):913–20.
82. Apisarnthanarak A, Kiratisin P, Mundy LM. Clinical and molecular epidemiology of healthcare-associated infections due to extended-spectrum beta-lactamase (ESBL)-producing strains of Escherichia coli and Klebsiella pneumoniae that harbor multiple ESBL genes. Infect Control Hosp Epidemiol 2008;29(11): 1026–34.
83. Doi Y, Adams-Haduch JM, Paterson DL. Escherichia coli isolate coproducing 16s rRNA methylase and ctx-m-type extended-spectrum beta-lactamase isolated from an outpatient in the united states. Antimicrob Agents Chemother 2008;52(3):1204–5.
84. Doi Y, Adams-Haduch JM, Shivannavar CT, et al. Faecal carriage of ctx-m-15-producing Klebsiella pneumoniae in patients with acute gastroenteritis. Indian J Med Res 2009;129(5):599–602.
85. Doi Y, Paterson DL, Egea P, et al. Extended-spectrum and cmy-type beta-lactamase-producing Escherichia coli in clinical samples and retail meat from Pittsburgh, USA and Seville, Spain. Clin Microbiol Infect 2010;16(1):33–8.
86. Livermore DM, Hawkey PM. Ctx-m: changing the face of ESBLs in the UK. J Antimicrob Chemother 2005;56(3):451–4.
87. Livermore DM, Hope R, Reynolds R, et al. Declining cephalosporin and fluoroquinolone non-susceptibility among bloodstream enterobacteriaceae from the UK: links to prescribing change? J Antimicrob Chemother 2013;68(11):2667–74.
88. Paterson DL. Extended-spectrum beta-lactamases: the European experience. Curr Opin Infect Dis 2001;14(6):697–701.

89. Poirel L, Nordmann P, Ducroz S, et al. Extended-spectrum beta-lactamase ctx-m-15-producing Klebsiella pneumoniae of sequence type st274 in companion animals. Antimicrob Agents Chemother 2013;57(5):2372–5.
90. Arpin C, Quentin C, Grobost F, et al. Nationwide survey of extended-spectrum {beta}-lactamase-producing enterobacteriaceae in the French community setting. J Antimicrob Chemother 2009;63(6):1205–14.
91. Djamdjian L, Naas T, Tande D, et al. Ctx-m-93, a ctx-m variant lacking penicillin hydrolytic activity. Antimicrob Agents Chemother 2011;55(5):1861–6.
92. Bauernfeind A, Grimm H, Schweighart S. A new plasmidic cefotaximase in a clinical isolate of Escherichia coli. Infection 1990;18(5):294–8.
93. Canton R, Gonzalez-Alba JM, Galan JC. Ctx-m enzymes: origin and diffusion. Front Microbiol 2012;3:110.
94. Bonnet R. Growing group of extended-spectrum beta-lactamases: the ctx-m enzymes. Antimicrob Agents Chemother 2004;48(1):1–14.
95. Navon-Venezia S, Chmelnitsky I, Leavitt A, et al. Dissemination of the ctx-m-25 family beta-lactamases among Klebsiella pneumoniae, Escherichia coli and Enterobacter cloacae and identification of the novel enzyme ctx-m-41 in Proteus mirabilis in Israel. J Antimicrob Chemother 2008;62(2):289–95.
96. Lytsy B, Lindback J, Torell E, et al. A case-control study of risk factors for urinary acquisition of Klebsiella pneumoniae producing ctx-m-15 in an outbreak situation in Sweden. Scand J Infect Dis 2010;42(6–7):439–44.
97. Azap OK, Arslan H, Serefhanoglu K, et al. Risk factors for extended-spectrum beta-lactamase positivity in uropathogenic Escherichia coli isolated from community-acquired urinary tract infections. Clin Microbiol Infect 2010;16(2):147–51.
98. Apisarnthanarak A, Kiratisin P, Saifon P, et al. Clinical and molecular epidemiology of community-onset, extended-spectrum beta-lactamase-producing Escherichia coli infections in Thailand: a case-case-control study. Am J Infect Control 2007;35(9):606–12.
99. Calbo E, Romani V, Xercavins M, et al. Risk factors for community-onset urinary tract infections due to Escherichia coli harbouring extended-spectrum beta-lactamases. J Antimicrob Chemother 2006;57(4):780–3.
100. Rodriguez-Bano J, Navarro MD, Romero L, et al. Clinical and molecular epidemiology of extended-spectrum beta-lactamase-producing Escherichia coli as a cause of nosocomial infection or colonization: implications for control. Clin Infect Dis 2006;42(1):37–45.
101. Association AU. Best practice policy statement on urologic surgery antimicrobial prophylaxis. 2011.
102. Urology EAo. Guidelines on urological infections; 2013.
103. Lo E, Nicolle L, Classen D, et al. Strategies to prevent catheter-associated urinary tract infections in acute care hospitals. Infect Control Hosp Epidemiol 2008;29(Suppl 1):S41–50.
104. Wolf JS Jr, Bennett CJ, Dmochowski RR, et al. Best practice policy statement on urologic surgery antimicrobial prophylaxis. J Urol 2008;179(4):1379–90.
105. Grabe M, Botto H, Cek M, et al. Preoperative assessment of the patient and risk factors for infectious complications and tentative classification of surgical field contamination of urological procedures. World J Urol 2012;30(1):39–50.
106. Botelho LA, Kraychete GB, Costa ESJL, et al. Widespread distribution of ctx-m and plasmid-mediated AmpC beta-lactamases in Escherichia coli from Brazilian chicken meat. Mem Inst Oswaldo Cruz 2015;110(2):249–54.

107. Nagy B, Szmolka A, Smole Mozina S, et al. Virulence and antimicrobial resistance determinants of verotoxigenic Escherichia coli (VTEC) and of multidrug-resistant E. Coli from foods of animal origin illegally imported to the EU by flight passengers. Int J Food Microbiol 2015;209:52–9.
108. Wong MH, Liu L, Yan M, et al. Dissemination of inci2 plasmids that harbor the blactx-m element among clinical salmonella isolates. Antimicrob Agents Chemother 2015;59(8):5026–8.
109. Xi M, Wu Q, Wang X, et al. Characterization of extended-spectrum beta-lactamase-producing Escherichia coli strains isolated from retail foods in Shaanxi Province, China. J Food Prot 2015;78(5):1018–23.
110. Capita R, Alonso-Calleja C. Antibiotic-resistant bacteria: a challenge for the food industry. Crit Rev Food Sci Nutr 2013;53(1):11–48.
111. Koluman A, Dikici A. Antimicrobial resistance of emerging foodborne pathogens: status quo and global trends. Crit Rev Microbiol 2013;39(1):57–69.
112. US supermarkets redefine antibiotic misuse. Lancet Infect Dis 2009;9(5):265.
113. Endimiani A, Bertschy I, Perreten V. Escherichia coli producing cmy-2 beta-lactamase in bovine mastitis milk. J Food Prot 2012;75(1):137–8.
114. Bortolaia V, Guardabassi L, Trevisani M, et al. High diversity of extended-spectrum beta-lactamases in Escherichia coli isolates from Italian broiler flocks. Antimicrob Agents Chemother 2010;54(4):1623–6.
115. Kluytmans JA, Overdevest IT, Willemsen I, et al. Extended-spectrum beta-lactamase-producing Escherichia coli from retail chicken meat and humans: comparison of strains, plasmids, resistance genes, and virulence factors. Clin Infect Dis 2013;56(4):478–87.
116. Huijbers PM, de Kraker M, Graat EA, et al. Prevalence of extended-spectrum beta-lactamase-producing enterobacteriaceae in humans living in municipalities with high and low broiler density. Clin Microbiol Infect 2013;19(6):E256–9.
117. Leverstein-van Hall MA, Dierikx CM, Cohen Stuart J, et al. Dutch patients, retail chicken meat and poultry share the same ESBL genes, plasmids and strains. Clin Microbiol Infect 2011;17(6):873–80.
118. Jensen LB, Hasman H, Agerso Y, et al. First description of an oxyimino-cephalosporin-resistant, ESBL-carrying Escherichia coli isolated from meat sold in Denmark. J Antimicrob Chemother 2006;57(4):793–4.
119. Politi L, Tassios PT, Lambiri M, et al. Repeated occurrence of diverse extended-spectrum beta-lactamases in minor serotypes of food-borne salmonella enterica subsp. enterica. J Clin Microbiol 2005;43(7):3453–6.
120. Leistner R, Meyer E, Gastmeier P, et al. Risk factors associated with the community-acquired colonization of extended-spectrum beta-lactamase (ESBL) positive Escherichia coli. An exploratory case-control study. PLoS One 2013;8(9):e74323.
121. Jourdan-da Silva N, Watrin M, Weill FX, et al. Outbreak of haemolytic uraemic syndrome due to shiga toxin-producing Escherichia coli o104:H4 among French tourists returning from turkey, September 2011. Euro Surveill 2012;17(4).
122. Ullrich S, Bremer P, Neumann-Grutzeck C, et al. Symptoms and clinical course of EHEC o104 infection in hospitalized patients: a prospective single center study. PLoS One 2013;8(2):e55278.
123. Aurass P, Prager R, Flieger A. EHEC/EAEC o104:H4 strain linked with the 2011 German outbreak of haemolytic uremic syndrome enters into the viable but non-culturable state in response to various stresses and resuscitates upon stress relief. Environ Microbiol 2011;13(12):3139–48.

124. Costa D, Vinue L, Poeta P, et al. Prevalence of extended-spectrum beta-lactamase-producing Escherichia coli isolates in faecal samples of broilers. Vet Microbiol 2009;138(3–4):339–44.
125. Guenther S, Aschenbrenner K, Stamm I, et al. Comparable high rates of extended-spectrum-beta-lactamase-producing Escherichia coli in birds of prey from Germany and Mongolia. PLoS One 2012;7(12):e53039.
126. Guenther S, Bethe A, Fruth A, et al. Frequent combination of antimicrobial multiresistance and extraintestinal pathogenicity in Escherichia coli isolates from urban rats (Rattus norvegicus) in Berlin, Germany. PLoS One 2012;7(11):e50331.
127. Guenther S, Grobbel M, Beutlich J, et al. Ctx-m-15-type extended-spectrum beta-lactamases-producing Escherichia coli from wild birds in Germany. Environ Microbiol Rep 2010;2(5):641–5.
128. Hiroi M, Yamazaki F, Harada T, et al. Prevalence of extended-spectrum beta-lactamase-producing Escherichia coli and Klebsiella pneumoniae in food-producing animals. J Vet Med Sci 2012;74(2):189–95.
129. Liu BT, Yang QE, Li L, et al. Dissemination and characterization of plasmids carrying oqxab-bla ctx-m genes in Escherichia coli isolates from food-producing animals. PLoS One 2013;8(9):e73947.
130. Hordijk J, Schoormans A, Kwakernaak M, et al. High prevalence of fecal carriage of extended spectrum beta-lactamase/AmpC-producing enterobacteriaceae in cats and dogs. Front Microbiol 2013;4:242.
131. Dierikx C, van Essen-Zandbergen A, Veldman K, et al. Increased detection of extended spectrum beta-lactamase producing salmonella enterica and Escherichia coli isolates from poultry. Vet Microbiol 2010;145(3–4):273–8.
132. Overdevest I, Willemsen I, Rijnsburger M, et al. Extended-spectrum beta-lactamase genes of Escherichia coli in chicken meat and humans, the Netherlands. Emerg Infect Dis 2011;17(7):1216–22.
133. Wassenberg MW, Bootsma MC, Troelstra A, et al. Transmissibility of livestock-associated methicillin-resistant staphylococcus aureus (st398) in Dutch hospitals. Clin Microbiol Infect 2011;17(2):316–9.
134. Laupland KB, Church DL, Vidakovich J, et al. Community-onset extended-spectrum beta-lactamase (ESBL) producing Escherichia coli: importance of international travel. J Infect 2008;57(6):441–8.
135. Lewis JS 2nd, Herrera M, Wickes B, et al. First report of the emergence of ctx-m-type extended-spectrum beta-lactamases (ESBLs) as the predominant ESBL isolated in a U.S. health care system. Antimicrob Agents Chemother 2007; 51(11):4015–21.
136. Moland ES, Black JA, Hossain A, et al. Discovery of ctx-m-like extended-spectrum beta-lactamases in Escherichia coli isolates from five US states. Antimicrob Agents Chemother 2003;47(7):2382–3.
137. Nicolas-Chanoine MH, Blanco J, Leflon-Guibout V, et al. Intercontinental emergence of Escherichia coli clone o25:H4-st131 producing ctx-m-15. J Antimicrob Chemother 2008;61(2):273–81.
138. Coque TM, Novais A, Carattoli A, et al. Dissemination of clonally related Escherichia coli strains expressing extended-spectrum beta-lactamase ctx-m-15. Emerg Infect Dis 2008;14(2):195–200.
139. Rodriguez-Bano J, Picon E, Gijon P, et al. Community-onset bacteremia due to extended-spectrum beta-lactamase-producing Escherichia coli: risk factors and prognosis. Clin Infect Dis 2010;50(1):40–8.
140. Cagnacci S, Gualco L, Debbia E, et al. European emergence of ciprofloxacin-resistant Escherichia coli clonal groups o25:H4-st 131 and o15:K52:H1 causing

community-acquired uncomplicated cystitis. J Clin Microbiol 2008;46(8): 2605–12.
141. Lau SH, Reddy S, Cheesbrough J, et al. Major uropathogenic Escherichia coli strain isolated in the northwest of England identified by multilocus sequence typing. J Clin Microbiol 2008;46(3):1076–80.
142. Dahbi G, Mora A, Lopez C, et al. Emergence of new variants of st131 clonal group among extraintestinal pathogenic Escherichia coli producing extended-spectrum beta-lactamases. Int J Antimicrob Agents 2013;42(4):347–51.
143. Peirano G, Pitout JD. Molecular epidemiology of Escherichia coli producing ctx-m beta-lactamases: the worldwide emergence of clone st131 o25:H4. Int J Antimicrob Agents 2010;35(4):316–21.
144. Clermont O, Bonacorsi S, Bingen E. Rapid and simple determination of the Escherichia coli phylogenetic group. Appl Environ Microbiol 2000;66(10):4555–8.
145. Clermont O, Johnson JR, Menard M, et al. Determination of Escherichia coli o types by allele-specific polymerase chain reaction: application to the o types involved in human septicemia. Diagn Microbiol Infect Dis 2007;57(2):129–36.
146. Pitout JD, Gregson DB, Campbell L, et al. Molecular characteristics of extended-spectrum-beta-lactamase-producing Escherichia coli isolates causing bacteremia in the Calgary health region from 2000 to 2007: emergence of clone st131 as a cause of community-acquired infections. Antimicrob Agents Chemother 2009;53(7):2846–51.
147. Rogers BA, Sidjabat HE, Paterson DL. Escherichia coli o25b-st131: a pandemic, multiresistant, community-associated strain. J Antimicrob Chemother 2011; 66(1):1–14.
148. Petty NK, Ben Zakour NL, Stanton-Cook M, et al. Global dissemination of a multidrug resistant Escherichia coli clone. Proc Natl Acad Sci U S A 2014;111(15): 5694–9.
149. Lopez-Cerero L, Navarro MD, Bellido M, et al. Escherichia coli belonging to the worldwide emerging epidemic clonal group o25b/st131: risk factors and clinical implications. J Antimicrob Chemother 2014;69(3):809–14.
150. Sherchan JB, Hayakawa K, Miyoshi-Akiyama T, et al. Clinical epidemiology and molecular analysis of extended-spectrum-beta-lactamase-producing Escherichia coli in Nepal: characteristics of sequence types 131 and 648. Antimicrob Agents Chemother 2015;59(6):3424–32.
151. Rattinger GB, Mullins CD, Zuckerman IH, et al. A sustainable strategy to prevent misuse of antibiotics for acute respiratory infections. PLoS One 2012;7(12): e51147.
152. Harris AD, Kotetishvili M, Shurland S, et al. How important is patient-to-patient transmission in extended-spectrum beta-lactamase Escherichia coli acquisition. Am J Infect Control 2007;35(2):97–101.
153. Arpin C, Dubois V, Coulange L, et al. Extended-spectrum beta-lactamase-producing enterobacteriaceae in community and private health care centers. Antimicrob Agents Chemother 2003;47(11):3506–14.
154. Arpin C, Dubois V, Maugein J, et al. Clinical and molecular analysis of extended-spectrum {beta}-lactamase-producing Enterobacteria in the community setting. J Clin Microbiol 2005;43(10):5048–54.
155. Rodriguez-Bano J, Navarro MD, Romero L, et al. Epidemiology and clinical features of infections caused by extended-spectrum beta-lactamase-producing Escherichia coli in nonhospitalized patients. J Clin Microbiol 2004;42(3): 1089–94.

156. Banerjee R, Strahilevitz J, Johnson JR, et al. Predictors and molecular epidemiology of community-onset extended-spectrum beta-lactamase-producing Escherichia coli infection in a Midwestern community. Infect Control Hosp Epidemiol 2013;34(9):947–53.
157. Soraas A, Sundsfjord A, Sandven I, et al. Risk factors for community-acquired urinary tract infections caused by ESBL-producing enterobacteriaceae–a case-control study in a low prevalence country. PLoS One 2013;8(7):e69581.
158. Freeman JT, Williamson DA, Heffernan H, et al. Comparative epidemiology of ctx-m-14 and ctx-m-15 producing Escherichia coli: association with distinct demographic groups in the community in New Zealand. Eur J Clin Microbiol Infect Dis 2012;31(8):2057–60.
159. Valverde A, Grill F, Coque TM, et al. High rate of intestinal colonization with extended-spectrum-beta-lactamase-producing organisms in household contacts of infected community patients. J Clin Microbiol 2008;46(8):2796–9.
160. Skippen I, Shemko M, Turton J, et al. Epidemiology of infections caused by extended-spectrum beta-lactamase-producing Escherichia coli and Klebsiella spp.: a nested case-control study from a tertiary hospital in London. J Hosp Infect 2006;64(2):115–23.
161. Pena C, Gudiol C, Tubau F, et al. Risk-factors for acquisition of extended-spectrum beta-lactamase-producing Escherichia coli among hospitalised patients. Clin Microbiol Infect 2006;12(3):279–84.
162. Graffunder EM, Preston KE, Evans AM, et al. Risk factors associated with extended-spectrum beta-lactamase-producing organisms at a tertiary care hospital. J Antimicrob Chemother 2005;56(1):139–45.
163. Friedman ND, Kaye KS, Stout JE, et al. Health care–associated bloodstream infections in adults: a reason to change the accepted definition of community-acquired infections. Ann Intern Med 2002;137(10):791–7.
164. Bratzler DW, Dellinger EP, Olsen KM, et al. Clinical practice guidelines for antimicrobial prophylaxis in surgery. Surg Infect (Larchmt) 2013;14(1):73–156.
165. Martin ET, Tansek R, Collins V, et al. The carbapenem-resistant enterobacteriaceae score: a bedside score to rule out infection with carbapenem-resistant enterobacteriaceae among hospitalized patients. Am J Infect Control 2013;41(2):180–2.
166. Marchaim D, Chopra T, Bhargava A, et al. Recent exposure to antimicrobials and carbapenem-resistant enterobacteriaceae: the role of antimicrobial stewardship. Infect Control Hosp Epidemiol 2012;33(8):817–30.
167. Abbo A, Carmeli Y, Navon-Venezia S, et al. Impact of multi-drug-resistant Acinetobacter baumannii on clinical outcomes. Eur J Clin Microbiol Infect Dis 2007;26(11):793–800.
168. Cosgrove SE, Sakoulas G, Perencevich EN, et al. Comparison of mortality associated with methicillin-resistant and methicillin-susceptible staphylococcus aureus bacteremia: a meta-analysis. Clin Infect Dis 2003;36(1):53–9.
169. Aloush V, Navon-Venezia S, Seigman-Igra Y, et al. Multidrug-resistant pseudomonas aeruginosa: risk factors and clinical impact. Antimicrob Agents Chemother 2006;50(1):43–8.
170. Carmeli Y, Samore MH, Huskins C. The association between antecedent vancomycin treatment and hospital-acquired vancomycin-resistant enterococci: a meta-analysis. Arch Intern Med 1999;159(20):2461–8.
171. Bogan C, Kaye KS, Chopra T, et al. Outcomes of carbapenem-resistant enterobacteriaceae isolation: matched analysis. Am J Infect Control 2014;42(6):612–20.

172. Melzer M, Eykyn SJ, Gransden WR, et al. Is methicillin-resistant staphylococcus aureus more virulent than methicillin-susceptible s. Aureus? a comparative cohort study of British patients with nosocomial infection and bacteremia. Clin Infect Dis 2003;37(11):1453–60.
173. Sahly H, Navon-Venezia S, Roesler L, et al. Extended-spectrum beta-lactamase production is associated with an increase in cell invasion and expression of fimbrial adhesins in Klebsiella pneumoniae. Antimicrob Agents Chemother 2008;52(9):3029–34.
174. Rodriguez-Bano J, Mingorance J, Fernandez-Romero N, et al. Outcome of bacteraemia due to extended-spectrum beta-lactamase-producing Escherichia coli: impact of microbiological determinants. J Infect 2013;67(1):27–34.
175. Park YS, Adams-Haduch JM, Shutt KA, et al. Clinical and microbiologic characteristics of cephalosporin-resistant Escherichia coli at three centers in the United States. Antimicrob Agents Chemother 2012;56(4):1870–6.
176. Sidjabat HE, Paterson DL, Adams-Haduch JM, et al. Molecular epidemiology of ctx-m-producing Escherichia coli isolates at a tertiary medical center in western Pennsylvania. Antimicrob Agents Chemother 2009;53(11):4733–9.
177. Doi Y, Adams J, O'Keefe A, et al. Community-acquired extended-spectrum beta-lactamase producers, united states. Emerg Infect Dis 2007;13(7):1121–3.
178. Harris AD. Control group selection is an important but neglected issue in studies of antibiotic resistance. Ann Intern Med 2000;132(11):925.
179. Kaye KS, Harris AD, Samore M, et al. The case-case-control study design: addressing the limitations of risk factor studies for antimicrobial resistance. Infect Control Hosp Epidemiol 2005;26(4):346–51.
180. Rodriguez-Bano J, Pascual A. Clinical significance of extended-spectrum beta-lactamases. Expert Rev Anti Infect Ther 2008;6(5):671–83.
181. Tumbarello M, Sanguinetti M, Montuori E, et al. Predictors of mortality in patients with bloodstream infections caused by extended-spectrum-beta-lactamase-producing enterobacteriaceae: importance of inadequate initial antimicrobial treatment. Antimicrob Agents Chemother 2007;51(6):1987–94.
182. Tumbarello M, Spanu T, Sanguinetti M, et al. Bloodstream infections caused by extended-spectrum-beta-lactamase-producing Klebsiella pneumoniae: risk factors, molecular epidemiology, and clinical outcome. Antimicrob Agents Chemother 2006;50(2):498–504.
183. Paul M, Shani V, Muchtar E, et al. Systematic review and meta-analysis of the efficacy of appropriate empiric antibiotic therapy for sepsis. Antimicrob Agents Chemother 2010;54(11):4851–63.
184. Kumar A, Roberts D, Wood KE, et al. Duration of hypotension before initiation of effective antimicrobial therapy is the critical determinant of survival in human septic shock. Crit Care Med 2006;34(6):1589–96.
185. Tumbarello M, Trecarichi EM, Bassetti M, et al. Identifying patients harboring extended-spectrum-beta-lactamase-producing enterobacteriaceae on hospital admission: derivation and validation of a scoring system. Antimicrob Agents Chemother 2011;55(7):3485–90.
186. Naas T, Cuzon G, Truong H, et al. Evaluation of a DNA microarray, the check-points ESBL/KPC array, for rapid detection of TEM, SHV, and ctx-m extended-spectrum beta-lactamases and KPC carbapenemases. Antimicrob Agents Chemother 2010;54(8):3086–92.
187. Oviano M, Fernandez B, Fernandez A, et al. Rapid detection of enterobacteriaceae producing extended spectrum beta-lactamases directly from positive

blood cultures by matrix-assisted laser desorption ionization-time of flight mass spectrometry. Clin Microbiol Infect 2014;20(11):1146–57.

188. Johnson SW, Anderson DJ, May DB, et al. Utility of a clinical risk factor scoring model in predicting infection with extended-spectrum beta-lactamase-producing enterobacteriaceae on hospital admission. Infect Control Hosp Epidemiol 2013;34(4):385–92.
189. Vitkon-Barkay I, Yekutiel M, Martin ET, et al. Developing a score to shorten the time to initiation of appropriate therapy for extensively drug resistant gram-negative bacilli and avoid unnecessary use of polymixins. In: (ESCMID) ESoCMaID, editor. Barcelona (Spain): European Congress of Clinical Microbiology and Infectious Diseases (ECCMID); 2014.
190. Paterson DL, Ko WC, Von Gottberg A, et al. Antibiotic therapy for Klebsiella pneumoniae bacteremia: implications of production of extended-spectrum beta-lactamases. Clin Infect Dis 2004;39(1):31–7.
191. Vardakas KZ, Tansarli GS, Rafailidis PI, et al. Carbapenems versus alternative antibiotics for the treatment of bacteraemia due to enterobacteriaceae producing extended-spectrum beta-lactamases: a systematic review and meta-analysis. J Antimicrob Chemother 2012;67(12):2793–803.
192. Carmeli Y, Lidji SK, Shabtai E, et al. The effects of group 1 versus group 2 carbapenems on imipenem-resistant pseudomonas aeruginosa: an ecological study. Diagn Microbiol Infect Dis 2011;70(3):367–72.
193. Dellinger RP, Levy MM, Carlet JM, et al. Surviving sepsis campaign: international guidelines for management of severe sepsis and septic shock: 2008. Crit Care Med 2008;36(1):296–327.
194. Gutierrez-Gutierrez B, Bonomo RA, Carmeli Y, et al. Ertapenem for the treatment of bloodstream infections due to esbl-producing enterobacteriaceae: A multinational pre-registered cohort study. J Antimicrob Chemother 2016. [Epub ahead of print].
195. Schwaber MJ, Carmeli Y. Carbapenem-resistant enterobacteriaceae: a potential threat. JAMA 2008;300(24):2911–3.
196. Schwaber MJ, Lev B, Israeli A, et al. Containment of a country-wide outbreak of carbapenem-resistant Klebsiella pneumoniae in Israeli hospitals via a nationally implemented intervention. Clin Infect Dis 2011;52(7):848–55.
197. Bin C, Hui W, Renyuan Z, et al. Outcome of cephalosporin treatment of bacteremia due to ctx-m-type extended-spectrum beta-lactamase-producing Escherichia coli. Diagn Microbiol Infect Dis 2006;56(4):351–7.
198. Paterson DL, Ko WC, Von Gottberg A, et al. Outcome of cephalosporin treatment for serious infections due to apparently susceptible organisms producing extended-spectrum beta-lactamases: implications for the clinical microbiology laboratory. J Clin Microbiol 2001;39(6):2206–12.
199. Wong-Beringer A, Hindler J, Loeloff M, et al. Molecular correlation for the treatment outcomes in bloodstream infections caused by Escherichia coli and Klebsiella pneumoniae with reduced susceptibility to ceftazidime. Clin Infect Dis 2002;34(2):135–46.
200. Kang CI, Kim SH, Park WB, et al. Bloodstream infections due to extended-spectrum beta-lactamase-producing Escherichia coli and Klebsiella pneumoniae: risk factors for mortality and treatment outcome, with special emphasis on antimicrobial therapy. Antimicrob Agents Chemother 2004;48(12):4574–81.
201. Clinical and Laboratory Standards Institute (CLSI). Performance standards for antimicrobial susceptibility testing. In: Clinical and Laboratory Standards

Institute, editor. Nineteenth informational supplement. Approved standard m100–s20. Wayne (PA): Clinical and Laboratory Standards Institute; 2010.
202. Livermore DM, Andrews JM, Hawkey PM, et al. Are susceptibility tests enough, or should laboratories still seek ESBLs and carbapenemases directly? J Antimicrob Chemother 2012;67(7):1569–77.
203. Endimiani A, Luzzaro F, Perilli M, et al. Bacteremia due to Klebsiella pneumoniae isolates producing the tem-52 extended-spectrum beta-lactamase: treatment outcome of patients receiving imipenem or ciprofloxacin. Clin Infect Dis 2004; 38(2):243–51.
204. Rodriguez-Martinez JM, Diaz de Alba P, Briales A, et al. Contribution of oqxab efflux pumps to quinolone resistance in extended-spectrum-beta-lactamase-producing Klebsiella pneumoniae. J Antimicrob Chemother 2013;68(1):68–73.
205. Kritsotakis EI, Tsioutis C, Roumbelaki M, et al. Antibiotic use and the risk of carbapenem-resistant extended-spectrum-{beta}-lactamase-producing Klebsiella pneumoniae infection in hospitalized patients: results of a double case-control study. J Antimicrob Chemother 2011;66(6):1383–91.
206. Lee CH, Su LH, Tang YF, et al. Treatment of ESBL-producing Klebsiella pneumoniae bacteraemia with carbapenems or flomoxef: a retrospective study and laboratory analysis of the isolates. J Antimicrob Chemother 2006;58(5):1074–7.
207. Lopez-Cerero L, Picon E, Morillo C, et al. Comparative assessment of inoculum effects on the antimicrobial activity of amoxycillin-clavulanate and piperacillin-tazobactam with extended-spectrum beta-lactamase-producing and extended-spectrum beta-lactamase-non-producing Escherichia coli isolates. Clin Microbiol Infect 2010;16(2):132–6.
208. Thomson KS, Moland ES. Cefepime, piperacillin-tazobactam, and the inoculum effect in tests with extended-spectrum beta-lactamase-producing enterobacteriaceae. Antimicrob Agents Chemother 2001;45(12):3548–54.
209. Zimhony O, Chmelnitsky I, Bardenstein R, et al. Endocarditis caused by extended-spectrum-beta-lactamase-producing Klebsiella pneumoniae: emergence of resistance to ciprofloxacin and piperacillin-tazobactam during treatment despite initial susceptibility. Antimicrob Agents Chemother 2006;50(9): 3179–82.
210. Rodriguez-Bano J, Navarro MD, Retamar P, et al. Beta-lactam/beta-lactam inhibitor combinations for the treatment of bacteremia due to extended-spectrum beta-lactamase-producing Escherichia coli: a post hoc analysis of prospective cohorts. Clin Infect Dis 2012;54(2):167–74.
211. Perez F, Bonomo RA. Can we really use ss-lactam/ss-lactam inhibitor combinations for the treatment of infections caused by extended-spectrum ss-lactamase-producing bacteria? Clin Infect Dis 2012;54(2):175–7.
212. Dedeic-Ljubovic A, Hukic M, Pfeifer Y, et al. Emergence of ctx-m-15 extended-spectrum beta-lactamase-producing Klebsiella pneumoniae isolates in Bosnia and Herzegovina. Clin Microbiol Infect 2010;16(2):152–6.
213. Pfundstein J, Roghmann MC, Schwalbe RS, et al. A randomized trial of surgical antimicrobial prophylaxis with and without vancomycin in organ transplant patients. Clin Transplant 1999;13(3):245–52.
214. Hall JC, Christiansen K, Carter MJ, et al. Antibiotic prophylaxis in cardiac operations. Ann Thorac Surg 1993;56(4):916–22.
215. Tissera S, Lee SM. Isolation of extended spectrum beta-lactamase (ESBL) producing bacteria from urban surface waters in Malaysia. Malays J Med Sci 2013; 20(3):14–22.

216. Ofer-Friedman H, Shefler C, Sharma S, et al. Carbapenems versus piperacillin-tazobactam for bloodstream infections of nonurinary source caused by extended-spectrum beta-lactamase-producing enterobacteriaceae. Infect Control Hosp Epidemiol 2015;36(8):981–5.
217. Tamma PD, Han JH, Rock C, et al. Carbapenem therapy is associated with improved survival compared with piperacillin-tazobactam for patients with extended-spectrum beta-lactamase bacteremia. Clin Infect Dis 2015;60(9):1319–25.
218. Lu PL, Liu YC, Toh HS, et al. Epidemiology and antimicrobial susceptibility profiles of gram-negative bacteria causing urinary tract infections in the Asia-Pacific region: 2009-2010 results from the study for monitoring antimicrobial resistance trends (SMART). Int J Antimicrob Agents 2012;40(Suppl):S37–43.
219. Hawser SP, Bouchillon SK, Lascols C, et al. Susceptibility of European Escherichia coli clinical isolates from intra-abdominal infections, extended-spectrum beta-lactamase occurrence, resistance distribution, and molecular characterization of ertapenem-resistant isolates (SMART 2008-2009). Clin Microbiol Infect 2012;18(3):253–9.
220. Hoban DJ, Bouchillon SK, Hawser SP, et al. Susceptibility of gram-negative pathogens isolated from patients with complicated intra-abdominal infections in the United States, 2007-2008: results of the study for monitoring antimicrobial resistance trends (SMART). Antimicrob Agents Chemother 2010;54(7):3031–4.
221. Rotschafer JC, Zabinski RA, Walker KJ. Pharmacodynamic factors of antibiotic efficacy. Pharmacotherapy 1992;12(6 Pt 2):64S–70S.
222. Gupta K, Hooton TM, Naber KG, et al. International clinical practice guidelines for the treatment of acute uncomplicated cystitis and pyelonephritis in women: a 2010 update by the Infectious Diseases Society of America and the European Society for Microbiology and Infectious Diseases. Clin Infect Dis 2011;52(5):e103–20.
223. Pakyz AL, MacDougall C, Oinonen M, et al. Trends in antibacterial use in US academic health centers: 2002 to 2006. Arch Intern Med 2008;168(20):2254–60.
224. Klastersky J, Thys JP, Mombelli G. Comparative studies of intermittent and continuous administration of aminoglycosides in the treatment of bronchopulmonary infections due to gram-negative bacteria. Rev Infect Dis 1981;3(1):74–83.
225. Falagas ME, Maraki S, Karageorgopoulos DE, et al. Antimicrobial susceptibility of multidrug-resistant (MDR) and extensively drug-resistant (XDR) enterobacteriaceae isolates to fosfomycin. Int J Antimicrob Agents 2010;35(3):240–3.
226. FDA. Drug safety communication - increased risk of death with tygacil (tigecycline) compared to other antibiotics used to treat similar infections. FDA; 2010.
227. Pogue JM, Lee J, Marchaim D, et al. Incidence of and risk factors for colistin-associated nephrotoxicity in a large academic health system. Clin Infect Dis 2011;53(9):879–84.
228. Pogue JM, Cohen DA, Marchaim D. Editorial commentary: polymyxin-resistant Acinetobacter baumannii: urgent action needed. Clin Infect Dis 2015;60(9):1304–7.
229. Chen PC, Chang LY, Lu CY, et al. Drug susceptibility and treatment response of common urinary tract infection pathogens in children. J Microbiol Immunol Infect 2014;47(6):478–83.
230. Kurtaran B, Candevir A, Tasova Y, et al. Antibiotic resistance in community-acquired urinary tract infections: prevalence and risk factors. Med Sci Monit 2010;16(5):CR246–51.

231. Yamamoto S, Higuchi Y, Nojima M. Current therapy of acute uncomplicated cystitis. Int J Urol 2010;17(5):450–6.
232. Kim ME, Ha US, Cho YH. Prevalence of antimicrobial resistance among uropathogens causing acute uncomplicated cystitis in female outpatients in South Korea: a multicentre study in 2006. Int J Antimicrob Agents 2008;31(Suppl 1):S15–8.
233. Ilic T, Gracan S, Arapovic A, et al. Changes in bacterial resistance patterns in children with urinary tract infections on antimicrobial prophylaxis at university hospital in split. Med Sci Monit 2011;17(7):CR355–61.
234. Lowe CF, McGeer A, Muller MP, et al. Decreased susceptibility to noncarbapenem antimicrobials in extended-spectrum-beta-lactamase-producing Escherichia coli and Klebsiella pneumoniae isolates in Toronto, Canada. Antimicrob Agents Chemother 2012;56(7):3977–80.
235. Puerto AS, Fernandez JG, del Castillo Jde D, et al. In vitro activity of beta-lactam and non-beta-lactam antibiotics in extended-spectrum beta-lactamase-producing clinical isolates of Escherichia coli. Diagn Microbiol Infect Dis 2006;54(2):135–9.
236. de Cueto M, Lopez L, Hernandez JR, et al. In vitro activity of fosfomycin against extended-spectrum-beta-lactamase-producing Escherichia coli and Klebsiella pneumoniae: comparison of susceptibility testing procedures. Antimicrob Agents Chemother 2006;50(1):368–70.
237. Arslan H, Azap OK, Ergonul O, et al. Risk factors for ciprofloxacin resistance among Escherichia coli strains isolated from community-acquired urinary tract infections in Turkey. J Antimicrob Chemother 2005;56(5):914–8.

Multidrug-Resistant Bacteria in the Community

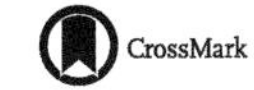

Trends and Lessons Learned

David van Duin, MD, PhD[a,*], David L. Paterson, MBBS, PhD[b]

KEYWORDS

- Carbapenem-resistant Enterobacteriaceae • *Klebsiella pneumoniae* • Readmission • Transmission • Tigecycline

KEY POINTS

- Wide variability is observed in community spread of common nosocomial MDR pathogens.
- This variability is likely secondary to several factors that include the natural habitats of the bacteria, and the competition present in those niches.
- In addition, certain strains of bacteria seem to be much more able to maintain their MDR phenotype and spread throughout the community.
- This is most likely secondary to additional genetic content that compensates for the relative fitness cost of the expression of genes associated with antibacterial resistance.
- Community spread of MDR bacteria is an important public health threat that should be approached urgently and proactively.

INTRODUCTION

Multidrug resistant (MDR) bacteria are well-recognized to be one of the most important current public health problems. The Infectious Diseases Society of America recognizes antimicrobial resistance as "one of the greatest threats to human health worldwide" (**Table 1**).[1] Several issues underlie the critical danger that is posed by the rise of MDR bacteria. First and most importantly, outcomes in patients infected with MDR bacteria tend to be worse compared with patients infected with more susceptible organisms.[2,3] In this way, rising rates of antibacterial resistance have an impact on all aspects of modern medicine, and threaten to decrease the yield of many accomplishments, such as cancer care, transplantation, and surgical procedures.[4] Second, tremendous added costs are associated with these infections. In

[a] Division of Infectious Diseases, University of North Carolina, CB 7030, 130 Mason Farm Road, Chapel Hill, NC 27599, USA; [b] The University of Queensland, Building 71/918 RBWH, Herston, QLD 4029, Australia
* Corresponding author.
E-mail address: david_vanduin@med.unc.edu

Infect Dis Clin N Am 30 (2016) 377–390
http://dx.doi.org/10.1016/j.idc.2016.02.004
id.theclinics.com
0891-5520/16/$ – see front matter

Table 1
Multidrug-resistant bacteria observed in the community

MDR Phenotype	Epidemiologic Setting of Community-Onset Infections
MRSA	Household colonization; farm animal exposure (emerging)
VRE	Typically health care–associated
ESBL + *Escherichia coli*	Endemic in Asia; in low-prevalence areas travel to Asia
CRE	Rare at present; emerging in India and China
CR-PA	Extremely rare
CR-AB	Extremely rare

Abbreviations: AB, acinetobacter baumanii; CR, carbapenem resistant; CRE, carbapenem-resistant Enterobacteriaceae; ESBL, extended-spectrum β-lactamases; MRSA, methicillin-resistant *Staphylococcus aureus*; PA, pseudomonas aeruginosa; VRE, vancomycin-resistant enterococci.

the United States, associated annual additional costs of infections caused by resistant organisms compared with susceptible organisms are estimated between $21 billion and $34 billion.[1] Third, the prevalence of specific MDR bacteria is closely linked to the use of broad-spectrum antibiotics, both for empiric and for definitive therapy.[5] This increased use in turn leads to even higher rates of MDR bacteria, thus creating a vicious cycle.

Typically, MDR bacteria are associated with nosocomial infections. However, some MDR bacteria have become quite prevalent causes of community-acquired infections. This is an important development because community spread of MDR bacteria leads to a large increase of the population-at-risk, and subsequently an increase in the number of infections caused by MDR bacteria. In addition, when the incidence of a certain resistance pattern in bacteria causing community-acquired infections exceeds a specific threshold, broader spectrum antibacterials and/or combination antibacterial therapy are indicated for the empiric treatment of community-acquired infections. This article outlines the trends in and epidemiology of community prevalence of various MDR bacteria.

COMMUNITY-ASSOCIATED, HEALTH CARE–ASSOCIATED, AND NOSOCOMIAL INFECTIONS

Infections can be divided into community-onset and nosocomial acquisition. The widely used cutoff to distinguish between these two categories is whether the onset of infection was within the first 48 hours of hospitalization (community-onset) or later (nosocomial). Limitations of this division include the arbitrary nature of the 48-hour time point, and the dependence on the timing of diagnosis. If cultures are performed earlier during hospitalization, more infections are likely to be labeled as community-onset.

The category of community-onset can then be further subdivided into community-acquired and health care–associated, based on work pioneered by Morin and Hadler[6] and Friedman and colleagues.[7] Generally, an infection is deemed to be health care–associated if a patient was hospitalized in an acute care hospital for 2 or more days within 90 days of the infection; resided in a nursing home or long-term care facility; received recent intravenous antibiotic therapy, chemotherapy, or wound care within the past 30 days of the current infection; or attended a hospital or hemodialysis clinic.[8]

The remaining category includes those patients who have a community-onset infection, and who do not meet any of the previously mentioned criteria for health care–associated infection. These infections are considered to be community-acquired. However, for the purposes of evaluating MDR bacteria in the community, these definitions may not tell the whole story. Patients tend to get infected with organisms with which they were previously colonized. Therefore, it is the timing of colonization, rather than the timing of diagnosis of infection, that is crucially important to determine the origin of the MDR bacteria. Studies that have used screening of noninfected individuals have addressed these questions for some MDR bacteria in certain populations.

REQUIREMENTS FOR TRANSITION FROM NOSOCOMIAL PATHOGEN TO COMMUNITY-ASSOCIATED PATHOGEN

The commonality of risk factors of MDR organisms, and opportunistic organisms, such as *Clostridium difficile* and *Candida* sp, was described by Safdar and Maki.[9] Many studies have explored specific risk factors for MDR bacteria and for the most part have found overlapping sets of risk factors. Exposure to antibiotics is a risk factor that is almost always found in studies with sufficient power to evaluate this risk. The specific antibiotic class associated with the risk for developing a specific antimicrobial resistance pattern may vary. Often, a simple association between the use of a specific antibacterial and resistance to that antibiotic is described. For instance, tigecycline use in patients with carbapenem-resistant *Klebsiella pneumoniae* was found to subsequently lead to tigecycline resistance in the same bacteria of those same patients.[10] Specific types of epidemiologic studies (case-case-control studies) often are needed to determine the true extent of the risk of use of an antibiotic contributing to resistance to itself.[11,12] Sometimes, patterns are more complicated. For example, the use of ceftriaxone, but not other cephalosporins, was associated with the incidence of bloodstream infections caused by vancomycin-resistant enterococci (VRE).[13] These examples are clear indications of the importance of antimicrobial stewardship at all levels (in hospitalized patients, in patients treated in the community, and nonmedical antibiotic use) for the control of antimicrobial resistance.

Health care exposure is an additional key risk factor for MDR bacteria. The presence of indwelling medical devices, such as urinary catheters, feeding tubes, endotracheal tubes, and vascular lines, is also a commonly identified risk factor.[9] Other categories of risk factors for infection with or colonization by MDR bacteria includes immunosuppressed states, such as solid organ or hematopoietic stem cell transplant recipients, and other comorbid conditions, such as renal failure. The impact of these last two categories is often difficult to definitively establish because there is usually considerable overlap with the first three categories.

For MDR bacteria to become widespread in the community, these traditional risk factors and their implied role in the pathophysiology of colonization have to become of lesser importance. First, the MDR phenotype has to be stable in the absence of antibiotic pressure of the type normally observed in hospitals or nursing homes. The potential implications of this requirement include an ability to compete with wild-type, antibiotic-susceptible bacteria, and a genetic stability of genes conferring the antibiotic resistance phenotype of interest. This means that resistance genes that are associated with a fitness cost to the organism are unlikely to become widespread in the community, unless compensatory genetic content also is accumulated, or if resistance gene expression is fully inducible on antibiotic exposure. Examples of such inducible genes are the erythromycin resistance methylase (*erm*) genes, which are found in mycobacteria and *Staphylococcus aureus*. The products of these genes are only made if the bacteria are exposed to specific antibiotic classes, leading to rapid phenotypic resistance to those antibiotics.

Furthermore, MDR bacteria that are successful in the community have to be able to persist without having to form biofilms on nonorganic matter. This involves competition with other microbial flora in specific microbiome settings, such as the skin, nares, mouth, and gut. Of course, even in the absence of foreign material, biofilm formation remains an important component of bacterial persistence. Biofilm formation is an essential pathophysiologic component of periodontal infections, gastric infection with *Helicobacter pylori*, middle ear infection, urinary cystitis, and many other common infections.[14] MDR bacteria with the ability to form biofilms in the absence of foreign material are more likely to become common in community settings.

In addition, community-associated MDR bacteria have to be able to coexist with the immune systems of otherwise healthy human hosts in the absence of obvious immunosuppression. Nonetheless, specific polymorphisms in immunity genes of the host may facilitate colonization of select bacteria. In persistent *S aureus* nasal carriage, human host genetics were even postulated to be the predominant determinant.[15]

In summary, it is clear that genetic content encoding for several distinct functions needs to be accumulated for a specific strain of MDR bacteria to become community-associated.

METHICILLIN-RESISTANT *STAPHYLOCOCCUS AUREUS*

Methicillin-resistant *S aureus* (MRSA) is the best example of a prevalent and important MDR bacterium that has successfully transitioned from an almost exclusively nosocomial setting to being widespread in the community. The epidemiology of community-associated MRSA (CA-MRSA) has been extensively reviewed elsewhere.[16,17] Here, we give a brief overview of MRSA in the community because it may be predictive of the behavior of other MDR bacteria.

In 1982 an outbreak of CA-MRSA was reported in Detroit.[18] In this outbreak, more than half of patients were intravenous drug users, and the remaining patients had several comorbidities that put them at risk. Importantly, various different strains were found in this outbreak.[18] It was not until the early 1990s that more genuine CA-MRSA outbreaks began to be reported. These outbreaks occurred in populations without specific risk factors. The MRSA strains involved were generally monoclonal or oligoclonal and rather than being extensively MDR, such as nosocomial MRSA strains at that time, these CA-MRSA strains were susceptible to many non-β-lactam antibiotics. In the early 2000s, a new strain of CA-MRSA (USA300) became the predominant CA-MRSA in the United States, effectively replacing the previous USA400 CA-MRSA strain.[16] This USA300 strain is characterized by the presence of the staphylococcal cassette chromosome mec type IV and of genes encoding for Panton-Valentine leucocidin toxins.[19] Households are an important reservoir for the USA300 strain. In a recent study that used whole genome sequencing data, USA300 MRSA was shown to persist in households between 2 and 8 years before admission of a symptomatic patient from that household, and to continue to persist for at least another year after that.[20] This and other evidence shows conclusively that this specific strain of MRSA has been able to become entrenched in a community setting in the absence of ongoing antibiotic pressure. In addition, specific strains of CA-MRSA have been shown to be associated with exposure to livestock, so-called livestock-associated (LA) MRSA. The ST398 LA-MRSA is predominantly found in Europe and America, whereas ST9 LA-MRSA is encountered in Asia.[21]

VANCOMYCIN-RESISTANT ENTEROCOCCI

VRE emerged in the late 1980s, and became a common cause of nosocomial infections in the 1990s.[22] Studies in the 1990s did not detect the presence of vancomycin resistance in enterococci isolated from subjects without health care exposure in the United States.[23,24] In contrast, in European studies from the same time period, VRE was detected in the stool of healthy volunteers.[25] In addition, VRE was commonly found in European food animals.[26,27] The underlying reason for this difference between Europe and the United States is the use of avoparcin, a glycopeptide antibiotic, for the purpose of promoting growth in food animals. Avoparcin was never approved for use in the United States or Canada, but its use was widespread in Europe up to 1997.[27] After a ban on avoparcin in animal husbandry, rates of VRE in animal samples and in samples from human volunteers started to decrease.[25,27] These important data illustrate the critical link between antibiotic use in the food industry and antimicrobial resistance rates in humans. It also indicates that it is never too late to make a change and that banning antimicrobials from the food chain may have an almost instantaneous positive and cost-saving effect.

Around 2000, community-associated VRE began to appear in the United States. In a screening study of patients attending an ambulatory care clinic in Nashville, Tennessee, three patients tested positive for VRE out of 100 patients screened. One of these patients came in for her annual check-up and had no prior health care exposures.[28] Also, VRE was found in wastewater from a semiclosed agrifood system.[29] Nonetheless, VRE remains an uncommon pathogen in community-associated infections. In 289 patients with community-onset VRE, 85% of patients had been hospitalized, and 71% had antimicrobial exposure in the last 3 months, respectively.[30] In another study that included 81 patients with community-onset VRE bacteremia, 79% of patients had prior hospitalizations.[31] These data indicate that even in those patients where VRE is detected on admission or early during hospitalization, acquisition likely occurred in the health care setting. This acquisition was driven by traditional risk factors of antimicrobial exposure, health care exposure, chronic illness, indwelling devices, malignancies, and immunosuppression.[30,31]

The discrepancy between the community spread of MRSA and VRE is notable, because *S aureus* and enterococci are common human colonizers. However, overall colonization with enterococci is much more universal than with *S aureus*, and *S aureus* is not truly a commensal. Apparently in contrast to MRSA, high prevalence of current strains of VRE in the community requires either an ongoing incoming supply of VRE into the shared community gut microbiome through the food chain, or a high level of antibiotic pressure. Fitness cost of maintaining a vancomycin-resistant phenotype would be an intuitive explanation for the relative lack of true community-associated VRE infections. However, the fitness cost of vancomycin resistance seems to be minimal for enterococci, especially in the context of inducible resistance.[32,33] A recent study suggests that pheromone-mediated killing of VRE may account for why vancomycin-susceptible commensal enterococci outcompete VRE in the human gut.[34] In this study, the prototype MDR clinical isolate strain *Enterococcus faecalis* V583 was killed by human fecal flora, whereas commensal antibiotic-susceptible *E faecalis* was able to survive in the presence of flora. The killing effect was traced to pheromone production by commensal *E faecalis* strains.[34]

CARBAPENEM-RESISTANT *ACINETOBACTER BAUMANNII*

Acinetobacter baumannii infections are commonly encountered in hospitalized patients, especially in the intensive care unit.[35] However, community-associated *A baumannii* infections have been well-described especially in tropical and subtropical climates, including Asia and Australia.[36] These are generally associated with pharyngeal carriage and are linked to alcohol abuse and smoking.[36] These are serious infections and the attributable mortality in 80 patients with bacteremia and/or pneumonia from various case series was reported at 56%.[36] Community reservoirs for *A baumannii* include environmental sources, such as soil and vegetables, and human and animal skin and throat carriage. Furthermore, *A baumannii* has also been recovered from human lice.[37]

A.baumannii is intrinsically resistant to several antibiotic classes. In addition, carbapenem resistance may occur through acquisition of carbapenemases, such as IMP-like carbapenemases and/or oxacillinases.[38] The rate of carbapenem resistance in clinical isolates of *A baumannii* rose sharply from 9% to 40% between 1995 and 2004 in the United States.[35] More recent studies suggest that this rate has remained around 40%.[39,40] In contrast, the rate of carbapenem resistance in *Acinetobacter* infections isolated from community-dwelling patients has remained around 4%.[39] Similarly, resistance to carbapenems was detected in only 1 out of 23 community-dwelling volunteers who had *A baumannii* isolated from their hands.[41] In an Australian study on 36 patients with community-onset bacteremic *Acinetobacter* pneumonia, all tested isolates were susceptible to carbapenems.[42] A more worrisome report from China described 32 patients with community-acquired pneumonia caused by *A baumannii*. Three and six isolates were nonsusceptible to meropenem and imipenem, respectively. In addition, $bla_{OXA\text{-}23}$ was found in 12 of 15 tested isolates, some of which tested susceptible to both meropenem and imipenem.[43] Of note, 87% of patients with MDR *A baumannii* had a "hospitalization history," suggesting that these did not truly represent community-associated infections.[43]

In summary, community-associated carbapenem-resistant *A baumannii* seems to remain uncommon, likely reflecting the natural habitats of *Acinetobacter* species, and the differences between true community strains found to cause infections in Asia and Australia and hospital-associated strains. Of concern is the potential for acquisition of carbapenemases by such a community strain, especially in high antibiotic use areas in Asia.

MULTIDRUG-RESISTANT *PSEUDOMONAS AERUGINOSA*

Pseudomonas aeruginosa is a common cause of nosocomial infections, including bloodstream infections and pneumonia. It prefers moist environments and is found in a large variety of places in the hospital, including sink traps and aerators, various equipment, such as scopes and respiratory gear, and contaminated solutions.[44] In addition, *P aeruginosa* may be present on fresh fruits and vegetables and on the fingernails of health care providers.[44]

Similar to *A baumannii*, *P aeruginosa* is intrinsically resistant to many antibiotic classes. Furthermore, additional acquired antibiotic resistance arises easily and quickly after antibiotic exposure. Some patients have chronic biofilm-mediated pseudomonal colonization; patients with cystic fibrosis are an important example.[45] In these patients, repeated antibiotic courses are the rule, as is the subsequent development of MDR strains. Although these patients are often community-dwelling, these infections are clearly health care–associated. Nonetheless, spread of MDR isolates between patients with cystic fibrosis has been well described and is an important infection control risk.[46]

True community-associated infections with MDR *P aeruginosa* fortunately remain uncommon.[47,48] In a cohort of 60 patients with community-acquired bloodstream infections with *P aeruginosa*, 100% of isolates were meropenem susceptible, and 95% were susceptible to piperacillin/tazobactam and ceftazidime.[49] A case report from Turkey describes a young man without health care exposure who presented with a pyogenic liver abscess caused by a *P aeruginosa* strain that was only susceptible to imipenem, amikacin, and colistin.[50]

ENTEROBACTERIACEAE THAT PRODUCE EXTENDED SPECTRUM β-LACTAMASES

Enterobacteriaceae are very common causes of community-associated infections, including urinary tract infections and bacteremia. Unfortunately, in contrast to the situation described previously with *P aeruginosa* and *A baumannii*, there is widespread resistance in community-associated Enterobacteriaceae isolates mediated by extended-spectrum β-lactamases (ESBL).[51] This is a global phenomenon and involves patients of all ages including pediatric populations. In a multicenter, prospective US study over a 1-year period in 2009 to 2010, 4% of *Escherichia coli* community-onset isolates were ESBL producers.[52] Most reflected urinary tract infections, such as cystitis or pyelonephritis. The most common ESBL encountered were of the CTX-M group (91%), the remaining ESBLs were either SHV (8%) or CMY-2 (1%). Most isolates (54%) belonged to the ST131 clonal group.[52] *E coli* ST131 is a globally disseminated MDR clone, and is characterized by resistance to fluoroquinolones in addition to production of CTX-M type ESBL.[53]

In Asia, the Middle East, South America, and some parts of Europe, community-onset infection with ESBL-producing *E coli* is extraordinarily frequent. Lower prevalence regions include North America, some parts of Northern Europe, Australia, and New Zealand. Specific risk factors for community-onset ESBL-producing *E coli* infections have been found in these low-prevalence regions. Reported risk factors from a Chicago-based study for ESBL-producing *E coli* included travel to India (odds ratio [OR], 14.4), increasing age (OR, 1.04 per year), and prior use of ciprofloxacin (OR, 3.92).[54] In a German survey-based study, risk factors for ESBL-positive *E coli* colonization included an Asian language being the primary language spoken in the household (OR, 13.4) and frequent pork consumption (OR, 3.5).[55] A population-based study in London also suggested South-Asian ethnicity and older age as risk factors for ESBL-positive *E coli* bacteriuria.[56] A study performed in Australia and New Zealand also found that birth on the Indian subcontinent or travel to Southeast Asia, China, India, Africa, or the Middle East were risk factors for community-onset third-generation cephalosporin-resistant *E coli* infections.[57]

A significant problem in Asia is disseminated infection with hypervirulent *K pneumoniae* strains. These "hypermucoviscous" strains have a propensity to cause community-onset pyogenic liver abscess and sometimes metastatic infections, including meningitis.[58] Although these strains were typically susceptible to multiple antibiotics, community-onset ESBL-producing strains are now well described and seem to be increasing.[59]

Community-associated ESBL-producing Enterobacteriaceae are of specific concern because treatment requires broad-spectrum antibiotics. Whether carbapenems are always indicated for severe infections caused by ESBL-producing organisms remains controversial. Retrospective studies suggest that carbapenem treatment is either superior or equivalent to treatment with alternatives, such as piperacillin/tazobactam.[60,61] Nevertheless, most clinicians consider a carbapenem the drug of choice for serious infections caused by ESBL-producing Enterobacteriaceae. Therefore, widespread infections from the community with these organisms is likely to lead to a dramatic increase in empiric carbapenem use. A randomized controlled trial is ongoing to address the question of comparative efficacy of piperacillin-tazobactam versus meropenem to treat bloodstream infections caused by ceftriaxone nonsusceptible *E coli* and *Klebsiella* sp, and has enrolled more than 100 patients at the time of writing (MERINO trial, NCT02176122).

CARBAPENEMASE-PRODUCING ENTEROBACTERIACEAE

Carbapenem-resistant Enterobacteriaceae (CRE) represent an immediate public health threat that requires urgent and aggressive action.[1,62] CRE are resistant to most antibiotics and clinical outcomes after CRE infections are generally poor.[63–68] Although less frequent than carbapenem-resistant *K pneumoniae*, carbapenem-resistant *E coli* constitute an important subset of CRE, and are on the rise globally and outbreaks have been reported in the United States.[69,70] To date, most CRE infections in the United States and Europe are health care–associated, with patients from long-term care facilities at especially high risk.[71] Although data from Asia are somewhat sparse, carbapenemases have been found in bacteria recovered from drinking water in India and in food-producing animals in China.[72,73] This raises the specter of huge numbers of people in these large countries being colonized with CRE. Clinical reports of the consequences of this are awaited.

Given the rapid global spread of ESBL-producing *E coli* ST131, the obvious concern is for this highly successful clone to acquire a carbapenemase. Indeed, several reports of carbapenemase-producing *E coli* ST131 have been published.[74–76] In a study from India, ST131 clinical isolates were compared with non-ST131 clinical isolates. Overall 20% of clinical isolates were positive for metallo-β-lactamases, such as $bla_{\text{NDM-1}}$, which was evenly distributed between ST131 and non-ST131 *E coli*.[75] Because the epidemiology of ESBL is estimated to be about 10 years ahead of that of the carbapenemases, it is likely that community-associated carbapenem-resistant ST131 *E coli* will become a major threat in the near future.

PREVENTION

Prevention of further spread of MDR bacteria in the community is one of the most urgent public health challenges. Unfortunately, national or even regional data on antibiotic susceptibilities are often limited. In addition, when these data are available in some form, the accompanying epidemiologic metadata are usually too restricted to determine which isolates are truly community-associated. Furthermore, clinical infections are generally the tip of the proverbial iceberg and once a signal is generated that is sufficient in amplitude to get the attention of policy-makers, subclinical spread has already occurred.

Any successful prevention strategy has to consist of a multipronged approach and involve all stakeholders. In addition to human clinical antimicrobial stewardship, antibiotics must be removed from the food chain. Furthermore, the amount of xenobiotics, such as quaternary ammonium compounds, that reach the environment must be limited.[77] Another challenging step in limiting exposure of bacteria to antibiotics is the treatment of contaminated wastewater, such as that generated by pharmaceutical factories and medical facilities. For instance, a study evaluated samples collected from a wastewater treatment plant in India that received water from 90 regional bulk drug manufacturers containing, among other compounds, higher concentrations of ciprofloxacin than are generally found in the blood of patients who are being treated with this agent. Bacteria recovered from this water were tested against 39 antibiotics. Approximately 30% of bacteria were resistant to 29 to 32 antibiotics tested, and another approximately 20% were resistant to 33 to 36 antibiotics.[78] The magnitude of this effect, combined with the knowledge that soil-dwelling bacteria pass on resistance genes to more clinically relevant bacteria, illustrates the importance of limiting this contamination.[79]

Antimicrobial stewardship is developing rapidly as a hospital specialty. Stewardship teams often combine strengths from infectious disease medical specialists and doctors of pharmacy to evaluate the appropriateness of choice and duration of antibiotic strategies.[80] However, most antibiotics are prescribed in ambulatory care and more attention is needed in this realm to really impact overall community antibiotic exposure.[81] This not only requires a paradigm shift in the behavior of prescribers, but also a cultural shift in the public on the risks and benefits of antibiotics. Rapid diagnostic testing to identify MDR bacteria more quickly and thus limit the empiric use of unnecessarily broad antibiotics is of great significance. Also, rapid testing to diagnose alternative, nonbacterial etiologies is important.

An important question is whether any interventions can address the issue of chronic colonization with MDR bacteria. Obviously, decolonizing these patients would decrease the risk of transmission. Also, the burden on the individual patient of this condition should not be underestimated. In many health care systems, patients with MRSA or CRE are "labeled" as carriers for life, resulting in the institution of isolation precautions whenever they are admitted to the hospital. This has multiple adverse effects and leads to decreased patient satisfaction.[82] For these reasons, decolonization is a theoretically attractive option. However, most decolonizing strategies involve the use of antibiotics. For MRSA decolonization, most strategies involve some combination of intranasal mupirocin with topical chlorhexidine.[83] This approach has been shown to be effective in decreasing infections after surgery.[84] However, the effect is generally short-lived and recurrence of colonization is generally the rule. For enteric bacteria, no good options are currently available. Various selective gut decontamination strategies have been described, but none have shown true promise. In addition, with growing knowledge of the role of the gut microbiome in the defense against MDR bacteria, it seems counterintuitive to give even more antibiotics. Modulating the gut microbiome either through probiotics or through fecal microbiota transplantation is a promising, but as of yet experimental method of decolonizing patients.

SUMMARY

Wide variability is observed in community spread of common nosocomial MDR pathogens. This variability is likely secondary to several factors that include the natural habitats of the bacteria, and the competition present in those niches. In addition, certain strains of bacteria seem to be much more able to maintain their MDR phenotype and spread throughout the community. This is most likely secondary to additional genetic content that compensates for the relative fitness cost of the expression of genes associated with antibacterial resistance. Community spread of MDR bacteria is an important public health threat that should be approached urgently and proactively.

REFERENCES

1. Spellberg B, Blaser M, Guidos RJ, et al. Combating antimicrobial resistance: policy recommendations to save lives. Clin Infect Dis 2011;52(Suppl 5):S397–428.
2. Vardakas KZ, Rafailidis PI, Konstantelias AA, et al. Predictors of mortality in patients with infections due to multi-drug resistant gram negative bacteria: the study, the patient, the bug or the drug? J Infect 2013;66:401–14.
3. Bodi M, Ardanuy C, Rello J. Impact of gram-positive resistance on outcome of nosocomial pneumonia. Crit Care Med 2001;29:N82–6.

4. Perez F, van Duin D. Carbapenem-resistant Enterobacteriaceae: a menace to our most vulnerable patients. Cleve Clin J Med 2013;80:225–33.
5. Ena J, Dick RW, Jones RN, et al. The epidemiology of intravenous vancomycin usage in a university hospital. A 10-year study. JAMA 1993;269:598–602.
6. Morin CA, Hadler JL. Population-based incidence and characteristics of community-onset *Staphylococcus aureus* infections with bacteremia in 4 metropolitan Connecticut areas, 1998. J Infect Dis 2001;184:1029–34.
7. Friedman ND, Kaye KS, Stout JE, et al. Health care–associated bloodstream infections in adults: a reason to change the accepted definition of community-acquired infections. Ann Intern Med 2002;137:791–7.
8. American Thoracic Society and Infectious Diseases Society of America. Guidelines for the management of adults with hospital-acquired, ventilator-associated, and healthcare-associated pneumonia. Am J Respir Crit Care Med 2005;171:388–416.
9. Safdar N, Maki DG. The commonality of risk factors for nosocomial colonization and infection with antimicrobial-resistant *Staphylococcus aureus*, enterococcus, gram-negative bacilli, *Clostridium difficile*, and *Candida*. Ann Intern Med 2002;136:834–44.
10. Van Duin D, Cober E, Richter S, et al. Tigecycline therapy for carbapenem-resistant *Klebsiella pneumoniae* (CRKP) bacteriuria leads to tigecycline resistance. Clin Microbiol Infect 2014;20(12):O1117–20.
11. Kaye KS, Harris AD, Samore M, et al. The case-case-control study design: addressing the limitations of risk factor studies for antimicrobial resistance. Infect Control Hosp Epidemiol 2005;26:346–51.
12. Harris AD, Carmeli Y, Samore MH, et al. Impact of severity of illness bias and control group misclassification bias in case-control studies of antimicrobial-resistant organisms. Infect Control Hosp Epidemiol 2005;26:342–5.
13. McKinnell JA, Kunz DF, Chamot E, et al. Association between vancomycin-resistant enterococci bacteremia and ceftriaxone usage. Infect Control Hosp Epidemiol 2012;33:718–24.
14. Costerton JW, Stewart PS, Greenberg EP. Bacterial biofilms: a common cause of persistent infections. Science 1999;284:1318–22.
15. Ruimy R, Angebault C, Djossou F, et al. Are host genetics the predominant determinant of persistent nasal *Staphylococcus aureus* carriage in humans? J Infect Dis 2010;202:924–34.
16. DeLeo FR, Otto M, Kreiswirth BN, et al. Community-associated meticillin-resistant *Staphylococcus aureus*. Lancet 2010;375:1557–68.
17. Witte W. Community-acquired methicillin-resistant *Staphylococcus aureus*: what do we need to know? Clin Microbiol Infect 2009;15(Suppl 7):17–25.
18. Saravolatz LD, Pohlod DJ, Arking LM. Community-acquired methicillin-resistant *Staphylococcus aureus* infections: a new source for nosocomial outbreaks. Ann Intern Med 1982;97:325–9.
19. Thurlow LR, Joshi GS, Richardson AR. Virulence strategies of the dominant USA300 lineage of community-associated methicillin-resistant *Staphylococcus aureus* (CA-MRSA). FEMS Immunol Med Microbiol 2012;65:5–22.
20. Alam MT, Read TD, Petit RA 3rd, et al. Transmission and microevolution of USA300 MRSA in U.S. households: evidence from whole-genome sequencing. MBio 2015;6:e00054.
21. Graveland H, Duim B, van Duijkeren E, et al. Livestock-associated methicillin-resistant *Staphylococcus aureus* in animals and humans. Int J Med Microbiol 2011;301:630–4.

22. Murray BE. Vancomycin-resistant enterococcal infections. N Engl J Med 2000; 342:710–21.
23. Coque TM, Tomayko JF, Ricke SC, et al. Vancomycin-resistant enterococci from nosocomial, community, and animal sources in the United States. Antimicrob Agents Chemother 1996;40:2605–9.
24. Silverman J, Thal LA, Perri MB, et al. Epidemiologic evaluation of antimicrobial resistance in community-acquired enterococci. J Clin Microbiol 1998;36:830–2.
25. Bruinsma N, Stobberingh E, de Smet P, et al. Antibiotic use and the prevalence of antibiotic resistance in bacteria from healthy volunteers in the Dutch community. Infection 2003;31:9–14.
26. Bates J. Epidemiology of vancomycin-resistant enterococci in the community and the relevance of farm animals to human infection. J Hosp Infect 1997;37:89–101.
27. Klare I, Badstubner D, Konstabel C, et al. Decreased incidence of VanA-type vancomycin-resistant enterococci isolated from poultry meat and from fecal samples of humans in the community after discontinuation of avoparcin usage in animal husbandry. Microb Drug Resist 1999;5:45–52.
28. D'Agata EM, Jirjis J, Gouldin C, et al. Community dissemination of vancomycin-resistant *Enterococcus faecium*. Am J Infect Control 2001;29:316–20.
29. Poole TL, Hume ME, Campbell LD, et al. Vancomycin-resistant *Enterococcus faecium* strains isolated from community wastewater from a semiclosed agri-food system in Texas. Antimicrob Agents Chemother 2005;49:4382–5.
30. Omotola AM, Li Y, Martin ET, et al. Risk factors for and epidemiology of community-onset vancomycin-resistant *Enterococcus faecalis* in southeast Michigan. Am J Infect Control 2013;41:1244–8.
31. Wolfe CM, Cohen B, Larson E. Prevalence and risk factors for antibiotic-resistant community-associated bloodstream infections. J Infect Public Health 2014;7:224–32.
32. Foucault ML, Depardieu F, Courvalin P, et al. Inducible expression eliminates the fitness cost of vancomycin resistance in enterococci. Proc Natl Acad Sci U S A 2010;107:16964–9.
33. Johnsen PJ, Townsend JP, Bohn T, et al. Retrospective evidence for a biological cost of vancomycin resistance determinants in the absence of glycopeptide selective pressures. J Antimicrob Chemother 2011;66:608–10.
34. Gilmore MS, Rauch M, Ramsey MM, et al. Pheromone killing of multidrug-resistant *Enterococcus faecalis* V583 by native commensal strains. Proc Natl Acad Sci U S A 2015;112:7273–8.
35. Munoz-Price LS, Weinstein RA. Acinetobacter infection. N Engl J Med 2008;358: 1271–81.
36. Falagas ME, Karveli EA, Kelesidis I, et al. Community-acquired *Acinetobacter* infections. Eur J Clin Microbiol Infect Dis 2007;26:857–68.
37. Eveillard M, Kempf M, Belmonte O, et al. Reservoirs of *Acinetobacter baumannii* outside the hospital and potential involvement in emerging human community-acquired infections. Int J Infect Dis 2013;17:e802–5.
38. Poirel L, Nordmann P. Carbapenem resistance in *Acinetobacter baumannii*: mechanisms and epidemiology. Clin Microbiol Infect 2006;12:826–36.
39. Sengstock DM, Thyagarajan R, Apalara J, et al. Multidrug-resistant *Acinetobacter baumannii*: an emerging pathogen among older adults in community hospitals and nursing homes. Clin Infect Dis 2010;50:1611–6.
40. Queenan AM, Pillar CM, Deane J, et al. Multidrug resistance among *Acinetobacter* spp. in the USA and activity profile of key agents: results from CAPITAL Surveillance 2010. Diagn Microbiol Infect Dis 2012;73:267–70.

41. Zeana C, Larson E, Sahni J, et al. The epidemiology of multidrug-resistant *Acinetobacter baumannii*: does the community represent a reservoir? Infect Control Hosp Epidemiol 2003;24:275–9.
42. Davis JS, McMillan M, Swaminathan A, et al. A 16-year prospective study of community-onset bacteremic *Acinetobacter* pneumonia: low mortality with appropriate initial empirical antibiotic protocols. Chest 2014;146:1038–45.
43. Peng C, Zong Z, Fan H. *Acinetobacter baumannii* isolates associated with community-acquired pneumonia in West China. Clin Microbiol Infect 2012;18: E491–3.
44. Paterson DL. The epidemiological profile of infections with multidrug-resistant *Pseudomonas aeruginosa* and *Acinetobacter* species. Clin Infect Dis 2006; 43(Suppl 2):S43–8.
45. Hassett DJ, Sutton MD, Schurr MJ, et al. *Pseudomonas aeruginosa* hypoxic or anaerobic biofilm infections within cystic fibrosis airways. Trends Microbiol 2009;17:130–8.
46. O'Malley CA. Infection control in cystic fibrosis: cohorting, cross-contamination, and the respiratory therapist. Respir Care 2009;54:641–57.
47. Rodriguez-Bano J, Lopez-Prieto MD, Portillo MM, et al. Epidemiology and clinical features of community-acquired, healthcare-associated and nosocomial bloodstream infections in tertiary-care and community hospitals. Clin Microbiol Infect 2010;16:1408–13.
48. Anderson DJ, Moehring RW, Sloane R, et al. Bloodstream infections in community hospitals in the 21st century: a multicenter cohort study. PLoS One 2014;9: e91713.
49. Hattemer A, Hauser A, Diaz M, et al. Bacterial and clinical characteristics of health care- and community-acquired bloodstream infections due to *Pseudomonas aeruginosa*. Antimicrob Agents Chemother 2013;57:3969–75.
50. Ulug M, Gedik E, Girgin S, et al. Pyogenic liver abscess caused by community-acquired multidrug resistance *Pseudomonas aeruginosa*. Braz J Infect Dis 2010; 14:218.
51. Pitout JD. Enterobacteriaceae that produce extended-spectrum beta-lactamases and AmpC beta-lactamases in the community: the tip of the iceberg? Curr Pharm Des 2013;19:257–63.
52. Doi Y, Park YS, Rivera JI, et al. Community-associated extended-spectrum beta-lactamase-producing *Escherichia coli* infection in the United States. Clin Infect Dis 2013;56:641–8.
53. Petty NK, Ben Zakour NL, Stanton-Cook M, et al. Global dissemination of a multidrug resistant *Escherichia coli* clone. Proc Natl Acad Sci U S A 2014;111:5694–9.
54. Banerjee R, Strahilevitz J, Johnson JR, et al. Predictors and molecular epidemiology of community-onset extended-spectrum beta-lactamase-producing *Escherichia coli* infection in a Midwestern community. Infect Control Hosp Epidemiol 2013;34:947–53.
55. Leistner R, Meyer E, Gastmeier P, et al. Risk factors associated with the community-acquired colonization of extended-spectrum beta-lactamase (ESBL) positive *Escherichia Coli*. An exploratory case-control study. PLoS One 2013;8: e74323.
56. Gopal Rao G, Batura D, Batura N, et al. Key demographic characteristics of patients with bacteriuria due to extended spectrum beta-lactamase (ESBL)-producing Enterobacteriaceae in a multiethnic community, in North West London. Infect Dis (Lond) 2015;47(10):719–24.

57. Rogers BA, Ingram PR, Runnegar N, et al. Community-onset *Escherichia coli* infection resistant to expanded-spectrum cephalosporins in low-prevalence countries. Antimicrob Agents Chemother 2014;58:2126–34.
58. Ko WC, Paterson DL, Sagnimeni AJ, et al. Community-acquired *Klebsiella pneumoniae* bacteremia: global differences in clinical patterns. Emerg Infect Dis 2002; 8:160–6.
59. Li W, Sun G, Yu Y, et al. Increasing occurrence of antimicrobial-resistant hypervirulent (hypermucoviscous) *Klebsiella pneumoniae* isolates in China. Clin Infect Dis 2014;58:225–32.
60. Tamma PD, Han JH, Rock C, et al. Carbapenem therapy is associated with improved survival compared with piperacillin-tazobactam for patients with extended-spectrum beta-lactamase bacteremia. Clin Infect Dis 2015;60: 1319–25.
61. Rodriguez-Bano J, Navarro MD, Retamar P, et al, Extended-Spectrum Beta-Lactamases–Red Española de Investigación en Patología Infecciosa/Grupo de Estudio de Infección Hospitalaria Group. β-Lactam/β-lactam inhibitor combinations for the treatment of bacteremia due to extended-spectrum β-lactamase-producing *Escherichia coli*: a post hoc analysis of prospective cohorts. Clin Infect Dis 2012;54:167–74.
62. Centers for Disease Control and Prevention. Antibiotic resistance threats in the United States, 2013. 2013. Available at: http://www.cdc.gov/drugresistance/threat-report-2013/. Accessed July 10, 2015.
63. Yigit H, Queenan AM, Anderson GJ, et al. Novel carbapenem-hydrolyzing beta-lactamase, KPC-1, from a carbapenem-resistant strain of *Klebsiella pneumoniae*. Antimicrob Agents Chemother 2001;45:1151–61.
64. Nordmann P, Cuzon G, Naas T. The real threat of *Klebsiella pneumoniae* carbapenemase-producing bacteria. Lancet Infect Dis 2009;9:228–36.
65. Schwaber MJ, Carmeli Y. Carbapenem-resistant Enterobacteriaceae: a potential threat. JAMA 2008;300:2911–3.
66. Hirsch EB, Tam VH. Detection and treatment options for *Klebsiella pneumoniae* carbapenemases (KPCs): an emerging cause of multidrug-resistant infection. J Antimicrob Chemother 2010;65(6):1119–25.
67. Neuner EA, Yeh JY, Hall GS, et al. Treatment and outcomes in carbapenem-resistant *Klebsiella pneumoniae* bloodstream infections. Diagn Microbiol Infect Dis 2011;69:357–62.
68. van Duin D, Kaye KS, Neuner EA, et al. Carbapenem-resistant Enterobacteriaceae: a review of treatment and outcomes. Diagn Microbiol Infect Dis 2013;75: 115–20.
69. Epstein L, Hunter JC, Arwady MA, et al. New Delhi metallo-beta-lactamase-producing carbapenem-resistant *Escherichia coli* associated with exposure to duodenoscopes. JAMA 2014;312:1447–55.
70. Khajuria A, Praharaj AK, Kumar M, et al. Emergence of *Escherichia coli*, co-producing NDM-1 and OXA-48 carbapenemases, in urinary isolates, at a tertiary care centre at Central India. J Clin Diagn Res 2014;8:DC01–4.
71. Bhargava A, Hayakawa K, Silverman E, et al. Risk factors for colonization due to carbapenem-resistant Enterobacteriaceae among patients exposed to long-term acute care and acute care facilities. Infect Control Hosp Epidemiol 2014;35: 398–405.
72. Walsh TR, Weeks J, Livermore DM, et al. Dissemination of NDM-1 positive bacteria in the New Delhi environment and its implications for human health: an environmental point prevalence study. Lancet Infect Dis 2011;11:355–62.

73. Wang Y, Wu C, Zhang Q, et al. Identification of New Delhi metallo-beta-lactamase 1 in *Acinetobacter lwoffii* of food animal origin. PLoS One 2012;7:e37152.
74. Pannaraj PS, Bard JD, Cerini C, et al. Pediatric carbapenem-resistant Enterobacteriaceae in Los Angeles, California, a high-prevalence region in the United States. Pediatr Infect Dis J 2015;34:11–6.
75. Hussain A, Ranjan A, Nandanwar N, et al. Genotypic and phenotypic profiles of *Escherichia coli* isolates belonging to clinical sequence type 131 (ST131), clinical non-ST131, and fecal non-ST131 lineages from India. Antimicrob Agents Chemother 2014;58:7240–9.
76. Peirano G, Schreckenberger PC, Pitout JD. Characteristics of NDM-1-producing *Escherichia coli* isolates that belong to the successful and virulent clone ST131. Antimicrob Agents Chemother 2011;55:2986–8.
77. Hawkey PM, Jones AM. The changing epidemiology of resistance. J Antimicrob Chemother 2009;64(Suppl 1):i3–10.
78. Marathe NP, Regina VR, Walujkar SA, et al. A treatment plant receiving waste water from multiple bulk drug manufacturers is a reservoir for highly multi-drug resistant integron-bearing bacteria. PLoS One 2013;8:e77310.
79. Forsberg KJ, Reyes A, Wang B, et al. The shared antibiotic resistome of soil bacteria and human pathogens. Science 2012;337:1107–11.
80. Wagner B, Filice GA, Drekonja D, et al. Antimicrobial stewardship programs in inpatient hospital settings: a systematic review. Infect Control Hosp Epidemiol 2014;35:1209–28.
81. Gangat MA, Hsu JL. Antibiotic stewardship: a focus on ambulatory care. S D Med 2015;Spec No:44–8.
82. Vinski J, Bertin M, Sun Z, et al. Impact of isolation on hospital consumer assessment of healthcare providers and systems scores: is isolation isolating? Infect Control Hosp Epidemiol 2012;33:513–6.
83. Coates T, Bax R, Coates A. Nasal decolonization of *Staphylococcus aureus with* mupirocin: strengths, weaknesses and future prospects. J Antimicrob Chemother 2009;64:9–15.
84. Chen AF, Wessel CB, Rao N. *Staphylococcus aureus* screening and decolonization in orthopaedic surgery and reduction of surgical site infections. Clin Orthop Relat Res 2013;471:2383–99.

Agents of Last Resort

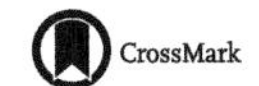

Polymyxin Resistance

Keith S. Kaye, MD, MPH[a,*], Jason M. Pogue, PharmD[b], Thien B. Tran[c], Roger L. Nation, PhD[c], Jian Li, PhD[c]

KEYWORDS

• Colistin • Polymyxin *B* • Polymyxins • Resistance • Gram-negative

KEY POINTS

- Polymyxin resistance is a major public health threat, as the polymyxins represent "last-line" therapeutics for Gram-negative pathogens resistant to essentially all other antibiotics.
- Improved understanding of mechanisms of, and risk factors for, polymyxin resistance, as well as infection prevention and stewardship strategies, together with optimization of dosing of polymyxins including in combination regimens, can help to limit the emergence and dissemination of polymyxin resistance.

INTRODUCTION

The polymyxins, colistin (also known as polymyxin E) and polymyxin B, have a unique and interesting history. Originally introduced in the 1950s for the treatment of infections due to Gram-negative organisms, the polymyxins fell out of favor by the mid-1970s because of high rates of nephrotoxicity (approaching 50%) and neurotoxicity and the advent of less toxic alternatives, notably the antipseudomonal aminoglycosides. By the mid-1990s the polymyxins were reintroduced into clinical practice, not because of an enhanced safety profile, but rather due to the development of extensively drug-resistant (XDR) Gram-negative bacilli resistant to all other treatment options.[1,2] The polymyxins now serve a critical role in the antimicrobial armamentarium, as they are one of few, and sometimes the only, antimicrobial agent retaining activity against carbapenem-resistant *Pseudomonas aeruginosa*, *Acinetobacter baumannii*, and Enterobacteriaceae (CRE), organisms that frequently cause life-threatening infections in the most vulnerable of patient populations. These pathogens have been recognized by the Centers for Disease Control and Prevention as serious or

[a] Division of Infectious Diseases, Department of Medicine, Detroit Medical Center, Wayne State University, 3990 John R, Detroit, MI 48201, USA; [b] Department of Pharmacy Services, Sinai-Grace Hospital, Detroit Medical Center, Wayne State University School of Medicine, Detroit, MI, USA; [c] Drug Delivery, Disposition and Dynamics, Monash Institute of Pharmaceutical Sciences, Monash University, Melbourne, Australia
* Corresponding author.
E-mail address: kkaye@dmc.org

Infect Dis Clin N Am 30 (2016) 391–414
http://dx.doi.org/10.1016/j.idc.2016.02.005
id.theclinics.com
0891-5520/16/$ – see front matter

urgent threats to human health and mortality rates in invasive infections due to these pathogens can exceed 50%.[2,3] The relatively dry antimicrobial pipeline for the treatment of infections caused by these organisms magnifies the importance of the polymyxins. Given the critical role of the polymyxins in the care of hospitalized patients, an understanding of both the epidemiology of polymyxin resistance as well as strategies to prevent resistance are paramount. Therefore, this article introduces similarities and differences between the two clinically available polymyxins, discusses the mechanism of action and resistance to these agents, describes the clinical epidemiology of polymyxin-resistant organisms, and finally suggests strategies to minimize the development and spread of polymyxin resistance.

Colistin (also known as polymyxin E) and polymyxin B are nearly structurally identical, differing by only one amino acid at position 6 (**Fig. 1**). They are considered to be very similar microbiologically and cross-resistance exists. Both polymyxins are products of fermentation and therefore are multicomponent mixtures. Colistin and polymyxin B have two major components (colistin A and B; polymyxin B1 and B2) that slightly differ at the site of the *N*-terminal fatty acyl tail.[4] The polymyxins are

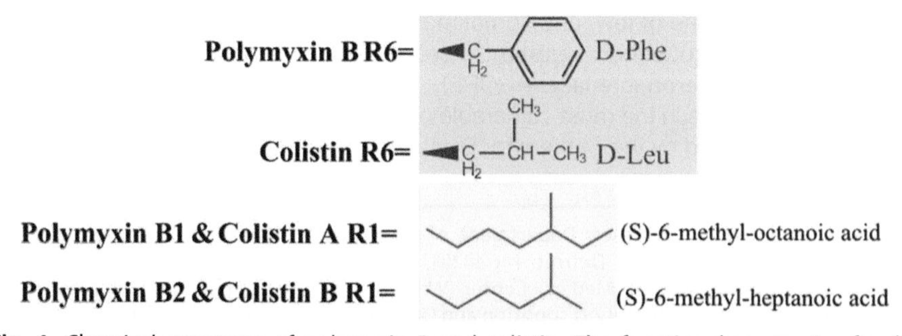

Fig. 1. Chemical structures of polymyxin B and colistin. The functional segments of polymyxins are colored as follows: yellow, fatty acyl chain; green, linear tripeptide segment; red, the polar residues of the heptapeptide; blue, the hydrophobic motif within the heptapeptide ring. (*Reprinted* with permission from Velkov T, Thompson PE, Nation RL, et al. Structure–activity relationships of polymyxin antibiotics. J Med Chem 2010;53(5):1898. Copyright © 2010 American Chemical Society.)

amphipathic molecules, consisting of both hydrophilic and hydrophobic regions (see **Fig. 1**) and these properties are essential to their antimicrobial activity (described later in this article). Although polymyxin B is administered directly as its sulfate salt, colistin is administered in the form of its inactive prodrug colistimethate sodium (CMS, also known as colistin methanesulfonate).[5] CMS is synthesized by sulfomethylation of active colistin, and although CMS is considered to exist in its fully penta-methanesulfonated form, recent analyses have shown that the material reconstituted for use in patients likely exists as a combination of up to 32 fully or partially methanesulfonated derivatives.[6] As is described in detail later in this article, the administration of colistin as an inactive prodrug has a significant impact on the pharmacokinetics of colistin in patients and is an important differentiator between the two polymyxins. Both polymyxins are associated with nephrotoxicity rates in the 30% to 50% range,[1] and all strategies for optimal use need to be taken in the context of the dose, and subsequent concentration-dependent toxicity that may be seen.

MECHANISM OF ACTION

The precise mechanism of antibacterial activity of polymyxins is not completely understood; however, the general current view is that polymyxins kill bacteria by disrupting the bacterial outer and inner membranes through the "self-promoted uptake" pathway.[7] The initial binding target of polymyxins is the lipopolysaccharides (LPS) in the outer membrane of Gram-negative bacteria, with both electrostatic and hydrophobic interactions being important.[4] Electrostatic interaction via the positively charged diaminobutyric acid (Dab) residues of the polymyxin (see **Fig. 1**) and the negatively charged phosphate groups on the lipid A moiety of LPS leads to displacement of divalent cations (Mg^{2+} and Ca^{2+}) that bridge the lipid A phosphoesters, thereby destabilizing the outer membrane.[8] This event allows the polymyxin to insert its hydrophobic regions (fatty acyl tail and amino acids at positions 6 and 7) into the bacterial outer membrane to interact with the fatty acyl chains of lipid A; this hydrophobic interaction causes further outer membrane disruption that promotes the uptake of the polymyxin.[7,9] It has been proposed that after transiting the outer membrane, polymyxins mediate the fusion of the inner leaflet of the outer membrane with the outer leaflet of the cytoplasmic membrane, which induces phospholipid exchange and causes osmotic imbalance that leads to cell death.[10] The amphipathic property of polymyxins (ie, presence of both cationic and hydrophobic regions) is necessary for the killing of Gram-negative bacteria. Polymyxin B nonapeptide (ie, polymyxin B lacking the fatty acyl tail and the Dab residue at position 1) and colistimethate (in which the Dab residues are masked by negatively charged methanesulfonate moieties) do not possess antibacterial activity.[5,11] In addition to their membrane-disrupting effect in Gram-negative bacteria, binding of polymyxins to lipid A also neutralizes the toxicity of endotoxins.[12,13]

A secondary antibacterial mechanism of polymyxins is thought to be via inhibition of the nicotinamide adenine dinucleotide oxidase enzyme family. This inhibitory activity has been observed in *Escherichia coli*, *Klebsiella pneumoniae*, *A baumannii*,[14] and *Mycobacterium smegmatis.*[15]

MECHANISMS OF RESISTANCE

As reviewed previously, the interaction of polymyxins with LPS is essential for their antimicrobial activity. This explains why polymyxin B and colistin are not active against Gram-positive bacteria. In Gram-negative bacteria, which are intrinsically resistant to polymyxins, this interaction is diminished due to LPS that has lower binding affinity for polymyxins. In these LPS molecules, lipid A usually contains modified phosphate groups, thereby decreasing their overall net negative charge.[16–18] Likewise, in bacteria that are susceptible to polymyxins, resistance is usually acquired through LPS modifications.[19]

Arguably, the modification of LPS that most commonly leads to polymyxin resistance in *P aeruginosa* involves the addition of 4-amino-4-deoxy-L-arabinose (L-Ara4N) to the phosphate groups in lipid A.[19] This modification is usually controlled by the *arn* (*pmr*) operon, which is regulated by the PmrA/PmrB and PhoP/PhoQ 2-component systems (TCSs).[20] These systems can also be activated by changes in the environment (eg, high Fe^{3+} concentration, low Mg^{2+} or Ca^{2+} concentrations, and low pH) and the lipid A modification can lead to decreased bridging of adjacent lipid A molecules via divalent cations.[21–23] PmrB and PhoQ are cytoplasmic membrane-bound sensor kinases that phosphorylate their respective regulator proteins PmrA and PhoP on activation. Once phosphorylated, PmrA and PhoP promote the upregulation of the *arn* operon leading to the addition of L-Ara4N to the phosphate groups of lipid A.[24] Resistance to polymyxins can develop when mutations occur in the PmrA/PmrB and PhoP/PhoQ systems.[25] Addition of phosphoethanolamine (PEtN) to lipid A, which also decreases the negative charge has also been identified in the modification of LPS of polymyxin-resistant *P aeruginosa*. This modification is controlled by the ColR/ColS TCS, which is upregulated in the presence of excess extracellular Zn^{2+}.[26]

In *A baumannii*, where L-Ara4N biosynthesis and attachment genes are generally lacking, polymyxin resistance is often achieved from the modification of LPS by the addition of PEtN to lipid A.[27] This modification can be caused by mutations in *pmrA* and/or *pmrB* that induce the autoregulation of the promoter region of the *pmrCAB* operon.[25] Recent findings from polymyxin-resistant *A baumannii* clinical isolates indicate that the modification of LPS with galactosamine (GalN) also contributes to polymyxin resistance, although the precise regulatory pathway is not yet understood.[28] Apart from LPS modifications, *A baumannii* also possesses a unique polymyxin resistance mechanism that involves the complete loss of LPS.[29] This phenotype can be caused by mutations in lipid A biosynthesis genes. In these polymyxin-resistant *A baumannii* isolates, genes responsible for transport of phospholipids/lipoproteins and production of poly-β-1,6-*N*-acetylglucosamine are upregulated to compensate for the missing LPS in the outer leaflet of the outer membrane.[30]

In *K pneumoniae*, resistance to polymyxins may involve several different strategies. One of these involves the modification of lipid A by the addition of either L-Ara4N or PEtN.[25] These modifications are caused by mutations in *pmrA*, *pmrB*, or *phoQ* genes that upregulate the PhoP/PhoQ and PmrA/PmrB systems.[31–33] It has also been reported that the upregulation of the PhoP/PhoQ and PmrA/PmrB systems can be caused by deletion in the *mgrB* locus.[34] Another polymyxin resistance mechanism in *K pneumoniae* is overproduction of surface capsular polysaccharides (CPS). It is believed that the CPS may act as a barrier to limit the interaction of polymyxins with lipid A,[35] by "trapping" polymyxins.[36] It is also reported that the AcrAB-TolC efflux pump may play a role in polymyxin resistance in *K pneumoniae*.[37]

Phenotypically, resistance to polymyxins also can be developed from polymyxin-heteroresistant bacteria. The minimum inhibitory concentrations (MICs) of polymyxins in these bacteria are $\leq$2 mg/L; however, there is a subpopulation of bacterial cells that can survive in the presence of more than 2 mg/L polymyxins. This leads to the amplification of the resistant subpopulation in the presence of polymyxin alone and the eventual development of polymyxin resistance.[38] Recent studies indicate that polymyxin heteroresistance in *P aeruginosa* is infrequent[39]; however, it is very common in both multidrug-resistant *K pneumoniae*[40] and *A baumannii*.[38,41]

Laboratory studies have indicated that resistance to polymyxins may compromise the resistance to other classes of antibiotics.[42,43] In a study with *A baumannii* that compared the antibiograms of multi-drug resistant (MDR) colistin-susceptible clinical isolates with those of the respective laboratory-generated colistin-resistant paired strains,[42] the polymyxin-resistant strains were more susceptible to other antibiotics compared with their parent polymyxin-susceptible strains. These findings suggested that polymyxin combinations may be useful to prevent polymyxin resistance in MDR bacteria. However, the clinical relevance of this finding remains to be determined, as in clinical practice most polymyxin-resistant isolates are usually resistant to a broad range of other antibiotics.

Resistance to polymyxins may also come at a fitness cost. *A baumannii* isolates with polymyxin resistance usually grow at a much slower rate and are less capable of causing infection.[44,45] Studies that compared the fitness cost of lipid A modification and LPS loss in *A baumannii* isolates showed that reduction in biological fitness associated with LPS loss was greater than with PEtN addition.[44,46] Impaired virulence in *A baumannii* is also linked to reduced expression of metabolic proteins and of the OmpA porin.[47] Significant biological fitness cost due to polymyxin resistance has yet to be observed in *P aeruginosa* and *K pneumoniae*.

CLINICAL EPIDEMIOLOGY OF POLYMYXIN-RESISTANT GRAM-NEGATIVE BACILLI

As previously discussed, the primary clinical role for the polymyxins is for the treatment of infections due to carbapenem-resistant *A baumannii, P aeruginosa*, or CRE (most notably carbapenem-resistant *K pneumoniae*), as no other reliable treatment options are available. Fortunately, colistin has excellent in vitro activity in this setting, and most isolates are susceptible at the susceptibility breakpoint of 2 mg/L or lower concentration. However, there are regional variations in susceptibility rates and clinicians should be aware of local susceptibility data. Although it is not the focus of this article, it is important for the reader to be aware of a few important points. First, not all published analyses have used the same susceptibility breakpoint for colistin to define resistance. Second, the current susceptibility breakpoints might not be ideal from a pharmacokinetic/pharmacodynamic standpoint. Third, there are unique complexities that exist with regards to the determination of the colistin MIC via conventional methods.[48] Because of these issues, Clinical and Laboratory Standards Institute (CLSI) and The European Committee on Antimicrobial Susceptibility Testing (EUCAST) have formed a joint Working Group to examine MIC testing methods and breakpoints for the polymyxins, and the work of that group is being informed by data from recent preclinical and clinical pharmacokinetic/pharmacodynamic studies.[49] For the purposes of this section, a susceptibility breakpoint of 2 mg/L is used. Polymyxin B susceptibility is not routinely performed and colistin is used as a categorical surrogate for susceptibility.

Published data regarding rates of colistin-resistant *P aeruginosa* are scarce; however, most published rates are between 0% and 4%.[50,51] Nonetheless, this finding is not universal and there are notable variations regionally. A recent analysis from India assessing *P aeruginosa* isolates found that 8 (8%) of 95 were resistant to colistin.[52] Furthermore, in 2002 Schulin[53] published susceptibility data to colistin from 385 *P aeruginosa* isolates in patients with cystic fibrosis from Germany and found colistin resistance (MIC >2 mg/L) in 35 (15%) of 229 nonmucoid strains and 5 (3%) of 156 mucoid strains, for an overall resistance rate of 10.4%.

Despite the widespread nature of carbapenem resistance in A baumannii and the increasingly common use of polymyxins as one of the only therapeutic options, widespread polymyxin resistance in this organism has not been reported. Data from the Sentry Antimicrobial Surveillance database, which include isolates from the United

States, Europe, Latin America, and the Asia-Pacific region, have shown resistance between 0.9% and 3.3% from 2001 to 2011.[54–56] Although some individual reports have shown higher numbers, rarely do rates exceed 5%,[57] and when they do, there are notable limitations. Many studies reporting high rates of colistin resistance include isolates that are carbapenem susceptible and/or are not all-inclusive studies of every *Acinetobacter* isolate in the institution. For example, a frequently cited report that showed colistin resistance to be 16.7% is limited because it included only 18 isolates, 3 of which were colistin resistant.[58] Additionally, the vast majority (17/18) were actually susceptible to carbapenems. Similarly, although Ko and colleagues[59] reported an extremely high rate of colistin resistance of 31% in 214 *A baumannii* isolates in Korea, of the 83 polymyxin-resistant strains, only 5 were resistant to imipenem. Although Arroyo and colleagues[60] reported a rate of colistin resistance of 19.1% in Spain (21/115 isolates), it is unclear how these isolates were selected and whether or not they represented all isolates in their institution. Similarly, in another report published by the same group in Spain that described a 41% rate of colistin resistance, the analysis did not consist of all *Acinetobacter* isolates from their institution and was specifically chosen to assess the in vitro activities of various other antimicrobials against both multidrug and pan-drug–resistant isolates.[61] Although these studies might overstate the incidence of colistin resistance in carbapenem-resistant *A baumannii*, they clearly demonstrate that colistin-resistant *A baumannii* exists in various geographic locales and some reports have shown the incidence to be increasing, albeit still at low overall numbers.[62] The most alarming epidemiologic trend with regard to carbapenem-resistant Gram-negative bacilli has been the rise and worldwide spread of CRE, primarily, but not exclusively, driven by the *K pneumoniae* carbapenemase (KPC) enzyme.[63] Although KPC is most commonly produced in *K pneumoniae*, it can be produced by other Enterobacteriaceae as well as nonfermenting organisms. Rates of KPC production among clinical isolates of *K pneumoniae* vary worldwide, but staggering numbers have been reported in some regions. For example, in Italy, surveillance data pertaining to *K pneumoniae* bloodstream isolates demonstrated a rise in carbapenem resistance from 1% to 2% in 2006 to 2009, to 30% in 2011.[63] Furthermore, a recent publication from Italy showed a continual climb in rates of carbapenem resistance in *K pneumoniae* bloodstream infections from a rate of 3% in 2009 to 42% in 2011 and to 66% in 2013.[64] Similar rates have been reported in neighboring Greece.[63]

Unfortunately, but perhaps unsurprisingly, immediately following the rise of KPCs worldwide, case reports and series describing clusters and outbreaks of colistin-resistant KPC-producers began to appear in the literature.[65] Additionally, rates of colistin resistance in *Klebsiella* spp from surveillance studies have varied greatly and interpretation of these studies is complicated because many of them do not focus solely on KPC-producing isolates.[65] However, the rates of colistin resistance in *K pneumoniae*, unlike what has been described with other carbapenem-resistant organisms, appear to be increasing at a much higher rate. Surveillance data examining rates of colistin resistance among carbapenem-resistant as well as carbapenem-susceptible *Klebsiella* isolates generally place the rate at ≤7%.[65] However, data from Greece from the mid to late 2000s place the rate at 10.5% to 20.0%.[66,67] Additionally, 2 reports, 1 from Austria, and 1 from the Netherlands, showed rates of approximately 50% of colistin resistance in extended-spectrum β-lactamase (ESBL)-producing *Klebsiella*, although these studies were done in the setting of oral colistin administration for selective gut decontamination.[68,69] Most concerning, however, have been reports of extremely high rates of colistin resistance from regions in which KPC-producers have become endemic. Rates of colistin resistance in carbapenemase-producing *Klebsiella* have ranged from 14% to 25% in

Greece.[70–74] In Italy, reported rates have been even higher. Multiple publications have reported colistin resistance exceeding 30% in carbapenem-resistant *K pneumoniae*.[65] One recent study of *Klebsiella* resistance in bloodstream infections in an Italian hospital reported 66% of strains to be carbapenem resistant, and 57% to 65% of those carbapenem-resistant *K pneumoniae* strains were also resistant to colistin.[64] To put these resistant rates in clinical perspective, if a patient was to develop a *Klebsiella* spp bloodstream infection, there would be approximately a 43% chance that it would be both colistin-resistant and carbapenem-resistant. Similarly, data examining 191 carbapenemase-producing Enterobacteriaceae in 21 hospitals in Italy (187 *K pneumoniae*, 4 *E coli*) from November 2013 to April 2014 reported 76 (43%) to also be colistin-resistant.[75]

Although most available data assessing rates of colistin resistance in Gram-negative bacilli represent nonclinical surveillance data, there are a few reports assessing risk factors for isolation of colistin-resistant Gram-negative bacilli. Although polymyxin exposure is frequently identified as a risk factor, this finding is not universal. Qureshi and colleagues[76] described the characteristics of 20 patients with colistin-resistant *A baumannii* isolated from their institution over a 7-year period. Nineteen (95%) of 20 patients had prior genetically related colistin-susceptible isolates and significant prior intravenous and inhaled colistin exposure was present in all but 1 of the 20 patients. Similarly, Papadimitriou-Olivgeris and colleagues[74] described their experience in 254 patients who were not colonized with colistin-resistant KPC-producing isolates on admission to the intensive care unit (ICU). Of the patients, 62 (24.4%) became colonized with colistin-resistant KPC-producing (CRKPC) organisms while in the ICU, with the primary risk factor for isolation being colistin exposure (odds ratio 13.5, 95% confidence interval 6.1–30.2). Other risk factors for isolation of colistin-resistant KPC producers were corticosteroid use and number of CRKPC-positive patients treated in nearby beds per day, suggesting the importance of horizontal transmission as well. Interestingly, Meletis and colleagues[77] evaluated colistin use over time and its association with colistin-resistant Gram-negative bacilli. Colistin use increased significantly over the period of the study from 7 defined daily doses (DDD) per 1000 patient days in 2007 to 27 DDD per 1000 patient days in 2013 and a likewise significant increase in colistin-resistant KPC was seen from 0% in 2007 to 2010, to 16% in 2010 to 2013. This increase was most notable among ICU isolates, where CRKPC was reported in 20 (22%) of 92 isolates. What is most interesting is that although there was a dramatic increase in colistin-resistant KPC over the study period, there was no parallel increase in colistin resistance in carbapenem-resistant *A baumannii* or *P aeruginosa*. Rates of colistin-resistant carbapenem-resistant *A baumannii* were 0% over the entire study period, and rates of colistin resistance in *P aeruginosa* actually decreased from 5% in 2007 to 2010, to 2% in 2010 to 2013. This finding is consistent with the overall data presented in this section that colistin resistance in KPC producers seems to be developing at an alarming rate, whereas colistin resistance rates in the nonfermenters remain relatively low and stable.

These findings are interesting in light of a recent publication by Giani and colleagues[64] in which the investigators described their experience with an outbreak of 93 bloodstream infections with colistin-resistant KPC over a 4-year period, in an area in Italy where KPC is endemic (the investigators report that two-thirds of all *Klebsiella* were carbapenem resistant, and carbapenem resistance was largely mediated by KPC). Data on previous colistin exposure were available for 38 patients, 35 (92%) of whom did not receive colistin before isolation of their colistin-resistant pathogen. Of the 59 patients in whom genotyping was performed, the mgrB gene deletion was present in 50 (85%) of 59 isolates; and in a subset of 19 subjects for whom colistin data were available,

18 (95%) had not had prior colistin exposure. Although the outbreak was initially tied to increased colistin utilization at the institution, the continued spread in the absence of colistin exposure suggested clonal expansion of a single strain (ie, patient-to-patient spread) and also suggested that this particular mechanism may not have been associated with decreased strain fitness of survival. This finding is in line with another report that associates mgrB inactivation with a lack of fitness cost in *A baumannii*.[46] Taken together, these results suggest that colistin-resistant carbapenem-resistant *K pneumoniae* could become more widespread.

In summary, although rates of colistin resistance among carbapenem-resistant *A baumannii*, *P aeruginosa*, and *K pneumoniae* remain relatively low, there are trends emerging that increased polymyxin exposure in institutions for the treatment of these pathogens is leading to the predictable emergence of resistance. Additionally, particularly in *K pneumoniae*, there is mounting evidence that a stable form of resistance is emerging that might be seen in the absence of polymyxin exposure with clonal expansion throughout a given unit or hospital. These findings, when taken together, stress the critical need for optimal strategies for the use of polymyxins, as well as infection control and antimicrobial stewardship programs to preserve these critical, last-line agents. Therefore, the rest of this article focuses on such strategies.

STRATEGIES TO MINIMIZE POLYMYXIN RESISTANCE

As discussed previously, there are two polymyxins currently being used in the clinic: colistin and polymyxin B.[78] Colistin is more widely used and is administered parenterally in the form of an inactive prodrug, the sodium salt of colistin methanesulfonate (CMS, also known as colistimethate).[78] A parenteral formulation of polymyxin B (as its sulfate salt) is available in a number of countries, including the United States, but is not available in Europe, Australia, and several other countries.[9,79] Polymyxin B is administered directly in its active antibacterial form, whereas CMS requires conversion in vivo to generate the active entity, colistin. This difference in the form administered to patients has a major effect on the clinical pharmacologic profile of the 2 polymyxins, an understanding of which is critical to their optimal clinical use.[80]

Because of the lack of new antibiotics and potential for development of resistance with polymyxin monotherapy, it is important that both polymyxins are used optimally to maximize their efficacy and minimize resistance and nephrotoxicity. Unfortunately, as polymyxins were approved for clinical use before the introduction of the contemporary drug development and regulatory approval processes, the prescribing information of both polymyxin products has been limited and not supported by solid pharmacologic data. Fortunately, this situation has been changing over the past decade. Indeed, the polymyxins have been the first of the “old” antibiotics to be subjected to a “redevelopment” process, largely led by academic and clinical researchers. To optimize their dosage regimens, it is essential to understand their pharmacokinetics (PK), pharmacodynamics (PD), and toxicodynamics (TD), and the relationships between exposure and desired/undesired responses (ie, PK/PD and PK/TD).[81–84] There are a number of approaches to minimize resistance development to polymyxins, in particular optimizing their dosage regimens in patients using PK/PD/TD, employment of rational combinations, and limiting clinical use to patients with MDR/XDR Gram-negative infections.

OPTIMIZING DOSING REGIMENS

Currently, there are two different labeling systems in use for parenteral CMS.[78] In Europe, the international unit (IU) is used for CMS, whereas colistin base activity

(CBA) is used in North America, South America, and Southeast Asia. For more information on the conversion between the number of IU and milligrams of CBA, please refer to our reviews and a recent editorial.[78,85,86] One million IU is equivalent to approximately 30 mg of CBA. It is crucial that clinicians are aware of the labeling differences and proper conversions are achieved before implementing at the local level dosage regimens reported in journal articles.[85,86]

Over the past decade, significant preclinical and clinical pharmacologic data have been generated to inform clinicians on optimizing the use of colistin and polymyxin B in patients. The PK/PD index that best predicts the activity of colistin was recently identified as the ratio of the area under the plasma concentration versus time curve across 24 hours to the minimum inhibitory concentration (AUC/MIC). This was first described using an in vitro PK/PD study with colistin against *P aeruginosa*.[82] In vivo studies using murine thigh and lung infection models have confirmed this finding.[81] The data from the recent mouse thigh infection studies, when translated to the clinic after accounting for interspecies differences in plasma protein binding, suggest that the average steady-state plasma colistin concentration ($C_{ss,avg}$) required for good antibacterial effect in a patient corresponds to the MIC of the organism causing the infection.[81] It is important, however, to keep in mind that the risk of nephrotoxicity in patients increases as the plasma colistin concentration increases, especially at concentrations above approximately 2.5 mg/L.[83,84,87] Thus, there is substantial overlap in the plasma concentrations associated with the desired and undesired effects of the drug; it is very clear that colistin is an antibiotic with a very narrow therapeutic window. Because the colistin MIC may not be known at initiation of therapy, a "target" plasma colistin $C_{ss,avg}$ of 2 mg/L would seem appropriate, especially in view of the known link between inadequate initial antibiotic therapy and clinical outcome.[88]

In terms of PK of colistin, as mentioned previously, it is important to note that colistin is used parenterally as the inactive prodrug CMS. Because CMS converts to colistin in vitro and in vivo,[78,89] it was not possible in the past to accurately determine the PK of CMS and formed colistin using microbiological assays. Liquid chromatographic analytical methods made possible the separate measurement of CMS and formed colistin in biological fluids.[90,91] It is evident now that CMS and colistin have very different PK; CMS is eliminated mainly by the kidney, whereas the colistin formed in the body is eliminated via nonrenal pathway(s).[78,89,92] An analysis of patients in the ICU who were given intravenous CMS for treatment of infections caused by Gram-negative bacteria showed that, due to the slow conversion of CMS to colistin, the plasma concentration of formed colistin increased slowly following the first few intravenous doses.[93] In these patients, in whom 3×10^6 IU (ie, ~90 mg CBA) CMS was given every 8 hours, a plasma colistin $C_{ss,avg}$ of 2 mg/L was not reached until after 3 doses or more. In a subsequent study, patients who received a higher first dose (ie, a loading dose) of 6×10^6 IU (~180 mg CBA) achieved the desired bactericidal concentration much faster than those who did not.[94] These findings indicate that a loading dose may contribute to improvement of the clinical outcomes.

The largest study on the population PK of CMS and formed colistin in critically ill patients to date was conducted by Garonzik and colleagues.[95] The study included 105 patients; 89 not receiving renal support and with large variation in creatinine clearance (range 3–169 mL/min/1.73 m^2), 12 on intermittent hemodialysis, and 4 on continuous renal replacement therapy (CRRT). The physician-selected daily intravenous dose among all patients ranged from 75 to 410 mg CBA. The plasma colistin $C_{ss,avg}$ ranged from 0.48 to 9.38 mg/L. The findings in this study highlighted several key points. First, a high daily dose of CMS did not always produce desirable colistin plasma concentrations, because of the influence of renal function on the disposition of CMS and the fraction of each dose of the prodrug available for conversion to colistin in the body. The plasma concentration of formed colistin was generally lower in patients with good renal function, as CMS was more rapidly cleared by the kidney and only a small fraction of the dose was retained in the body and available for conversion to colistin. In patients with good renal function, it is important to consider active combination therapy with colistin (discussed later in this article), especially if the MIC of the infecting pathogen is near the current susceptibility breakpoint. Second, there was a large degree of interpatient variability in the apparent clearance of formed colistin and, consequently, the plasma colistin $C_{ss,avg}$ achieved from the same daily dose. This large variability was observed even among patients with similar renal function, possibly related to brand-to-brand and batch-to-batch variability across CMS parenteral products in the rate and extent of conversion of CMS to colistin.[6] Third, the findings supported previous PK data from patients on CRRT and intermittent hemodialysis, which indicated that renal replacement therapy has significant impact on the plasma concentration of formed colistin.[96,97] As a result, patients receiving CRRT require daily doses of CMS similar to those used in patients with normal kidney function; and patients on intermittent hemodialysis should be dosed on nondialysis days, as for an anuric patient, but receive a supplemental dose at the end of each dialysis session.[95] In summary, the most important outcome of the largest population PK study was the development of dosing algorithms to calculate the loading and daily maintenance doses of CMS to be administered to patients with various degrees of renal function and in those who require either intermittent or continuous renal supportive therapy.[95]

As noted previously, a major difference between polymyxin B and colistin is that the former is administered as its active form. To date, there is less information known about the clinical pharmacology of polymyxin B. In a study that involved 8 critically ill patients, polymyxin B was infused over 60 minutes with doses ranging from 0.5 to 1.5 mg/kg every 12 to 48 hours. The plasma polymyxin B concentrations were analyzed from blood samples of all patients and urine samples of 4 patients. In this study, the peak plasma concentrations of polymyxin B at the end of the infusion ranged from 2.38 to 13.9 mg/L. Only 0.04% to 0.86% of the dose was recovered as unchanged form in urine.[98] This study showed that, like colistin in rats,[99] polymyxin B is eliminated mainly by nonrenal pathway(s) and the status of the renal function would be expected to have little impact on the total body clearance of polymyxin B. In a more recent study on the population PK of polymyxin B, a total of 24 critically ill patients were included. Two patients received CRRT, whereas the rest exhibited a wide range of creatinine clearance (range 10–143 mL/min). The intravenous doses of polymyxin B administered ranged from 0.45 to 3.38 mg/kg per day. The total body clearance of polymyxin B was very similar among all patients, with the population mean of 0.0276 L/h/kg. Median urinary recovery of polymyxin B was very low at 4.04%. This study confirmed the previous finding from this research group that polymyxin B is largely nonrenally cleared and that the daily dose required to achieve a given average steady-state plasma concentration of polymyxin B is not dependent on renal function. The study also indicated that although a loading dose of polymyxin B is less critical than for CMS, steady-state can be achieved more quickly with the addition of a loading dose.[100]

Due to the different formulations of the parenteral products of colistin and polymyxin B, the 2 products are considered pharmacokinetically as “chalk and cheese” rather than “peas in a pod.”[80] In most clinical applications, polymyxin B would be regarded as having superior clinical pharmacologic properties; for example, it is possible to more quickly and reliably achieve and maintain plasma concentrations that are likely to be effective across a wide range of renal function. Relatively little pharmacodynamic and clinical work has been published with polymyxin B to date and comparative data between the two agents are lacking.[49] Colistin may be a better option for treatment of urinary tract infection, as CMS is extensively eliminated by the renal pathway and degrades to colistin within the urinary tract. For inhalation, CMS is less irritating than colistin[101] and very likely polymyxin B also, although there appear to be no direct comparisons of CMS and polymyxin B administered by inhalation. It is therefore important to optimize dosage regimens of each drug according to patient characteristics, as these factors will influence their distribution in the body.

Currently, there are limited data available regarding the impact of dosing of polymyxins and the development of polymyxin resistance. An in vitro study that examined the effect of once-daily, twice-daily, and thrice-daily dosing of colistin on the emergence of colistin resistance in *P aeruginosa* suggested the 8-hourly regimen to be the most effective at minimizing emergence of resistance.[102] Similar observations were obtained for another in vitro study that investigated polymyxin B against *P aeruginosa*.[103] These results, however, have not yet been confirmed in clinical studies.

Little information is available regarding the distribution of polymyxins into extravascular sites. In cerebral spinal fluid (CSF), colistin concentrations were found to be relatively low compared with the plasma concentration following intravenous administration of CMS.[104,105] Similar findings were also obtained for colistin concentrations in sputum and bronchoalveolar lavage fluid.[106–108] A combination of intravenous and intraventricular administration of CMS in critically ill patients with central nervous system infection showed an overall higher mean CSF colistin concentration than intravenous or intraventricular administration alone.[105] In cystic fibrosis and mechanically ventilated critically ill patients, inhalational delivery of CMS resulted in significantly higher colistin concentrations in the sputum and epithelial lining fluid, respectively, compared with intravenous administration.[108,109] Based on the current literature, alternative routes of dosing combined with intravenous administration of CMS may be useful for the treatment of extravascular infections.

COMBINATION THERAPY

Based on recent animal PK/PD and clinical PK data, colistin combination therapy is likely to be beneficial in patients infected by a causative pathogen with an MIC greater than 1 mg/L, or in patients with moderate-to-good renal function receiving intravenous CMS.[81,95] Given the high incidence of polymyxin heteroresistance in *K pneumoniae* and *A baumannii*,[40,41] polymyxin combinations may be useful in the prevention of polymyxin resistance development in these pathogens. The presence of a second antibiotic is potentially beneficial, as it may help eliminate the subpopulation that is resistant to the other antibiotic.[110] Additionally, when two antibiotics are used, they may target different cellular pathways that can lead to overall enhanced antimicrobial activity.[110] It has also been proposed that, as polymyxins disrupt the outer membrane of Gram-negative bacteria, they can promote the entry of other antibiotics into the Gram-negative bacterial cells.[111] Unfortunately, many polymyxin combinations used in the clinic have been chosen empirically. Such an approach does not take into consideration the rationalities of antibiotic combinations discussed previously. A more systematic and rational approach to the choice of a secondary antibiotic to use in the combination with polymyxins should include consideration of the following: the effect of the second antibiotic on the polymyxin-resistant subpopulation and vice versa; whether the target for the second antibiotic is intracellular; and the changes in global bacterial response to the combination treatment.

The synergistic activity of antibiotic combination therapy is often assessed in vitro with fractional inhibitory concentration (FIC) index and E-test methods.[112,113] These methods, however, only provide information regarding the activity for a single time point; therefore, they are not very informative and the results can be variable. The more desirable in vitro methods for the assessment of antibiotic combination therapy are static concentration or dynamic (ie, fluctuating concentrations to mimic dosage regimens in patients) killing kinetics assays; these assays are more useful than the FIC and E-test methods, as they examine the antimicrobial activity over time.[112,113]

A number of different antibiotics have been investigated for their combinations with polymyxins; however, the most common combinations are with carbapenems and rifampicin. A systematic review and meta-analysis of polymyxin combinations with carbapenems showed that in in vitro time-kill studies synergism occurred for *P aeruginosa*, *A baumannii*, and *K pneumoniae*; however, it occurred more frequently against *A baumannii* (143 [77%] of 186 isolates) than *P aeruginosa* (68 [50%] of 136 isolates) and *K pneumoniae* (64 [44%] of 146 isolates).[114] For all 3 species, polymyxins combined with doripenem produced the highest synergy. For *A baumannii*, the combination of polymyxins with meropenem was more active than with imipenem, whereas against *P aeruginosa* the converse was the case. In addition to enhanced initial bacterial killing, the combinations also suppressed the development of resistance to polymyxins.[114] For combinations of polymyxins with rifampicin, time-kill studies showed synergy against 14 (100%) of 14 carbapenemase-producing *K pneumoniae* isolates,[115] and 160 (57%) of 280 *A baumannii* isolates.[113] In a mouse pneumonia model with multidrug-resistant *P aeruginosa*, a combination of colistin (intranasal) and rifampicin (oral) provided maximum survival protection compared with either drug alone.[116]

Apart from the enhanced killing, in vitro studies have also demonstrated that the combinations of polymyxins and carbapenems or rifampicin successfully suppressed the emergence of polymyxin resistance. Suppression of polymyxin resistance development was observed for colistin combined with doripenem against *P aeruginosa*,[117] including biofilm-embedded MDR *P aeruginosa*,[118] and *K pneumoniae*.[119] The combination of colistin and rifampicin has been shown to suppress the development of polymyxin resistance in *A baumannii*.[120]

Although the results from preclinical studies are promising, the potential benefit of polymyxin combinations in patients remains unclear. Many reports relating to polymyxin combinations describe observational studies, usually involving small numbers of patients and being nonrandomized. For example, in a clinical study, the benefit of combining colistin with another antibiotic was evaluated in 70 patients with ventilator-associated pneumonia.[121] Of the total number of patients, 17 patients were administered intravenous colistin alone, 20 patients were administered intravenous colistin and sulbactam, and 33 patients were administered intravenous colistin and a carbapenem. The clinical and microbiological responses from the investigation showed no significant difference statistically ($P>.05$), although both responses were higher in the carbapenem combination group.[121] In a recent analysis conducted on all clinical studies that compared colistin monotherapy with colistin-based combination therapy for the treatment of carbapenem-resistant Gram-negative bacteria, the findings indicated that both colistin alone and colistin/carbapenem combination produced similar outcome.[122] The investigators of the analysis, however, indicated that there are potential sources of bias in the original studies, including selection bias (different criteria required for the selection of polymyxin monotherapy or combination therapy), small study size (does not permit adjustment for other risk factors), potentially suboptimal dosing strategies, and the appropriateness of the initial empirical antibiotic treatment.

Regarding the potential benefit of polymyxin and rifampicin combinations in patients, a recent multicenter randomized controlled trial (RCT) was conducted comparing the clinical outcome of colistin and rifampicin with colistin alone in 210 patients with serious infections due to extensively drug-resistant *A baumannii.*[123] In this study, the patients were randomly allocated (1:1) to either CMS alone (2 MIU [~60 mg CBA] every 8 hours intravenously), or CMS (at the same dose specified) plus rifampicin (600 mg intravenously every 12 hours). The primary end point of the study was overall 30-day mortality and the secondary end points were infection-related death, microbiologic eradication, and length of hospitalization. The results showed a significant increase in microbiologic eradication rate for the colistin/rifampicin combination group; however, no difference was observed for infection-related death and length of hospitalization.[123] The multicenter RCT conducted by Durante-Mangoni and colleagues[123] also included polymyxin resistance emergence as one of its secondary outcome measures, but no difference between the combination and monotherapy groups was found. In a single-center RCT, the benefit of using colistin combined with rifampicin over colistin alone was evaluated in 43 patients with ventilator-associated pneumonia.[124] In this study, 22 patients were administered only colistin intravenously (300 mg CBA [~10 MIU] per day), and the other 21 patients were administered colistin intravenously (at the same dose) combined with rifampicin (600 mg/day) nasogastrically. Similar to the multicenter RCT,[123] the time to microbiological clearance was significantly shorter in the combination group. The findings also showed that clinical, laboratory, radiological, and microbiological response rates were better in the combination group; however, they were not statistically significant ($P>.05$). At present, the available clinical data do not support the combination of colistin and rifampicin because of the lack of improved clinical outcomes with the combination therapy. Some degree of synergy between colistin and fosfomycin against *A baumannii* and *P aeruginosa* isolates, including those resistant to carbapenems, has been observed in in vitro studies, most typically using the checkerboard technique for determination of FIC index.[125–127] However, the role of this combination in the clinic remains unclear. A recent preliminary open-label RCT compared this combination against colistin alone in 94 patients (47 in each group) infected with carbapenem-resistant *A baumannii*; approximately 75% of patients in both groups had ventilator-associated pneumonia.[126,128] There was a significantly more favorable microbiological response for the colistin-fosfomycin group. However, favorable clinical outcomes, mortality at the end of study treatment, and mortality at 28 days were not significantly different, nor was there a significant difference in survival time between the patients who received combination therapy and monotherapy.

As noted previously, multiple factors may have contributed to the lack of significant benefit observed with polymyxin combinations in clinical studies. In addition, as previously discussed, colistin is administered in the clinic as CMS, thus often leads to suboptimal plasma exposure at initiation of therapy and during the treatment course. To rapidly achieve a desirable plasma colistin $C_{ss,avg}$ (ie, 2 mg/L), a loading dose is usually required. Most clinical studies that have compared colistin combination therapy with colistin monotherapy did not include a loading dose and many studies involved administration of daily maintenance doses that were most likely suboptimal. To understand the real benefit of polymyxin combination treatments, future RCTs should include a loading dose and/or use higher daily maintenance doses to achieve optimal plasma polymyxin concentrations throughout the treatment course. Furthermore, several clinical studies were underpowered and/or suffered from the ethical constraints involved in conducting RCTs in critically ill patients. With regard to the latter, in most studies, patients in both the polymyxin monotherapy and combination groups received multiple other antibiotics in addition to the index second antibiotic under consideration.[123] Because of the last-line status of the polymyxins, in many studies it is likely (but usually not reported) that the time from diagnosis of infection to the initiation of polymyxin in the polymyxin monotherapy and combination groups differed, very likely favoring the monotherapy group. Most studies have had multiple endpoints, but many have neglected to identify the potential benefit of polymyxin combinations to prevent the development of polymyxin resistance. Future studies should also be appropriately designed to evaluate the emergence of polymyxin resistance following combination and monotherapy. Although the clinical benefit of polymyxin combinations remains unproven, it may be beneficial to use polymyxin combination therapy considering the polymyxin-associated nephrotoxicity and PK/PD considerations as reviewed previously. Well-designed and appropriately powered RCTs are required to examine the potential advantage of polymyxin combination therapy versus polymyxin monotherapy. Currently, 2 such RCTs of the colistin and carbapenem combination are being conducted in Europe (NCT01732250) and the United States (NCT01597973). These studies are expected to be completed in approximately September 2016 for Europe and September 2017 for the United States.

PREVENTION OF POLYMYXIN RESISTANCE

Infection Control

Polymyxin MIC testing is typically performed only for XDR pathogens, and thus, most identified polymyxin-resistant pathogens are XDR and, as a result, patients often have already been placed in enhanced infection control precautions. As the polymyxins are a "last-line" therapeutic option, polymyxin-resistant XDR pathogens represent an urgent threat, and an outbreak could lead to temporary closure of a hospital ward or floor. Patients colonized with polymyxin-resistant MDR or XDR pathogens should be managed as an infection-control emergency and serious efforts should be made to prevent hospital spread of these pathogens.

In addition to standard precautions (eg, hand hygiene), enhanced infection control precautions for patients colonized with polymyxin-resistant MDR pathogens often involve contact precautions (ie, use of gowns and gloves and dedicated medical equipment, such as stethoscopes) and placement of a patient in a private room.[127,129] Extrapolating from experience in controlling CRE,[130] cohorting patients colonized with polymyxin-resistant MDR pathogens and when hospital resources permit, cohorting health care workers caring for those patients (so that certain health care workers care for colonized and/or infected patients only) are warranted in outbreaks or in hyperendemic settings. Active surveillance screening (eg, of rectal swabs for CRE), coupled with contact precautions, has been useful in containing MDR Gram-negative pathogens, including CRE,[131] and could be used in a similar way to identify patients asymptomatically colonized with polymyxin-resistant MDR pathogens. Chlorhexidine bathing of patients has also been reported to be effective in reducing risk for spread of MDR pathogens.[131,132] Prevention bundles used to effectively control CRE have included active surveillance, contact precautions, chlorhexidine bathing, and cohorting of patients. A similar bundle of strategies would likely be effective in preventing the spread of polymyxin-resistant Gram-negative pathogens.[131–133]

Antimicrobial Stewardship

Antimicrobial stewardship strategies are an important component of prevention strategies to limit the emergence of antimicrobial resistance among Gram-negative bacteria.[134] Although avoidance of polymyxin use whenever possible will likely help to prevent the emergence and spread of polymyxin resistance, timely and appropriate use can have a positive impact on clinical outcomes. In some instances, when patients are at increased risk for infection due to XDR-GNB pathogens, empiric polymyxin use is warranted. Certain patient characteristics, such as a prior history of XDR-GNB infection or admission from a long-term acute-care center where XDR-GNB pathogens are common, in addition to assessment of level of acute severity of illness, can help to identify patients who have increased risk for life-threatening XDR-GNB infection, and who might be appropriate candidates for empiric polymyxin therapy. Using formal clinical scores to identify patients at high risk for infection due to an XDR pathogen and who is an appropriate candidate for empiric polymyxin therapy have, unfortunately, not been shown to be accurate or effective.[134] As an alternative to empiric polymyxin therapy, rapid diagnostics can be used to more quickly identify XDR-GNB pathogens and more rapidly implement polymyxin therapy.

Additionally, negative results from rapid diagnostic tests can be used to quickly discontinue polymyxins. If polymyxins are empirically prescribed, then rapid de-escalation should be practiced whenever possible to limit unnecessary polymyxin use. De-escalation is modification of empiric therapy (when appropriate) based on a patient's clinical status and available culture results.[135] Typically, de-escalation occurs at approximately day 3 of antimicrobial therapy. If patients have microbiologic data indicating that an XDR pathogen is not present, then more often than not, polymyxin therapy can be stopped. De-escalation can help to limit unnecessary polymyxin use and prevent emergence of polymyxin resistance. If a full course of polymyxins is needed to treat an infection, then the duration of therapy should be monitored and the shortest effective duration should be prescribed. Careful attention to the "day of polymyxin therapy," and to the patient's clinical response to therapy, can help to minimize the duration of therapy whenever possible, to avoid unnecessarily long polymyxin courses and to prevent the emergence of polymyxin resistance.

Finally, as polymyxins represent a last-line therapeutic option, and resistance to these agents will in many cases leave clinicians with no viable treatment alternatives, the use of polymyxins for selective gut decontamination strategies for ESBL-producing organisms or other Gram-negative pathogens, should be avoided. Multiple analyses looking at ESBL gut decontamination strategies with colistin showed both a failure to eradicate the ESBL-producing pathogens and even more concerning, an astounding rise in the rate of colistin resistance from essentially zero to greater than 50%.[68,69]

SUMMARY

Polymyxin resistance is a major public health threat, as the polymyxins represent "last-line" therapeutics for Gram-negative pathogens resistant to essentially all other antibiotics. Improved understanding of mechanisms of, and risk factors for, polymyxin resistance, as well as infection prevention and stewardship strategies, together with optimization of dosing of polymyxins including in combination regimens, can help to limit the emergence and dissemination of polymyxin resistance.

REFERENCES

1. Ortwine JK, Kaye KS, Li J, et al. Colistin: understanding and applying recent pharmacokinetic advances. Pharmacotherapy 2015;35(1):11–6.
2. Centers for Disease Control and Prevention. Antibiotic resistant threats in the United States, 2013. 2013. Available at: http://www.cdc.gov/drugresistance/pdf/ar-threats-2013-508.pdf. Accessed March 16, 2016.

3. Morrill HJ, Pogue JM, Kaye KS, et al. Treatment options for carbapenem-resistant Enterobacteriaceae infections. Open Forum Infect Dis 2015;2(2): ofv050.
4. Velkov T, Thompson PE, Nation RL, et al. Structure–activity relationships of polymyxin antibiotics. J Med Chem 2010;53(5):1898–916.
5. Bergen PJ, Li J, Rayner CR, et al. Colistin methanesulfonate is an inactive prodrug of colistin against *Pseudomonas aeruginosa.* Antimicrob Agents Chemother 2006;50(6):1953–8.
6. He H, Li JC, Nation RL, et al. Pharmacokinetics of four different brands of colistimethate and formed colistin in rats. J Antimicrob Chemother 2013;68(10): 2311–7.
7. Hancock RE. Peptide antibiotics. Lancet 1997;349(9049):418–22.
8. Hancock RE, Chapple DS. Peptide antibiotics. Antimicrob Agents Chemother 1999;43(6):1317–23.
9. Velkov T, Roberts KD, Nation RL, et al. Pharmacology of polymyxins: new insights into an 'old' class of antibiotics. Future Microbiol 2013;8(6):711–24.
10. Cajal Y, Rogers J, Berg OG, et al. Intermembrane molecular contacts by polymyxin B mediate exchange of phospholipids. Biochemistry 1996;35(1):299–308.
11. Dixon RA, Chopra I. Polymyxin B and polymyxin B nonapeptide alter cytoplasmic membrane permeability in *Escherichia coli.* J Antimicrob Chemother 1986;18(5):557–63.
12. Vincent JL, Laterre PF, Cohen J, et al. A pilot-controlled study of a polymyxin B-immobilized hemoperfusion cartridge in patients with severe sepsis secondary to intra-abdominal infection. Shock 2005;23(5):400–5.
13. Nishibori M, Takahashi HK, Katayama H, et al. Specific removal of monocytes from peripheral blood of septic patients by polymyxin B-immobilized filter column. Acta Med Okayama 2009;63(1):65–9.
14. Deris ZZ, Akter J, Sivanesan S, et al. A secondary mode of action of polymyxins against Gram-negative bacteria involves the inhibition of NADH-quinone oxidoreductase activity. J Antibiot 2014;67(2):147–51.
15. Mogi T, Murase Y, Mori M, et al. Polymyxin B identified as an inhibitor of alternative NADH dehydrogenase and malate: quinone oxidoreductase from the Gram-positive bacterium *Mycobacterium smegmatis.* J Biochem 2009;146(4): 491–9.
16. Basu S, Radziejewska-Lebrecht J, Mayer H. Lipopolysaccharide of *Providencia rettgeri.* Chemical studies and taxonomical implications. Arch Microbiol 1986; 144(3):213–8.
17. Boll M, Radziejewska-Lebrecht J, Warth C, et al. 4-Amino-4-deoxy-L-arabinose in LPS of enterobacterial R-mutants and its possible role for their polymyxin reactivity. FEMS Immunol Med Microbiol 1994;8(4):329–41.
18. Vinogradov E, Lindner B, Seltmann G, et al. Lipopolysaccharides from *Serratia marcescens* possess one or two 4-amino-4-deoxy-L-arabinopyranose 1-phosphate residues in the lipid A and D-glycero-D-talo-oct-2-ulopyranosonic acid in the inner core region. Chemistry 2006;12(25):6692–700.
19. Kline T, Trent MS, Stead CM, et al. Synthesis of and evaluation of lipid A modification by 4-substituted 4-deoxy arabinose analogs as potential inhibitors of bacterial polymyxin resistance. Bioorg Med Chem Lett 2008;18(4):1507–10.
20. Miller AK, Brannon MK, Stevens L, et al. PhoQ mutations promote lipid A modification and polymyxin resistance of *Pseudomonas aeruginosa* found in colistin-treated cystic fibrosis patients. Antimicrob Agents Chemother 2011;55(12): 5761–9.

21. Breazeale SD, Ribeiro AA, McClerren AL, et al. A formyltransferase required for polymyxin resistance in *Escherichia coli* and the modification of lipid A with 4-Amino-4-deoxy-L-arabinose. Identification and function of UDP-4-deoxy-4-formamido-L-arabinose. J Biol Chem 2005;280(14):14154–67.
22. McPhee JB, Lewenza S, Hancock RE. Cationic antimicrobial peptides activate a two-component regulatory system, PmrA-PmrB, that regulates resistance to polymyxin B and cationic antimicrobial peptides in *Pseudomonas aeruginosa*. Mol Microbiol 2003;50(1):205–17.
23. Gunn JS, Lim KB, Krueger J, et al. PmrA-PmrB-regulated genes necessary for 4-aminoarabinose lipid A modification and polymyxin resistance. Mol Microbiol 1998;27(6):1171–82.
24. McPhee JB, Bains M, Winsor G, et al. Contribution of the PhoP-PhoQ and PmrA-PmrB two-component regulatory systems to Mg2+-induced gene regulation in *Pseudomonas aeruginosa*. J Bacteriol 2006;188(11):3995–4006.
25. Olaitan AO, Morand S, Rolain JM. Mechanisms of polymyxin resistance: acquired and intrinsic resistance in bacteria. Front Microbiol 2014;5:643.
26. Nowicki EM, O'Brien JP, Brodbelt JS, et al. Extracellular zinc induces phosphoethanolamine addition to *Pseudomonas aeruginosa* lipid A via the ColRS two-component system. Mol Microbiol 2015;97(1):166–78.
27. Adams MD, Nickel GC, Bajaksouzian S, et al. Resistance to colistin in *Acinetobacter baumannii* associated with mutations in the PmrAB two-component system. Antimicrob Agents Chemother 2009;53(9):3628–34.
28. Pelletier MR, Casella LG, Jones JW, et al. Unique structural modifications are present in the lipopolysaccharide from colistin-resistant strains of *Acinetobacter baumannii*. Antimicrob Agents Chemother 2013;57(10):4831–40.
29. Moffatt JH, Harper M, Harrison P, et al. Colistin resistance in *Acinetobacter baumannii* is mediated by complete loss of lipopolysaccharide production. Antimicrob Agents Chemother 2010;54(12):4971–7.
30. Henry R, Vithanage N, Harrison P, et al. Colistin-resistant, lipopolysaccharide-deficient *Acinetobacter baumannii* responds to lipopolysaccharide loss through increased expression of genes involved in the synthesis and transport of lipoproteins, phospholipids, and poly-beta-1,6-N-acetylglucosamine. Antimicrob Agents Chemother 2012;56(1):59–69.
31. Cannatelli A, Di Pilato V, Giani T, et al. In vivo evolution to colistin resistance by PmrB sensor kinase mutation in KPC-producing *Klebsiella pneumoniae* is associated with low-dosage colistin treatment. Antimicrob Agents Chemother 2014; 58(8):4399–403.
32. Jayol A, Poirel L, Brink A, et al. Resistance to colistin associated with a single amino acid change in protein PmrB among *Klebsiella pneumoniae* isolates of worldwide origin. Antimicrob Agents Chemother 2014;58(8):4762–6.
33. Olaitan AO, Diene SM, Kempf M, et al. Worldwide emergence of colistin resistance in *Klebsiella pneumoniae* from healthy humans and patients in Lao PDR, Thailand, Israel, Nigeria and France owing to inactivation of the PhoP/PhoQ regulator mgrB: an epidemiological and molecular study. Int J Antimicrob Agents 2014;44(6):500–7.
34. Cannatelli A, Giani T, D'Andrea MM, et al. MgrB inactivation is a common mechanism of colistin resistance in KPC-producing *Klebsiella pneumoniae* of clinical origin. Antimicrob Agents Chemother 2014;58(10):5696–703.
35. Campos MA, Vargas MA, Regueiro V, et al. Capsule polysaccharide mediates bacterial resistance to antimicrobial peptides. Infect Immun 2004;72(12): 7107–14.

36. Llobet E, Tomas JM, Bengoechea JA. Capsule polysaccharide is a bacterial decoy for antimicrobial peptides. Microbiology 2008;154(Pt 12):3877–86.
37. Padilla E, Llobet E, Domenech-Sanchez A, et al. *Klebsiella pneumoniae* AcrAB efflux pump contributes to antimicrobial resistance and virulence. Antimicrob Agents Chemother 2010;54(1):177–83.
38. Li J, Rayner CR, Nation RL, et al. Heteroresistance to colistin in multidrug-resistant *Acinetobacter baumannii*. Antimicrob Agents Chemother 2006;50(9): 2946–50.
39. Hermes DM, Pormann Pitt C, Lutz L, et al. Evaluation of heteroresistance to polymyxin B among carbapenem-susceptible and -resistant *Pseudomonas aeruginosa*. J Med Microbiol 2013;62(Pt 8):1184–9.
40. Poudyal A, Howden BP, Bell JM, et al. In vitro pharmacodynamics of colistin against multidrug-resistant *Klebsiella pneumoniae*. J Antimicrob Chemother 2008;62(6):1311–8.
41. Barin J, Martins AF, Heineck BL, et al. Hetero- and adaptive resistance to polymyxin B in OXA-23-producing carbapenem-resistant *Acinetobacter baumannii* isolates. Ann Clin Microbiol Antimicrob 2013;12:15.
42. Li J, Nation RL, Owen RJ, et al. Antibiograms of multidrug-resistant clinical *Acinetobacter baumannii*: promising therapeutic options for treatment of infection with colistin-resistant strains. Clin Infect Dis 2007;45(5):594–8.
43. Vidaillac C, Benichou L, Duval RE. In vitro synergy of colistin combinations against colistin-resistant *Acinetobacter baumannii*, *Pseudomonas aeruginosa*, and *Klebsiella pneumoniae* isolates. Antimicrob Agents Chemother 2012; 56(9):4856–61.
44. Beceiro A, Moreno A, Fernandez N, et al. Biological cost of different mechanisms of colistin resistance and their impact on virulence in *Acinetobacter baumannii*. Antimicrob Agents Chemother 2014;58(1):518–26.
45. Hraiech S, Roch A, Lepidi H, et al. Impaired virulence and fitness of a colistin-resistant clinical isolate of *Acinetobacter baumannii* in a rat model of pneumonia. Antimicrob Agents Chemother 2013;57(10):5120–1.
46. Wand ME, Bock LJ, Bonney LC, et al. Retention of virulence following adaptation to colistin in *Acinetobacter baumannii* reflects the mechanism of resistance. J Antimicrob Chemother 2015;70(8):2209–16.
47. Lopez-Rojas R, Dominguez-Herrera J, McConnell MJ, et al. Impaired virulence and in vivo fitness of colistin-resistant *Acinetobacter baumannii*. J Infect Dis 2011;203(4):545–8.
48. Humphries RM. Susceptibility testing of the polymyxins: where are we now? Pharmacotherapy 2015;35(1):22–7.
49. Nation RL, Li J, Cars O, et al. Framework for optimisation of the clinical use of colistin and polymyxin B: the Prato polymyxin consensus. Lancet Infect Dis 2015;15(2):225–34.
50. Morrow BJ, Pillar CM, Deane J, et al. Activities of carbapenem and comparator agents against contemporary US *Pseudomonas aeruginosa* isolates from the CAPITAL surveillance program. Diagn Microbiol Infect Dis 2013;75(4):412–6.
51. Tunyapanit W, Pruekprasert P, Laoprasopwattana K, et al. In vitro activity of colistin against multidrug-resistant *Pseudomonas aeruginosa* isolates from patients in Songklanagarind Hospital, Thailand. Southeast Asian J Trop Med Public Health 2013;44(2):273–80.
52. Mohanty S, Maurya V, Gaind R, et al. Phenotypic characterization and colistin susceptibilities of carbapenem-resistant of *Pseudomonas aeruginosa* and *Acinetobacter* spp. J Infect Dev Ctries 2013;7(11):880–7.

53. Schulin T. In vitro activity of the aerosolized agents colistin and tobramycin and five intravenous agents against *Pseudomonas aeruginosa* isolated from cystic fibrosis patients in southwestern Germany. J Antimicrob Chemother 2002; 49(2):403–6.
54. Yau W, Owen RJ, Poudyal A, et al. Colistin hetero-resistance in multidrug-resistant *Acinetobacter baumannii* clinical isolates from the Western Pacific region in the SENTRY antimicrobial surveillance programme. J Infect 2009;58(2):138–44.
55. Gales AC, Jones RN, Sader HS. Global assessment of the antimicrobial activity of polymyxin B against 54 731 clinical isolates of Gram-negative bacilli: report from the SENTRY antimicrobial surveillance programme (2001-2004). Clin Microbiol Infect 2006;12(4):315–21.
56. Gales AC, Reis AO, Jones RN. Contemporary assessment of antimicrobial susceptibility testing methods for polymyxin B and colistin: review of available interpretative criteria and quality control guidelines. J Clin Microbiol 2001;39(1): 183–90.
57. Cai Y, Chai D, Wang R, et al. Colistin resistance of *Acinetobacter baumannii*: clinical reports, mechanisms and antimicrobial strategies. J Antimicrob Chemother 2012;67(7):1607–15.
58. Dobrewski R, Savov E, Bernards AT, et al. Genotypic diversity and antibiotic susceptibility of *Acinetobacter baumannii* isolates in a Bulgarian hospital. Clin Microbiol Infect 2006;12(11):1135–7.
59. Ko KS, Suh JY, Kwon KT, et al. High rates of resistance to colistin and polymyxin B in subgroups of *Acinetobacter baumannii* isolates from Korea. J Antimicrob Chemother 2007;60(5):1163–7.
60. Arroyo LA, Garcia-Curiel A, Pachon-Ibanez ME, et al. Reliability of the E-test method for detection of colistin resistance in clinical isolates of *Acinetobacter baumannii*. J Clin Microbiol 2005;43(2):903–5.
61. Arroyo LA, Mateos I, Gonzalez V, et al. In vitro activities of tigecycline, minocycline, and colistin-tigecycline combination against multi- and pandrug-resistant clinical isolates of *Acinetobacter baumannii* group. Antimicrob Agents Chemother 2009;53(3):1295–6.
62. Baadani AM, Thawadi SI, El-Khizzi NA, et al. Prevalence of colistin and tigecycline resistance in *Acinetobacter baumannii* clinical isolates from 2 hospitals in Riyadh Region over a 2-year period. Saudi Med J 2013;34(3):248–53.
63. Munoz-Price LS, Poirel L, Bonomo RA, et al. Clinical epidemiology of the global expansion of *Klebsiella pneumoniae* carbapenemases. Lancet Infect Dis 2013; 13(9):785–96.
64. Giani T, Arena F, Vaggelli G, et al. Large nosocomial outbreak of colistin-resistant KPC carbapenemase-producing *Klebsiella pneumoniae* by clonal expansion of an mgrB deletion mutant. J Clin Microbiol 2015;53(10):3341–4.
65. Ah YM, Kim AJ, Lee JY. Colistin resistance in *Klebsiella pneumoniae*. Int J Antimicrob Agents 2014;44(1):8–15.
66. Neonakis IK, Samonis G, Messaritakis H, et al. Resistance status and evolution trends of *Klebsiella pneumoniae* isolates in a university hospital in Greece: ineffectiveness of carbapenems and increasing resistance to colistin. Chemotherapy 2010;56(6):448–52.
67. Kontopidou F, Plachouras D, Papadomichelakis E, et al. Colonization and infection by colistin-resistant Gram-negative bacteria in a cohort of critically ill patients. Clin Microbiol Infect 2011;17(11):E9–11.
68. Strenger V, Gschliesser T, Grisold A, et al. Orally administered colistin leads to colistin-resistant intestinal flora and fails to prevent faecal colonisation with

extended-spectrum beta-lactamase-producing enterobacteria in hospitalised newborns. Int J Antimicrob Agents 2011;37(1):67–9.

69. Halaby T, Al Naiemi N, Kluytmans J, et al. Emergence of colistin resistance in Enterobacteriaceae after the introduction of selective digestive tract decontamination in an intensive care unit. Antimicrob Agents Chemother 2013;57(7):3224–9.
70. Meletis G, Tzampaz E, Sianou E, et al. Colistin heteroresistance in carbapenemase-producing *Klebsiella pneumoniae*. J Antimicrob Chemother 2011;66(4):946–7.
71. Samonis G, Maraki S, Karageorgopoulos DE, et al. Synergy of fosfomycin with carbapenems, colistin, netilmicin, and tigecycline against multidrug-resistant *Klebsiella pneumoniae*, *Escherichia coli*, and *Pseudomonas aeruginosa* clinical isolates. Eur J Clin Microbiol Infect Dis 2012;31(5):695–701.
72. Souli M, Galani I, Antoniadou A, et al. An outbreak of infection due to beta-Lactamase *Klebsiella pneumoniae* Carbapenemase 2-producing *K. pneumoniae* in a Greek University Hospital: molecular characterization, epidemiology, and outcomes. Clin Infect Dis 2010;50(3):364–73.
73. Souli M, Kontopidou FV, Papadomichelakis E, et al. Clinical experience of serious infections caused by Enterobacteriaceae producing VIM-1 metallo-beta-lactamase in a Greek University Hospital. Clin Infect Dis 2008;46(6):847–54.
74. Papadimitriou-Olivgeris M, Christofidou M, Fligou F, et al. The role of colonization pressure in the dissemination of colistin or tigecycline resistant KPC-producing *Klebsiella pneumoniae* in critically ill patients. Infection 2014;42(5):883–90.
75. Monaco M, Giani T, Raffone M, et al. Colistin resistance superimposed to endemic carbapenem-resistant *Klebsiella pneumoniae*: a rapidly evolving problem in Italy, November 2013 to April 2014. Euro Surveill 2014;19(42) [pii: 20939].
76. Qureshi ZA, Hittle LE, O'Hara JA, et al. Colistin-resistant *Acinetobacter baumannii*: beyond carbapenem resistance. Clin Infect Dis 2015;60(9):1295–303.
77. Meletis G, Oustas E, Botziori C, et al. Containment of carbapenem resistance rates of *Klebsiella pneumoniae* and *Acinetobacter baumannii* in a Greek hospital with a concomitant increase in colistin, gentamicin and tigecycline resistance. New Microbiol 2015;38(3):417–21.
78. Li J, Nation RL, Turnidge JD, et al. Colistin: the re-emerging antibiotic for multidrug-resistant Gram-negative bacterial infections. Lancet Infect Dis 2006;6(9):589–601.
79. Zavascki AP, Goldani LZ, Li J, et al. Polymyxin B for the treatment of multidrug-resistant pathogens: a critical review. J Antimicrob Chemother 2007;60(6):1206–15.
80. Nation RL, Velkov T, Li J. Colistin and polymyxin B: peas in a pod, or chalk and cheese? Clin Infect Dis 2014;59(1):88–94.
81. Cheah S, Wang J, Nguyen V, et al. New pharmacokinetic/pharmacodynamic studies of systemically administered colistin against *Pseudomonas aeruginosa* and *Acinetobacter baumannii* in mouse thigh and lung infection models: smaller response lung infection. J Antimicrob Chemother 2015;70(12):3291–7.
82. Bergen PJ, Bulitta JB, Forrest A, et al. Pharmacokinetic/pharmacodynamic investigation of colistin against *Pseudomonas aeruginosa* using an in vitro model. Antimicrob Agents Chemother 2010;54(9):3783–9.
83. Sorli L, Luque S, Grau S, et al. Trough colistin plasma level is an independent risk factor for nephrotoxicity: a prospective observational cohort study. BMC Infect Dis 2013;13:380.

84. Forrest A, Silveira FP, Thamlikitkul V, et al. Toxicodynamics for colistin-associated changes in creatinine clearance. Paper Presented at Interscience Conference on Antimicrobial Agents and Chemotherapy. Washington, DC, 2014.
85. Nation RL, Li J, Cars O, et al. Consistent global approach on reporting of colistin doses to promote safe and effective use. Clin Infect Dis 2014;58(1):139–41.
86. Nation RL, Li J, Turnidge JD. The urgent need for clear and accurate information on the polymyxins. Clin Infect Dis 2013;57(11):1656–7.
87. Forrest A, Silveira FP, Thamlikitkul V. Risk factors for colistin-associated nephrotoxicity. Paper Presented at 1st International Conference on Polymyxins. Prato (Italy), May 2–4, 2013.
88. Kumar A, Roberts D, Wood KE, et al. Duration of hypotension before initiation of effective antimicrobial therapy is the critical determinant of survival in human septic shock. Crit Care Med 2006;34(6):1589–96.
89. Nation RL, Li J. Optimizing use of colistin and polymyxin B in the critically ill. Semin Respir Crit Care Med 2007;28(6):604–14.
90. Li J, Milne RW, Nation RL, et al. A simple method for the assay of colistin in human plasma, using pre-column derivatization with 9-fluorenylmethyl chloroformate in solid-phase extraction cartridges and reversed-phase high-performance liquid chromatography. J Chromatogr B Biomed Sci Appl 2001;761(2): 167–75.
91. Li J, Milne RW, Nation RL, et al. Simple method for assaying colistin methanesulfonate in plasma and urine using high-performance liquid chromatography. Antimicrob Agents Chemother 2002;46(10):3304–7.
92. Landersdorfer CB, Nation RL. Colistin: how should it be dosed for the critically ill? Semin Respir Crit Care Med 2015;36(1):126–35.
93. Plachouras D, Karvanen M, Friberg LE, et al. Population pharmacokinetic analysis of colistin methanesulfonate and colistin after intravenous administration in critically ill patients with infections caused by Gram-negative bacteria. Antimicrob Agents Chemother 2009;53(8):3430–6.
94. Mohamed AF, Karaiskos I, Plachouras D, et al. Application of a loading dose of colistin methanesulfonate in critically ill patients: population pharmacokinetics, protein binding, and prediction of bacterial kill. Antimicrob Agents Chemother 2012;56(8):4241–9.
95. Garonzik SM, Li J, Thamlikitkul V, et al. Population pharmacokinetics of colistin methanesulfonate and formed colistin in critically ill patients from a multicenter study provide dosing suggestions for various categories of patients. Antimicrob Agents Chemother 2011;55(7):3284–94.
96. Li J, Rayner CR, Nation RL, et al. Pharmacokinetics of colistin methanesulfonate and colistin in a critically ill patient receiving continuous venovenous hemodiafiltration. Antimicrob Agents Chemother 2005;49(11):4814–5.
97. Marchand S, Frat JP, Petitpas F, et al. Removal of colistin during intermittent haemodialysis in two critically ill patients. J Antimicrob Chemother 2010;65(8): 1836–7.
98. Zavascki AP, Goldani LZ, Cao G, et al. Pharmacokinetics of intravenous polymyxin B in critically ill patients. Clin Infect Dis 2008;47(10):1298–304.
99. Li J, Milne RW, Nation RL, et al. Pharmacokinetics of colistin methanesulphonate and colistin in rats following an intravenous dose of colistin methanesulphonate. J Antimicrob Chemother 2004;53(5):837–40.
100. Sandri AM, Landersdorfer CB, Jacob J, et al. Population pharmacokinetics of intravenous polymyxin B in critically ill patients: implications for selection of dosage regimens. Clin Infect Dis 2013;57(4):524–31.

101. Westerman EM, Le Brun PP, Touw DJ, et al. Effect of nebulized colistin sulphate and colistin sulphomethate on lung function in patients with cystic fibrosis: a pilot study. J Cyst Fibros 2004;3(1):23–8.
102. Bergen PJ, Li J, Nation RL, et al. Comparison of once-, twice- and thrice-daily dosing of colistin on antibacterial effect and emergence of resistance: studies with *Pseudomonas aeruginosa* in an in vitro pharmacodynamic model. J Antimicrob Chemother 2008;61(3):636–42.
103. Tam VH, Schilling AN, Vo G, et al. Pharmacodynamics of polymyxin B against *Pseudomonas aeruginosa*. Antimicrob Agents Chemother 2005;49(9):3624–30.
104. Markantonis SL, Markou N, Fousteri M, et al. Penetration of colistin into cerebrospinal fluid. Antimicrob Agents Chemother 2009;53(11):4907–10.
105. Ziaka M, Markantonis SL, Fousteri M, et al. Combined intravenous and intraventricular administration of colistin methanesulfonate in critically ill patients with central nervous system infection. Antimicrob Agents Chemother 2013;57(4):1938–40.
106. Lee JY, Chung ES, Na IY, et al. Development of colistin resistance in pmrA-, phoP-, parR- and cprR-inactivated mutants of *Pseudomonas aeruginosa*. J Antimicrob Chemother 2014;69(11):2966–71.
107. Imberti R, Cusato M, Villani P, et al. Steady-state pharmacokinetics and BAL concentration of colistin in critically Ill patients after IV colistin methanesulfonate administration. Chest 2010;138(6):1333–9.
108. Yappa SWS, Li J, Patel K, et al. Pulmonary and systemic pharmacokinetics of inhaled and intravenous colistin methanesulfonate in cystic fibrosis patients: targeting advantage of inhalational administration. Antimicrob Agents Chemother 2014;58(5):2570–9.
109. Athanassa ZE, Markantonis SL, Fousteri MZ, et al. Pharmacokinetics of inhaled colistimethate sodium (CMS) in mechanically ventilated critically ill patients. Intensive Care Med 2012;38(11):1779–86.
110. Landersdorfer CB, Ly NS, Xu H, et al. Quantifying subpopulation synergy for antibiotic combinations via mechanism-based modeling and a sequential dosing design. Antimicrob Agents Chemother 2013;57(5):2343–51.
111. Delcour AH. Outer membrane permeability and antibiotic resistance. Biochim Biophys Acta 2009;1794(5):808–16.
112. White RL, Burgess DS, Manduru M, et al. Comparison of three different in vitro methods of detecting synergy: time-kill, checkerboard, and E test. Antimicrob Agents Chemother 1996;40(8):1914–8.
113. Ni W, Shao X, Di X, et al. In vitro synergy of polymyxins with other antibiotics for *Acinetobacter baumannii*: a systematic review and meta-analysis. Int J Antimicrob Agents 2015;45(1):8–18.
114. Zusman O, Avni T, Leibovici L, et al. Systematic review and meta-analysis of in vitro synergy of polymyxins and carbapenems. Antimicrob Agents Chemother 2013;57(10):5104–11.
115. Pankey GA, Ashcraft DS. Detection of synergy using the combination of polymyxin B with either meropenem or rifampin against carbapenemase-producing *Klebsiella pneumoniae*. Diagn Microbiol Infect Dis 2011;70(4):561–4.
116. Aoki N, Tateda K, Kikuchi Y, et al. Efficacy of colistin combination therapy in a mouse model of pneumonia caused by multidrug-resistant *Pseudomonas aeruginosa*. J Antimicrob Chemother 2009;63(3):534–42.
117. Ly NS, Bulitta JB, Rao GG, et al. Colistin and doripenem combinations against *Pseudomonas aeruginosa*: profiling the time course of synergistic killing and prevention of resistance. J Antimicrob Chemother 2015;70(5):1434–42.

118. Lora-Tamayo J, Murillo O, Bergen PJ, et al. Activity of colistin combined with doripenem at clinically relevant concentrations against multidrug-resistant *Pseudomonas aeruginosa* in an in vitro dynamic biofilm model. J Antimicrob Chemother 2014;69(9):2434–42.
119. Deris ZZ, Yu HH, Davis K, et al. The combination of colistin and doripenem is synergistic against *Klebsiella pneumoniae* at multiple inocula and suppresses colistin resistance in an in vitro pharmacokinetic/pharmacodynamic model. Antimicrob Agents Chemother 2012;56(10):5103–12.
120. Lee HJ, Bergen PJ, Bulitta JB, et al. Synergistic activity of colistin and rifampin combination against multidrug-resistant *Acinetobacter baumannii* in an in vitro pharmacokinetic/pharmacodynamic model. Antimicrob Agents Chemother 2013;57(8):3738–45.
121. Yilmaz GR, Guven T, Guner R, et al. Colistin alone or combined with sulbactam or carbapenem against *A. baumannii* in ventilator-associated pneumonia. J Infect Dev Ctries 2015;9(5):476–85.
122. Paul M, Carmeli Y, Durante-Mangoni E, et al. Combination therapy for carbapenem-resistant Gram-negative bacteria. J Antimicrob Chemother 2014; 69(9):2305–9.
123. Durante-Mangoni E, Signoriello G, Andini R, et al. Colistin and rifampicin compared with colistin alone for the treatment of serious infections due to extensively drug-resistant *Acinetobacter baumannii*: a multicenter, randomized clinical trial. Clin Infect Dis 2013;57(3):349–58.
124. Aydemir H, Akduman D, Piskin N, et al. Colistin vs. the combination of colistin and rifampicin for the treatment of carbapenem-resistant *Acinetobacter baumannii* ventilator-associated pneumonia. Epidemiol Infect 2013;141(6):1214–22.
125. Santimaleeworagun W, Wongpoowarak P, Chayakul P, et al. In vitro activity of colistin or sulbactam in combination with fosfomycin or imipenem against clinical isolates of carbapenem-resistant Acinetobacter baumannii producing OXA-23 carbapenemases. The Southeast Asian journal of tropical medicine and public health Jul 2011;42(4):890–900.
126. Di X, Wang R, Liu B, et al. In vitro activity of fosfomycin in combination with colistin against clinical isolates of carbapenem-resistant Pseudomas aeruginosa. The Journal of antibiotics Mar 25 2015.
127. Wei W, Yang H, Liu Y, et al. In vitro synergy of colistin combinations against extensively drug-resistant Acinetobacter baumannii producing OXA-23 carbapenemase. J Chemother May 15 2015:1973947815Y0000000030.
128. Sirijatuphat R, Thamlikitkul V. Preliminary study of colistin versus colistin plus fosfomycin for treatment of carbapenem-resistant Acinetobacter baumannii infections. Antimicrobial agents and chemotherapy Sep 2014;58(9):5598–601.
129. Centers for Disease Prevention. Management of Multidrug-Resistant Organisms In Healthcare Settings, 2006. 2009; http://www.cdc.gov/hicpac/mdro/mdro_glossary.html. Accessed August 26, 2015.
130. Schwaber MJ, Lev B, Israeli A, et al. Containment of a country-wide outbreak of carbapenem-resistant Klebsiella pneumoniae in Israeli hospitals via a nationally implemented intervention. Clinical infectious diseases : an official publication of the Infectious Diseases Society of America Apr 1 2011;52(7):848–55.
131. Hayden MK, Lin MY, Lolans K, et al. Prevention of colonization and infection by Klebsiella pneumoniae carbapenemase-producing enterobacteriaceae in long-term acute-care hospitals. Clinical infectious diseases : an official publication of the Infectious Diseases Society of America Apr 15 2015;60(8):1153–61.

132. Schwaber MJ, Carmeli Y. An ongoing national intervention to contain the spread of carbapenem-resistant enterobacteriaceae. Clinical infectious diseases : an official publication of the Infectious Diseases Society of America Mar 2014; 58(5):697–703.
133. Goel G, Hmar L, Sarkar De M, et al. Colistin-resistant Klebsiella pneumoniae: report of a cluster of 24 cases from a new oncology center in eastern India. Infection control and hospital epidemiology 2014;35(8):1076–7.
134. Pogue JM, Kaye KS, Cohen DA, et al. Appropriate antimicrobial therapy in the era of multidrug-resistant human pathogens. Clinical microbiology and infection : the official publication of the European Society of Clinical Microbiology and Infectious Diseases 2015;21(4):302–12.
135. Kaye KS. Antimicrobial de-escalation strategies in hospitalized patients with pneumonia, intra-abdominal infections, and bacteremia. Journal of hospital medicine 2012;7(Suppl 1):S13–21.

Vancomycin-Resistant Enterococci

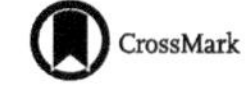

Therapeutic Challenges in the 21st Century

William R. Miller, MD[a], Barbara E. Murray, MD[a,b], Louis B. Rice, MD[c], Cesar A. Arias, MD, MSc, PhD[a,b,d,*]

KEYWORDS

- Vancomycin resistant enterococcus • Antibiotic resistance • Combination therapy

KEY POINTS

- Multidrug-resistant enterococcal infections continue to be a clinical challenge despite the advent of new therapeutic agents.
- The genetic plasticity of enterococci underscores the versatile nature of the organisms and has provided new insights into the mechanisms by which bacteria can become resistant to antibiotics and how commensal organisms evolve to become prominent hospital-associated opportunistic pathogens.
- Development of resistance to almost all antienterococcal antibiotics currently available in clinical practice highlights the difficulties facing clinicians in the setting of deep-seated enterococcal infections.
- Vancomycin-resistant enterococci infections in the 21st century will require the use of new or innovative therapeutic treatments that involve both old and new antimicrobials.

Disclosure Statement: Dr W.R. Miller has no relevant affiliations or financial disclosures. Dr B.E. Murray has grant support from Johnson & Johnson, Astellas, Palumed, Intercell and Cubist, and has served as consultant for Astellas (Theravance), Cubist, Targanta Therapeutics Corporation, Pfizer, Rib-X, AstraZeneca and Durata Therapeutics. Dr L.B. Rice has served as a consultant for Astra-Zeneca, Tetraphase Pharmaceuticals, MicuRx, Macrolide Pharmaceuticals and Adenium Pharmaceuticals. Dr C.A. Arias has received lecture fees, research support and consulting fees from Theravance, Bayer and Cubist; research support from Forrest Pharmaceuticals and Theravance Inc and has served as speaker for Forest, Theravance, Pfizer, Astra-Zeneca, Cubist, The Medicines Company and Norvartis.

[a] Division of Infectious Diseases, Department of Internal Medicine, University of Texas Medical School at Houston, 6431 Fannin Street, Houston, TX 77030, USA; [b] Department of Microbiology and Molecular Genetics, University of Texas Medical School at Houston, 6431 Fannin Street, Houston, TX 77030, USA; [c] Departments of Medicine, Microbiology and Immunology, Warren Alpert Medical School of Brown University, 593 Eddy Street, Providence, RI 02903, USA; [d] Molecular Genetics and Antimicrobial Resistance Unit, International Center for Microbial Genomics, Universidad El Bosque, Avenue Cra 9 No. 131 A - 02, Bogotá, Colombia
* Corresponding author. University of Texas Medical School, 6431 Fannin Street, Room MSB 2.112, Houston, TX 77030.
E-mail address: Cesar.Arias@uth.tmc.edu

Infect Dis Clin N Am 30 (2016) 415–439
http://dx.doi.org/10.1016/j.idc.2016.02.006 **id.theclinics.com**
0891-5520/16/$ – see front matter

INTRODUCTION: A REPORT FROM THE FRONT LINES

The year 1899 saw the first report of the bacterium *Micrococcus zymogenes* (thought today to be *Enterococcus faecalis*) as a cause of infective endocarditis (IE).[1] The patient, a 37-year-old German man, described a 2-month history of fever with an indolent, yet relentlessly progressive course. The medical staff could only watch helplessly as he died 18 days later from complications of his illness. One hundred fifteen years later, a man in his 40s with a hematologic malignancy was found to be colonized with vancomycin-resistant enterococci (VRE) on admission to the hospital for treatment of his cancer. During the admission, he became febrile, and *Enterococcus faecium* was isolated from the blood several times.[2] The medical team administered a progressive regimen of antimicrobials, including daptomycin, ampicillin, gentamicin, quinupristin-dalfopristin, tigecycline, and linezolid; however, after 3 months on therapy, blood cultures remained positive for VRE. Despite the availability of antibiotics, the eventual outcomes of both patients (separated by medical care that had evolved for 150 years) were not that different.

As the 21st century dawns, organisms such as multi–drug-resistant (MDR) *E faecium* present new challenges to clinicians. Medical science races to keep pace with the spread of resistance determinants and provide clinicians new drugs to combat an ever-changing enemy. The number of antibiotics in the therapeutic armamentarium that are active against enterococci has expanded over the last decade; however, there are little published clinical data to guide their most effective use. Below is a profile of the pathogen and its genomic plasticity, the attributes thought to be associated with its ability to colonize and infect the human host, and its strategies for resisting antimicrobial attack. This review concludes with a synthesis of the available therapeutic data to guide physicians in selecting the best treatment for these difficult infections.

PROFILE OF AN OPPORTUNISTIC PATHOGEN

From the Iron Age to the Antibiotic Age

Enterococci are facultative gram-positive cocci that live as commensals of the gastrointestinal (GI) tract of animals and humans. Enterococci are rugged and durable, able to survive in high salt concentrations and elevated temperatures, and able to resist chemical stress from chlorine and alcohol-based disinfectants.[3] Enterococci lack the cadre of virulence determinants of *Staphylococcus aureus* or the more pathogenic streptococci; however, their durability and commensal nature position them to not only survive but thrive in the modern medical setting. Surveys of organisms responsible for health care–associated infection have found that enterococci are second only to staphylococci in being isolated from health care–associated infections across the United States.[4]

Enterococcal infections, like most human diseases, have a history shaped not only by bacterial biology but also by the social, economic, and geographic factors that affect the human host. Whole genome sequencing and analyses of *E faecium* genomes have shed some light on the evolutionary history and adaptation of enterococci with the human host.[5,6] This story appears to emerge at the dawn of the Iron Age (ca. 3000 years ago) with the divergence of 2 genetic lineages (clades) of *E faecium*. One, designated clade B, would remain as a commensal of the human gastrointestinal tract with low potential for infectivity and general lack of antibiotic resistance determinants. The other (clade A) seems to have evolved and adapted to the gastrointestinal tract of livestock and domesticated animals. This bifurcation was driven, as Lebreton and colleagues[6] hypothesized, by the increasing contact between humans and domesticated animals owing to the spread of animal husbandry for agricultural and economic gain, the specialization of diets that resulted, and the changing patterns of hygiene that accompanied urbanization. Interestingly, the animal clade would go on to diverge again, this time a mere 75 years ago, at about the time antibiotics were introduced in clinical medicine. This occurrence gave rise to a hospital-associated lineage (designated clade A1), which seems to have a better ability to infect humans, disseminate in the hospital environment, and acquire a plethora of antibiotic resistance determinants, the hallmarks of the current VRE epidemic.

A cardinal feature of the members of the A1 clade is the remarkable adaptability of their genome. This plasticity stems from the large repertoire of mobile genetic elements capable of transferring pieces of DNA as small as a single gene to large pathogenicity islands and chromosomal fragments.[7] In both *E faecalis* and *E faecium*, the transmissibility of mobile elements and recruitment of a large number of antibiotic resistance determinants seem to be associated in part with a deficiency in the CRISPR (clustered regularly interspaced short palindromic repeats)–associated system (*cas*).[8] CRISPRs and the *cas* genes are present in a diverse number of archaea and bacteria.[9] Together, they encode an adaptive immunity against phages, plasmids, and other mobile genetic elements. Proteins encoded by the *cas* genes can process and integrate small sequences of foreign DNA between the clustered repeats, which serve as a template to create small RNAs that recognize and bind incoming foreign nucleic acid, targeting them for destruction by further components of the *cas* system. With an apparent limitation in the ability to degrade incoming DNA, it is thought the genomes of the A1 clade were primed to evolve and respond to the selective pressures of the hospital environment. This ability, when coupled with intrinsic resistance to several broad-spectrum antibiotics (eg, cephalosporins) and increases in the numbers of chronically and critically ill patients, set the stage for the emergence and dissemination of this multidrug-resistant clade.

Enterococcal Infections: A Tale of Two Species

From the late 1970s and into the early 1980s, *E faecalis* recorded a 3-fold surge in rates of nosocomial bacteremia, whereas rates of community-associated infection remained flat.[10] Although these isolates largely retained their sensitivity to ampicillin, their emergence would serve as a harbinger of the challenge to come. In the late 1970s, clinicians noted an increase in the minimum inhibitory concentration (MIC) of ampicillin from 4 to 64 μg/mL in isolates of *E faecium*, and over the next decade an alarming phenotype characterized by high-level resistance to ampicillin (>128 μg/mL) began to emerge.[11,12] This resistance depends on the chromosomally encoded penicillin-binding protein 5 (PBP5), a monofunctional transpeptidase capable of cross-linking peptidoglycan when all other PBPs are inactivated.[13] It was later recognized that differences in up to 5% of the amino acids between the PBP5 of resistant strains, compared with ampicillin-sensitive strains (PBP5-S), correlated with both the resistance phenotype and origin of the strain.[14] Most often, PBP5-resistance strains were found in the hospital-associated clade, whereas PBP5 ampicillin-sensitive strains predominated in community-associated strains, reflecting the shift from clade B to A1 within the hospital environment. At about the same time, the glycopeptide vancomycin entered widespread use against methicillin-resistant *S aureus*, setting the stage for the emergence of vancomycin resistance in enterococci.

The glycopeptide antibiotic vancomycin binds to the last 2 residues of the pentapeptide moiety of peptidoglycan (the terminal D-Ala-D-Ala), thereby inhibiting transglycosylation and transpeptidation reactions, leading to an arrest in cell wall synthesis.[15] Two species of enterococci, *Enterococcus gallinarum* and *Enterococcus casseliflavus*, possess related chromosomally encoded gene clusters designated *vanC1* and *vanC2* that can confer intrinsic low-level resistance to vancomycin (MICs of up to 2–32 μg/mL) via a change in the terminal precursor's residues to D-Ala-D-Ser.[16] In contrast, high-level resistance to vancomycin (MICs >64 μg/mL) is mediated by the production of pentadepsipeptides (ending in D-Ala-D-Lac) and destruction of the normal D-Ala-D-Ala ending precursors. The enzymatic machinery is encoded by the *vanA* gene cluster frequently found on transposons within plasmids (eg, Tn*1546*) and less often the *vanB* cluster integrated into the chromosome on Tn*5382*.[17,18] Of note, 7 other *van* clusters have been described so far, of which, *vanD* and *vanM* also allow synthesis of peptidoglycan ending in D-Ala-D-Lac and confer high levels of resistance to vancomycin.[17,19] The recent source of the genes implicated in vancomycin resistance in enterococci is likely environmental, as the genus *Paenibacillus* has a cluster nearly identical to that of *vanA* found in enterococci.[20]

Clinically relevant strains of VRE were first described from England in 1988.[21] It was later postulated that VRE in Europe arose first in livestock owing to the association of the emergence of VRE with the use of avoparcin, a glycopeptide antibiotic used as a growth promoter, a finding that led to the ban of this practice in 1997.[22] In the United States, vancomycin resistance in *E faecium* arose in clinical isolates and quickly came to dominate the landscape of enterococcal infections, with vancomycin resistance reported in more than 80% of *E faecium* and 8% to 9% of *E faecalis*.[4]

MASTER OF SURVIVAL

Host Colonization—Preamble to Infection

The first step toward infection with VRE appears to involve colonization of the host gastrointestinal tract. The normal flora of individuals in the United States consists of a diverse mixture of bacterial taxa, including *Enterobacteriaceae*, anaerobes, and gram-positive organisms, such as vancomycin-sensitive enterococci. However, in health care settings, VRE are often found colonizing the intestines of hospitalized patients (particularly the critically ill or patients with multiple comorbidities). This finding is reflected in the risk factors for hospital acquisition of VRE including prolonged stay in a hospital or other long-term care facility, solid organ or bone marrow transplantation, physical proximity to other patients with VRE, use of antibiotics, hemodialysis, and indwelling hardware such as urinary catheters.[23] A study of VRE colonization in patients from 2 intensive care units found, using multivariate analysis, that occupation of a room by a previous patient with VRE was an independent predictor of subsequent patients becoming colonized, an effect that persisted for 2 weeks.[24] Investigations conducted in outpatient dialysis units found up to 18% of patients colonized, with 15% acquiring VRE over a 6-month period. Further, evaluation of the chairs and gowns of staff at a dialysis unit found rates of VRE contamination of 58% and 30%, respectively.[25]

Once established as members of the gastrointestinal tract flora, VRE can take advantage of perturbations of microbial diversity to dominate the bacterial populations in the gut. Antibiotics play a large role in this transition, via direct inhibitory effects on the microbes themselves and the host's innate immune response. One consequence of therapy with broad-spectrum antimicrobials is the collateral damage they inflict on otherwise benign commensal flora, providing an opening for microbes resistant to these agents, such as VRE, to expand and fill the void. A study of 146 patients who were admitted to the intensive care unit with negative VRE surveillance cultures and who received treatment with either piperacillin-tazobactam or cefepime showed subsequent colonization rates of 26.4% and 31.1%, respectively.[26]

Disruption of the gram-negative intestinal flora by broad-spectrum antibiotics also has profound effects on the host innate immune response and alters the ability to control VRE. These pathways rely on signals from the toll-like receptor family of proteins, which recognize conserved pathogen-associated molecular patterns such as lipopolysaccharides. These signals, in turn, activate the MyD88-dependent signaling cascade resulting in the ultimate production of a variety of antimicrobial peptides. The peptide RegIIIγ, a lectin with potent anti–gram-positive activity, was shown to play an important role in controlling VRE colonization in mice.[27] Elimination of the normal intestinal anaerobic and gram-negative flora via the administration of metronidazole, neomycin, and vancomycin resulted in down regulation of the production of RegIIIγ by the murine intestinal epithelial cells. In the absence of this antimicrobial peptide, mice were unable to clear VRE from the intestine. Supplementing the mouse with oral lipopolysaccharide (a component of the gram-negative cell envelope), but not lipoteichoic acid (a component of the gram-positive cell wall), restored the production of RegIIIγ and allowed the mice to control the growth of VRE. In the human gastrointestinal tract, RegIIIα is thought to play a similar role.[28] By analogy, in the hospital setting, the administration of broad-spectrum antibiotics to patients can eliminate gram-negative organisms in the gastrointestinal tract, much as was shown in the mouse model. Without gram-negative bacteria, it seems likely that human production of RegIIIα would also decrease, allowing overgrowth of resistant colonizers such as VRE. Once established in the gut, VRE pose a risk of invasive infection in vulnerable patients. Clinical studies in recipients of hematopoietic stem cell transplants showed a clear progression from colonization to dominance and subsequent bacteremia in patients in whom dominance of VRE in their gastrointestinal tracts occurred.[29]

Virulence Factors

The shift from commensal to pathogen, while aided by resistance to antimicrobials, also depends on the ability of an organism to adhere to or invade tissues and evade host defenses. Although enterococci lack a robust repertoire of secreted toxins like those produced by the staphylococci or streptococci, a cadre of virulence determinants have been reported to help them to adhere to tissues and form biofilms.

Among the best studied of these determinants are proteins that harbor the LPxTG motif (which is the protein signature for attachment to the cell wall peptidoglycan). Several are found as a feature of the core genome of enterococci, including the collagen adhesins of *E faecalis* (Ace) and *E faecium* (Acm). Adherence to extracellular matrix molecules such as collagen and laminin would be an important first step in establishing an infection, and both Ace and Acm are thought to be involved in this process. The role of Ace and Acm in supporting infection was shown in a rat model of IE, as deletion mutants in both species were found to be attenuated as compared to the wild type.[30,31] In addition, antibodies against Ace provided protection against developing IE in this same model.[31] Further, in community-associated isolates of *E faecium*, the *acm* allele is often a pseudogene, which does not express a functional product, resulting in a phenotype that is unable to bind collagen.[32] Another major group of genes in the core genome encode the enterococcal pili. These multiprotein structures are long filamentous protrusions from the cell surface that are also shown to promote adherence to the matrix proteins fibrinogen and collagen and support biofilm formation.[33] The *E faecalis* Ebp pilus operon consists of 3 structural genes and a pilus-specific sortase; the individual subunits contain the LPxTG recognition motif that allows the pilus sortase to assemble the structural proteins into a complete pilus before it is anchored to the cell wall via a housekeeping sortase.[34,35] In *E faecium*, deletion of genes from a homologous operon, known as Ebp_{fm}, impaired bacterial adhesion and biofilm formation and resulted in impaired pathogenic potential compared with the wild type in a mixed infection model of murine urinary tract infection.[36]

Several other proteins possessing the LPxTG motif are acquired determinants and not present in all enterococcal isolates. Aggregation substance proteins are a family of plasmid-encoded surface adhesins that mediate adhesion to molecules of the extracellular matrix and promote clumping, biofilm formation, and high-frequency transfer of plasmid DNA.[37] In animal models of IE, *E faecalis* strains overexpressing aggregation substance were found to have larger vegetations with increased bacterial loads compared with mutants lacking the gene.[38] Esp (enterococcal surface protein) and Esp_{fm} (its homologue in *E faecium*) have been implicated in biofilm formation and in the pathogenesis of IE.[39,40] This determinant is often found within a pathogenicity island that seems to be associated with hospital-acquired isolates.[39]

Another important subset of cell envelope–located virulence factors contains the WxL motif, a signature sequence that is conserved among the low G + C gram-positive bacteria and binds to peptidoglycan.[41] ElrA (enterococcal leucine-rich repeat-containing protein A) is one of multiple WxL proteins in *E faecalis* and is located in a polycistronic operon; previous characterizations of a homologue in *Listeria* spp. showed its involvement in inducing uptake of the bacteria into nonphagocytic cells.[42] Deletion of the *elrA* gene attenuated lethality in a mouse peritonitis model and decreased the strain's ability to infect macrophages and induce an interleukin-6–mediated inflammatory response. *In silico* analysis of the *E faecium* genome identified 6 genes encoding potential WxL-containing proteins. The genes are organized in 3 operons, termed *WxL* locus *A*, *B*, and *C*. Using electron microscopy and enzyme-linked immunosorbent assays, locus A and C were found to be antigenic and expressed on the cell surface at much higher levels in clinical strains (as opposed to community-associated lineages). In addition, WxL proteins from locus A were able to bind collagen and fibronectin and deletion of all 3 loci-attenuated virulence in a mixed infection rat endocarditis model.[43]

Glycolipids and polysaccharides are also important components of the enterococcal cell envelope. Lipoteichoic acid is an antigenic component of gram-positive cell walls, and antibodies directed against this epitope were shown to enhance opsonization and killing of enterococci by complement and leukocytes.[44] Some isolates of *E faecalis*, particularly members of hospital-associated clades, possess a capsular polysaccharide gene locus that allows the bacteria to synthesize a polysaccharide shield for the antigenic lipoteichoic acid, enabling evasion of antibody-mediated opsonization.[45] Other polysaccharides are found shown to be important in the production of biofilm, which mediates persistence on environmental surfaces and reduces the effectiveness of many antimicrobials. Enterococcal polysaccharide antigen is the product of a 16-gene locus named *epa* that produces a rhamnose-containing polysaccharide important for the formation of biofilm.[46] It is present in all *E faecalis*, and antibodies directed against this antigen can be found in most samples of sera from patients with deep-seated *E faecalis* infections.[47] In animal models, deletion of this locus from the laboratory strain *E faecalis* OG1RF led to attenuation in both a mouse peritonitis and murine urinary tract infection model.[48] In addition to polysaccharides, glycolipids play a role in enterococcal pathogenesis. Deficiency of the glycolipid α-diglucosyldiacylglycerol has been described to reduce both biofilm formation and adherence to host cells in *E faecalis,* and this defect was associated with faster sterilization of blood cultures compared with a wild type strain in mouse model of bacteremia.[49]

Secreted virulence factors also play a role in the pathogenesis of experimental enterococcal infection. Approximately 30% of *E faecalis* produce the toxin cytolysin

(Cyl), which is encoded by an 8-gene operon carried on plasmids or chromosomal pathogenicity islands.[50,51] The toxin is a pore-forming multimer of 2 subunits, $CylL_L$ and $CylL_S$, which are activated by CylA, a serine protease. The spectrum of activity includes other gram-positive organisms and erythrocytes of humans, horses, and rabbits but not sheep or cows (a specificity thought to be conferred by membrane levels of phosphatidylcholine). Clinical data from a retrospective series of 190 patients found that those with Cyl-producing isolates had a 5-fold increased risk of mortality at 3 weeks as compared to Cyl negative isolates.[52] However, a subsequent larger prospective study of 398 cases of *E faecalis* bacteremia failed to confirm this association.[53] Two enterococcal proteases, gelatinase (GelE) and extracellular serine protease, mediate virulence under the control of the Fsr quorum sensor, a 2-component signaling system that bears homology to *agr* (accessory gene regulator) in *S aureus*.[54] GelE is able to digest host matrix proteins and also activates autolysin, which promotes biofilm formation caused by cell lysis and release of DNA into the extracellular space.[55] In a rabbit model of endocarditis, GelE deletion mutants were associated with decreased vegetation colony counts and increased migration of inflammatory cells (such as neutrophils) to the site of infection.[56] Similarly, in a rat model of IE, *E faecalis* with a disruption of GelE was attenuated and had a lower IE induction rate than the wild type.[57] Finally, a variety of other proteins involved in stress response and neutralization of reactive oxygen species has been associated with enterococcal virulence, presumably allowing the bacteria to survive the oxidative burst of human polymorphonuclear leukocytes and macrophages.[58]

Antibiotic Resistance—Beyond Vancomycin

The flexibility of the enterococcal genetic repertoire has given rise to a variety of resistance strategies as new antimicrobial compounds are deployed. A comprehensive look at these strategies has recently been described in depth elsewhere.[59,60] This section discusses the mechanisms mediating resistance to newer agents used to treat serious VRE infections.

Daptomycin

Daptomycin (DAP) is a lipopeptide antibiotic with in vitro bactericidal activity against both *E faecalis* and *E faecium*, including VRE.[61] DAP consists of a cyclic polypeptide core with a lipid tail that facilitates insertion into the bacterial membrane in a calcium-dependent manner, a characteristic shared with cationic peptides of the innate immune response.[62] The precise mechanism by which the antibiotic mediates cell death is not known, but DAP-treated bacteria rapidly lose membrane physicochemical properties with disruption of the ionic gradient used to drive many biosynthetic pathways.[63] It is postulated that DAP forms a multimeric pore structure in the presence of phosphatidylglycerol, with 2 tetramers aligned opposite each other on the inner and outer leaflet of the membrane.[64] Enrichment of the membrane with cardiolipin (CL), with its 4 bulky fatty acyl chains, stabilizes the membrane to local perturbations caused by the DAP insertion. This CL-DAP interaction seems to decrease the ability of the antibiotic to transition from the outer to the inner leaflet, preventing tetramer alignment and pore formation. Both *E faecalis* and *E faecium* have adopted strategies to avoid DAP-mediated membrane damage; however, the underlying mechanism seems to be species specific.

In *E faecalis*, diversion of the antibiotic from critical membrane locations such as the dividing septum is associated with daptomycin resistance (DAP-R). This resistance seems to be associated with redistribution of CL microdomains, which are suggested to act as decoys to sequester the antibiotic away from important septal areas and might also protect the membrane at these locations (the diversion hypothesis).[65] Changes associated with this redistribution were described in isolates both in vitro and in vivo and implicated genes involved in the cell envelope stress response (the 3-component regulatory system, LiaFSR) and phospholipid synthesis.[66,67] In contrast, *E faecium* does not exhibit the characteristic redistribution of cardiolipin microdomains seen in *E faecalis*. Instead, *E faecium* seems to repel the DAP molecule from the cell surface, changes more akin to the proposed repulsion strategy for DAP resistance described in staphylococci. In this scenario, the positively charged calcium-DAP complex is repelled from the cell surface owing to electrostatic changes (as the cell envelope becomes more positively charged).[68] Interestingly, despite the mechanistic differences in DAP resistance between *E faecalis* and *E faecium*, similar genes in both species (including *liaFSR*, see below) are involved.

The *lia* operon (for Lipid II Interacting Antibiotics) belongs to a family of 3-component signaling systems composed of a sensor histidine kinase (LiaS), its cognate response regulator (LiaR), and a putative transmembrane negative regulator protein (LiaF). The LiaFSR system is conserved in all gram-positive organisms of clinical relevance.[69] In the presence of cell envelope stress, the system seems to be activated either by phosphorylation of LiaR (via LiaS) or by mutations in LiaR that mimic phosphorylation.[70] In *E faecalis*, a mutation in *liaF* (resulting in a deletion of an isoleucine residue at position 177) seemed to activate the system leading to an increase in DAP MIC from 1 to 4 μg/mL. More importantly, this single change in LiaF resulted in loss of DAP bactericidal activity in vitro.[71] This increase in MIC and loss of bactericidal activity at a supposedly susceptible MIC questions the current DAP breakpoint for enterococci (4 μg/mL, which is 4 times higher that than for *S aureus*). DAP-susceptible *E faecium* isolates with DAP MICs close to the susceptibility breakpoint (3–4 μg/mL) often harbor mutations associated with DAP resistance (mostly in *liaFSR*),[72] and, like *E faecalis*, these isolates are tolerant (ie, even at 5x, MIC DAP is not bactericidal) to DAP in vitro.[73] In a recent report, a patient with recalcitrant *E faecium* bacteremia treated with DAP experienced failure with this antibiotic, and the initial bloodstream isolate harbored alterations in LiaRS, supporting the notion that changes in LiaFSR are clinically associated with DAP therapeutic failure.[2] Of note, mutations associated with DAP resistance have been described in isolates from patients who had never been exposed to DAP, and it is postulated that, in addition to spread from other patients, naturally occurring antimicrobial peptides (like those produced by the innate immune system) may trigger cell envelope adaptive responses similar to those observed with DAP.[74,75]

The *yycFG* operon is involved in cell wall homeostasis and is highly conserved among the low G + C gram-positive bacteria. The *yycFG* operon is known to be active in modification of peptidoglycan synthesis, modulating autolysin expression (including *pcsB* in streptococci), and mutations in this operon are found in vancomycin-intermediate *S aureus* and in vancomycin-resistant *S aureus* strains.[76] In addition, the *yycFG* operon has also been found to have indirect effects on fatty acid metabolism and membrane fluidity. The histidine kinase (YycG) of this 2-component system from *S aureus* is found to associate with the lipid bilayer via a transmembrane domain and responds to stress via a conserved sensing sequence known as the PAS domain.[77,78] Upon activation, the sensor kinase auto phosphorylates before passing the phosphate to its cognate response regulator (YycF) to induce transcription of the regulon. This system was associated with DAP-R in a clinical strain-pair of *E faecium* that developed resistance to therapy.[79] Changes found in the PAS domain were postulated to alter the sensing activity of the YycFG system, although it is not understood precisely how this effect is mediated. Further, in a genomic survey of resistant isolates of *E faecium*, changes in the *yycFG* operon were the second most commonly found changes associated with DAP-R, with changes in LiaFSR encountered most often.[73]

The contribution of alterations in enzymes involved in phospholipid metabolism to the DAP-resistance phenotype has not been fully elucidated, but such changes seem to act synergistically with those related to the cell envelope stress response mediated by LiaFSR (or other regulatory systems, see earlier discussion). Alterations involving enzymes such as cardiolipin synthase (Cls) appear to occur after changes in LiaFSR, potentiating the resistance phenotype.[80] Davlieva and colleagues[81] recently found that substitutions in one of the phospholipase domains of Cls increased the catalytic activity of the enzyme, albeit marginally. Experimental data have also found that when additional copies of Cls harboring changes found in DAP-R strains were introduced in *trans* on a plasmid into the laboratory strain of *E faecalis* OG1RF, they increased the DAP MICs.[67] These findings suggest that Cls substitutions are associated with a gain in function of the enzyme; however, how this change is linked to redistribution of CL microdomains is unknown.

Oxazolidinones

Linezolid and the recently approved tedizolid are the clinically available oxazolidinones. These compounds bind to the A site of ribosomes and disrupt the docking of the aminoacyl-transfer RNA, inhibiting the delivery of peptides and the subsequent elongation of the polypeptide chain.[82,83] Tedizolid differs from linezolid in that the former harbors a fourth D-ring constituent and also has a hydroxymethyl group on the oxazolidinone ring. These modifications greatly increase the binding affinity of tedizolid for its target compared with linezolid, with MICs 4- to 8-fold lower than those of linezolid.[84] A common mechanism that mediates resistance to both compounds is target modification, namely mutations in the 23S rRNA. The substitutions G2505A and G2576U are the most common changes observed in resistant clinical isolates. As enterococci possess multiple copies of the 23S rRNA gene, the number of mutated alleles correlates directly with the level of resistance.[85] The number of mutated copies has been associated with the length of drug exposure and is accelerated by recombination of mutant alleles with wild type alleles within the enterococcal genome.[86] This gene-dosage effect was demonstrated in vitro with a laboratory strain of *E faecalis* and its recombination-deficient mutant exposed to linezolid. The time to first G2576U mutation was similar for both strains, as expected for a spontaneous mutation rate, but the wild type developed subsequent mutations 6 passages sooner than the recombination deficient strain, indicating interallelic recombination within the cell played a role in the propagation of resistant alleles.[87]

The ribosomal proteins L3 and L4, which are part of the peptidyl-transferase center, have also been associated with resistance to oxazolidinones in both enterococci and staphylococci.[88,89] It was found in *Streptococcus pneumoniae* that changes in L3 not only confer oxazolidinone resistance, but also seem to have compensatory effects to balance the fitness cost associated with mutations in the 23S rRNA.[90] In a genetic survey to characterize linezolid-resistant versus susceptible *Staphylococcus epidermidis* clinical isolates, mutations in 23S rRNA genes were always accompanied by changes in L3, a finding the authors speculated may be caused by its compensatory nature.[91] Further, whole genome sequencing of 21 *S epidermidis* bloodstream isolates resistant to linezolid found 19 isolates harbored coexisting mutations in 23S rRNA and L3.[92] Whether these findings are generalizable to other gram-positive cocci, including enterococci, is not known.

Two transmissible oxazolidinone resistance determinants have been described to date, *cfr* and *optrA*. Cfr (for chloramphenicol-florfenicol resistance) is a methylase that modifies the adenine nucleotide at position 2503 of the 23S rRNA. It has been found in clinical isolates of *E faecalis* and in other clinically relevant gram-positive organisms such as staphylococci.[93,94] It has been postulated that *cfr* has spread from animal strains to humans, as this gene seems to be widespread in bacterial isolates recovered from livestock (where florfenicol use is widespread) and is usually found on plasmids or other mobile genetic elements that can readily transfer between bacterial cells.[95] Of note, the binding of tedizolid to the ribosome does not seem to be affected by Cfr-mediated methylation of the 23S rRNA, and this compound retains activity in vitro against enterococcal strains that carry the *cfr* gene.[96] The *optrA* gene encodes a putative ABC transporter associated with elevated MICs to the oxazolidinones in the absence of known 23S rRNA mutations or the gene *cfr* and has been recently identified in both *E faecalis* and *E faecium* from animal and human sources.[97]

Lipoglycopeptides

The lipoglycopeptides are a class of compounds based on the modified glycopeptide core to which a lipophilic side chain has been added. Several lipoglycopeptides are now in clinical use and include telavancin, dalbavancin, and oritavancin. These compounds, like vancomycin, bind to peptidoglycan precursors ending in D-Ala-D-Ala. However, unlike vancomycin, they harbor hydrophobic moieties that permit insertion into the cell membrane, which is likely to affect membrane homeostasis in addition to their effect on cell wall synthesis.[98,99] This double mechanism of action increases the in vitro activity against enterococci. Despite the improvement in activity, telavancin and dalbavancin still exhibit high MICs against VRE (4–8 and 16–32 μg/mL, respectively, although several-fold lower than those of vancomycin) that preclude their use in clinical settings against these organisms.[100] Indeed, telavancin and dalbavancin do not bind peptidoglycan precursors ending in D-Ala-D-Lac.[100]

More promising is oritavancin, which demonstrates in vitro activity against VRE mediated by both *vanA* and *vanB* gene clusters. This enhanced activity seems to be derived from its mechanism of binding to peptidoglycan precursors. Nuclear magnetic resonance spectroscopy data have shown that oritavancin has more interactions with the peptidoglycan precursors than vancomycin, spanning the third amino acid of the pentadepsipeptides (L-lysine) and amino acids present in the cross bridge of both staphylococci and enterococci, mitigating the effect of the D-Ala to D-Lac substitution.[101] In addition, the lipophilic 4'-chlorobiphenylmethyl side chain has greater binding affinity for lipid II, both concentrating the antibiotic near the site of active synthesis and disrupting transglycosylation.[102] This improved binding to the cell wall assembly apparatus coupled with its membrane effects mediate potent bactericidal activity against both growing cells and biofilms. As this compound has recently entered clinical practice, the degree and mechanisms of resistance are not fully characterized. Arthur and colleagues[103] found that high-level expression of the *vanA* gene cluster and an increase in D-Lac-ending precursors was associated with 16-fold higher MICs to oritavancin. Additionally, expression of the *vanZ* gene of the same cluster increased oritavancin MIC by 4-fold, although the mechanism is not known.[103] Thus, the role of oritavancin in the treatment of VRE infections remains to be established.

Streptogramins

Streptogramins are a class of compounds that inhibit protein synthesis by targeting the 50S subunit of the bacterial ribosome. Quinupristin-dalfopristin (Q/D) is a mixture of pristinamycin derivatives, streptogramin A (dalfopristin) and B (quinupristin), which exhibit in vitro bactericidal activity owing to the synergism between the 2 compounds. The binding of dalfopristin has been reported to induce a conformational change in the ribosome that unmasks a high affinity binding site for quinupristin, leading to irreversible inhibition of the ribosome complex.[104] Importantly, Q/D is effective against *E faecium* but not *E faecalis,* as the latter possesses a chromosomal gene named *lsa* (for lincosamide and streptogramin A resistance), which provides all *E faecalis* with intrinsic resistance to streptogramin A and lincosamides (eg, clindamycin). This gene encodes a putative protein with an adenosine triphosphate–binding cassette motif of transporter proteins but not the transmembrane region that would be expected for an efflux pump, and its exact mechanism of action remains unknown.[105]

Reduced susceptibility to Q/D in *E faecium* is mediated by several mechanisms. First, modification of dalfopristin via the acetyltransferases VatD and VatE reduces binding affinity owing to steric hindrance, disrupting the bactericidal synergy of the 2 compounds.[106] Enzymatic cleavage of the ring structure of quinupristin by the lactonases VgbA and VgbB, originally described in staphylococci, leads to inactivation of the compound.[107] The *ermB* gene involved in macrolide resistance is a ribosomal methyltransferase, which also affects the binding of quinupristin. It confers a phenotype, MLS_B (for Macrolide, Lincosamide, Streptogramin B), that results in resistance to these antibiotics and is widespread in enterococci.[108] Dalfopristin, a streptogramin A, remains active in vitro in the presence of the *erm* gene, but as a bacteriostatic agent.[106] In vivo, the presence of *erm* may compromise the activity of Q/D, as this compound exhibited decreased activity against MLS_B enterococci in a rat endocarditis model.[109]

Efflux of Q/D from the bacterial cell also plays a role in resistance, and some resistant isolates of *E faecium* have been found to contain a mutation in the *eatA* gene (for Enterococcus ABC Transporter) that was shown to confer resistance to Q/D when introduced into susceptible strains.[110]

Glycylcyclines

Tigecycline is a glycylcycline antibiotic and a synthetic derivative of minocycline with activity against both gram-negative and gram-positive bacteria, including methicillin-resistant *S aureus* and VRE. Similar to the tetracycline class of antimicrobials, tigecycline binds to the 16S rRNA of the 30S subunit of the ribosome and inhibits the docking of the aminoacyl-transfer RNA.[111] Unlike the tetracycline class of antibiotics, tigecycline MICs are not affected by typical tetracycline resistance determinants such as efflux pumps (*tetK*, *tetL*) or ribosomal protection proteins (*tetO*, *tetM*, *tetS*).[112] Resistance in *E faecalis* has been described in 2 case reports of patients with intra-abdominal infections treated with tigecycline and in antimicrobial surveys.[113–115] Decreased susceptibility in *E faecium* was recently described in both clinical isolates and strains passaged in vitro. Using genomic analysis, a mutation in the S10 protein, a constituent of the 30S ribosomal subunit, was found in 4 of the 5 isolates with decreased susceptibility.[116] Analysis of resistant strains found that the changes in S10 are clustered in an extended loop of the protein that lies in close proximity to the tigecycline binding site of the 16S rRNA, possibly interfering with access to or binding of its target.[117] Even modest increases in the tigecycline MIC are problematic in serious infections such as bacteremia or endocarditis because of the low achievable serum concentration of this antibiotic.

COMBINED ARMS—THERAPEUTIC STRATEGIES FOR THE TREATMENT OF VANCOMYCIN-RESISTANT ENTEROCOCCI

Managing deep-seated enterococcal infections has always been a clinical challenge. Even with the advent of penicillin, clinicians noted that IE caused by enterococci was much more difficult to treat than that caused by streptococci, with mortality rates of 60% with penicillin monotherapy in IE.[10] The discovery that aminoglycosides, when added to β-lactams (or vancomycin), resulted in better patient outcomes and in vitro synergism with bactericidal activity, led to this combination becoming the standard of care for enterococcal IE with cure rates increasing to 88%.[118] However, the spread of resistance determinants, including high-level resistance to ampicillin, aminoglycosides, and vancomycin led to a new era in which the cell wall synthesis inhibitor/aminoglycoside combination is obsolete in serious VRE infections.

In this scenario, the only compound with current US Food and Drug Administration (FDA) approval for treatment of VRE infections is linezolid (Q/D previously carried such an indication, but this approval has since been withdrawn). However, linezolid has the limitation that it is a bacteriostatic antibiotic (less desirable in endovascular infections) and that important hematologic and neurologic toxicity may emerge during prolonged therapy (ie, in the case of IE). The only reliably in vitro bactericidal options against multidrug-resistant VRE are DAP and oritavancin, although neither carry an FDA indication for VRE. The latter antibiotic (oritavancin) is only approved for soft tissue infections, and its use (including the dosing regimen) for deep seated infections remains to be established. As a result, DAP (despite also lacking an indication for VRE) has become almost the go-to antibiotic for severe VRE infections, including IE and other endovascular infections. The reason is that DAP generally seems to retain bactericidal activity against susceptible VRE strains, at least in vitro, and the toxicity profile is favorable in infections that require prolonged administration.[119] However, robust clinical evidence to support the use of DAP over linezolid (an FDA-approved drug) is lacking. Recent meta-analyses have tried to address this issue and attempted to summarize the available clinical data on the treatment of VRE bacteremia with linezolid compared with DAP.[120–122] In the analysis conducted by Whang and colleagues,[120] there was no statistical difference in clinical success between DAP and linezolid, although there was a trend favoring the latter. In the studies by Balli and colleagues,[121] and Chuang and colleagues,[122] linezolid compared favorably with DAP with regard to infection-related mortality (odds ratio, 3.61; 95% confidence interval [CI], 1.42–9.2) and pooled all-cause mortality (odds ratio, 1.43; 95% CI, 1.09–1.86), respectively. In contrast, a recent observational study of the largest cohort of patients with VRE bacteremia yet published provided important insights into this question.[123] Using the Veterans Affairs medical record database, 644 patients with VRE bacteremia treated exclusively with DAP or linezolid were identified. In this study, linezolid was associated with a significantly higher risk of treatment failure compared with DAP (risk ratio, 1.15; 95% CI, 1.02–1.3), which was defined as a composite endpoint of 30-day all-cause mortality, microbiologic failure, and 60-day recurrence of VRE bacteremia. Although retrospective and observational in nature, the use of predefined clinically relevant outcomes and propensity analysis strengthen the latter study conclusions. Despite these efforts, the lack of prospective randomized, controlled trials precludes definitive conclusions regarding optimal therapy for VRE bacteremia.

An important consideration when using DAP is that the approved dose seems to be suboptimal for the treatment of severe VRE infections. In a pharmacokinetic/pharmacodynamic model using simulated endocardial vegetations, DAP used at both 6 mg/kg and 10 mg/kg resulted in bactericidal activity against VR *E faecium* at 8 hours, but by 72 hours, bacteria from vegetations treated with 6 mg/kg showed regrowth.[124] Further analysis of DAP at doses of 6, 8, 10, and 12 mg/kg against 2 clinical strains of *E faecium* and one of *E faecalis* in the same pharmacokinetic/pharmacodynamic model showed sustained reductions in colony count at 96 hours only in the groups receiving 10 and 12 mg/kg.[125] Importantly, the *E faecalis* strain exposed to 6 and

8 mg/kg, but not 12 mg/kg, developed reduced susceptibility to DAP with a change in MIC from 0.5 μg/mL to 16 μg/mL. These experiments strongly suggest that DAP concentrations at the site of infection are likely to be of paramount importance for activity, and the consideration of higher doses in serious infections is warranted.

Dual β-lactam Combinations

Recent data originating in Spain indicate that the combination of ampicillin and ceftriaxone is equivalent to the standard β-lactam plus aminoglycoside combination with less toxicity in *E faecalis* IE.[126] The use of the double β-lactam combination was first explored in vitro by showing that differential inhibition of the enterococcal PBPs by cefotaxime and amoxicillin resulted in synergistic bactericidal effect.[127] In a nonrandomized observational study of *E faecalis* IE involving 246 patients across multiple centers in Spain and Italy, there were no significant differences in mortality during treatment at 3-month follow-up or in relapses between standard combination therapy of β-lactam plus aminoglycosides versus the dual β-lactam combination.[126] However, this study was not designed to assess noninferiority, and further experience is needed before abandoning aminoglycosides for susceptible isolates. In vitro data suggest a similar rationale with the use of ampicillin plus imipenem in *E faecium*, as this combination was able to reduce bacterial counts by 5 log when compared against single agents in a rabbit model of endocarditis.[128] It was also successfully used to cure a patient with IE caused by *E faecalis* with high-level resistance to aminoglycosides (HLRAg).[129]

Daptomycin Combinations

Combinations of DAP plus β-lactams are among the most promising and potent combinations against multidrug-resistant enterococcal isolates. Observations that resistance to cationic antimicrobial peptides (such as DAP and the human cathelicidin LL-37) sensitized various organisms (including staphylococci and enterococci) to β-lactam antibiotics emerged from the use of the combination of DAP and β-lactams as salvage therapy for recalcitrant enterococcal infections.[130,131] Subsequent investigations found in vitro synergistic effects between DAP plus β-lactams including ampicillin, ceftaroline, and ertapenem.[132–134] There is a lack of concrete clinical data as to which agent provides the greatest benefit when added to the regimen, but case reports most commonly feature the use of ampicillin or ceftaroline. Of note, the genetic pathway to DAP resistance seems to influence the activity of the DAP/β-lactam combination. Two recent publications[73,135] testing the combination of DAP-ampicillin and DAP-ceftaroline in vitro suggested that the presence of *liaFSR* mutations is indicative of synergistic activity with these combinations. In contrast, synergism was not observed in isolates that harbor mutations in *yycFG* (another regulatory system involved in cell wall homeostasis). Experimental data in vitro have also shown that the concomitant use of DAP and β-lactams (in this case amoxicillin and ampicillin) delayed or prevented the emergence of DAP resistance in both *E faecalis* and *E faecium*.[136] This finding suggests that combination therapy with DAP plus β-lactams may play a role in preventing emergence of DAP resistance, prolonging the usefulness of this antibiotic in complicated VRE infections. Clinical data are urgently needed to support the use of such a combination against enterococci.

In addition to β-lactams, DAP has been combined with a variety of other antimicrobial agents in challenging VRE infections. DAP plus tigecycline has been evaluated both in vitro and in vivo against VRE, with synergism shown via the checkerboard method, in time-kill curves, and in a mouse-wound model of enterococcal infection.[137] There are several case reports of MDR *E faecium* IE also treated with this same combination.[138] The use of DAP plus aminoglycosides (gentamicin or streptomycin) in the absence of HLRAg has also been reported[139] and was found to be synergistic in an animal model of endocarditis.[140] There are some conflicting laboratory data on the use of rifampin with DAP. One study found synergy between DAP and rifampin in 75% of the 24 isolates of linezolid-resistant VRE tested by time-kill curve, without any evidence of antagonism.[141] A second study, however, found that rifampin antagonized the action of both DAP and linezolid in time-kill studies against VRE, although this was apparent only at a high inoculum (1 x 10^9 colony-forming units per milliliter).[142] Further studies are needed to determine the role of DAP plus rifampin combinations, although mutations in the *rpoB* gene conferring rifampin resistance have been associated with DAP nonsusceptibility in other gram-positive organisms.[143] Fosfomycin, an agent currently available only in an oral formulation in the United States, is concentrated in the urine and may have a role in providing synergy with DAP against MDR VRE urinary tract infections.[144]

Other Combinations

Linezolid is a bacteriostatic agent, and combination therapy to enhance activity or prevent resistance would be of benefit, especially in deep-seated infections such as IE, or if source control is not feasible. However, linezolid seems not to have a synergistic effect when added to other antibiotics. For example, one study found that 99.2% of 1380 organism-drug combinations failed to show synergism with linezolid using the checkerboard broth microdilution method.[145] The combination of linezolid plus imipenem or doxycycline did display synergism, but each in only one of 23 VRE isolates. A second in vitro analysis determined that linezolid plus either doxycycline or Q/D (tested isolates were sensitive to both) provided a synergistic effect.[146] Therefore, limited data suggest that linezolid combinations are unlikely to be reliable for treatment of deep-seated VRE infections.

Q/D showed clinical response in 68.8% of patients infected with VRE in a prospective, noncomparative, multicenter study in which no other effective agents were available.[147] A series of 56 patients with VRE infection at a major oncology center treated with Q/D plus minocycline showed a similar response rate (68%).[148] In vivo data from a rabbit model of endocarditis showed that Q/D combined with imipenem or levofloxacin resulted in greater reductions in vegetation colony counts than did Q/D alone.[149] The combination of Q/D plus doxycycline was shown in vitro via the checkerboard method to achieve synergism in 36% of *E faecium* clinical isolates.[150] Clinically, case reports of Q/D plus doxycycline and rifampin or Q/D plus high-dose ampicillin (24 g/d) have also been successful in treating enterococcal IE.[138]

Therapeutic Approach

A framework for approaching complicated enterococcal infections is presented in **Fig. 1**. For *E faecalis* isolates susceptible to ampicillin, this agent plus either an aminoglycoside (if no HLRAg) or ceftriaxone (HLRAg) is still the treatment of choice. For patients with penicillin allergy, vancomycin may be substituted for ampicillin if the isolate is not VRE, although vancomycin plus aminoglycosides may increase nephrotoxicity.

E faecium are often resistant to ampicillin, vancomycin, and the aminoglycosides (gentamicin and streptomycin). Thus, in severe infections caused by these organisms, DAP and linezolid are likely to be the drugs of choice. We favor DAP (particularly in recalcitrant and endovascular infections) over linezolid because of the inherent bactericidal activity of the former. An important caveat is that particular attention should be paid to both the DAP MIC of the isolate and the DAP dosage. In the case of MICs near the breakpoint (eg, 3–4 μg/mL), and for deep-seated infections (endovascular or

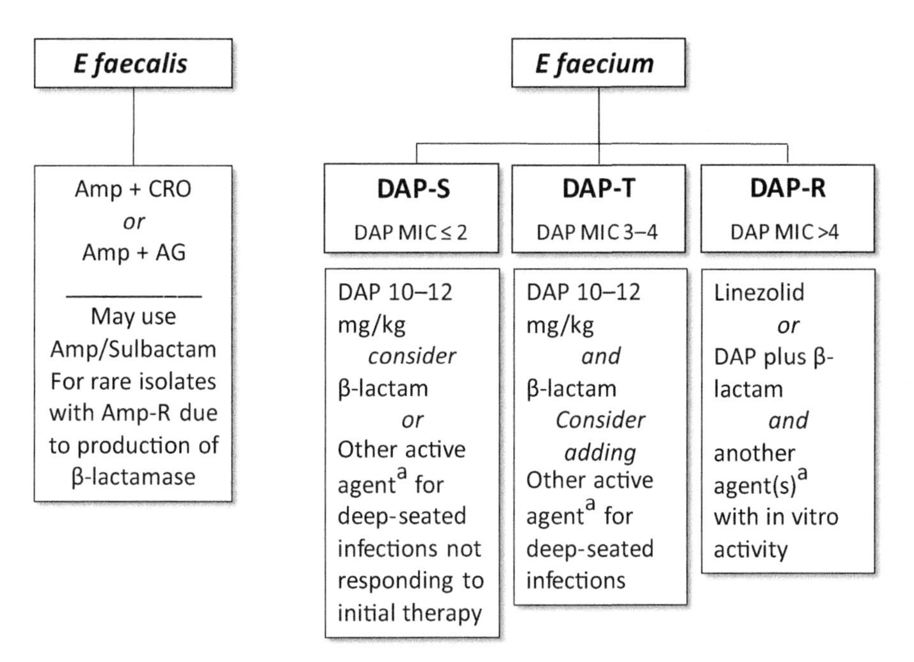

Fig. 1. Suggested approach to complicated VRE infections. For ampicillin-sensitive *E faecalis*, a combination of ampicillin plus either gentamicin or streptomycin, if no HLRAg, or ampicillin plus ceftriaxone if HLRAg is present, is the preferred therapy. For *E faecium*, the authors prefer DAP for its bactericidal action. For deep-seated infections or isolates with DAP MIC 3 to 4 μg/mL (DAP tolerant) we suggest the addition of a β-lactam for synergism. For isolates with DAP MIC greater than 4 linezolid may be used; however, if treating a deep-seated or endovascular infection, consider the addition of DAP plus a β-lactam or at least one other agent with demonstrated in vitro activity (eg, tigecycline, AG, or oritavancin). AG, aminoglycoside; Amp, ampicillin; Amp-R, ampicillin resistant; CRO, ceftriaxone; DAP-R daptomycin resistant; DAP-S, daptomycin susceptible; DAP-T, daptomycin tolerant.[a] Other active agents (confirm with in vitro testing): (1) tigecycline, (2) linezolid, (3) oritavancin, (4) Q/D (*E faecium* only), (5) AG (gentamicin or streptomycin) if no HLRAg.

source control not achievable), we favor the use of combination therapy (DAP plus ampicillin or ceftaroline), using DAP at high doses (10–12 mg/kg). Additional active agents may be required if bacteremia persists. In the case of resistance to both DAP and linezolid, DAP plus β-lactams, Q/D, or oritavancin (if available) may be considerations, in combination with at least 1 other active agent (eg, tigecycline).

SUMMARY—NEW MILLENNIUM, NEW STRATEGIES

Through the first decade of the 21st century, the emergence and spread of antibiotic resistance determinants is presenting a new clinical challenge to physicians. Antibiotics previously used for their reliability or low toxicity are being supplanted by newer agents active against MDR organisms; however, therapeutic decisions must be made at the bedside with limited clinical data available on how best to use these new drugs. Furthermore, the advances and expansion of the health care system have conspired to create an environment that allows the transmission and proliferation of MDR organisms such as VRE. There is concern that improper use of these new agents in this setting will compromise their effectiveness or possibly promote the development of resistance.

As we tackle the spread of resistant bacteria, we must be judicious in our use of antibiotics, the tools that make modern medicine possible. Novel combination therapies, with old agents and new, may help take back the health care setting from MDR organisms such as VRE. Strategies such as the use of daptomycin plus β-lactams offer the potential for synergism against a bacterium that is difficult to kill. Analogous to combination therapy in human immunodeficiency virus infection, such regimens may also delay or preclude the development of resistance in VRE infections. Clinical data are urgently needed to establish the effectiveness of such therapy and limit unnecessary increases in complexity of regimens, health care costs, and side effects associated with delivery.

REFERENCES

1. MacCallum W, Hastings T. A case of acute endocarditis caused by *Micrococcus zymogenes* (nov. spec.), with a description of the microorganism. J Exp Med 1899;4:521–34.
2. Munita JM, Mishra NN, Alvarez D, et al. Failure of high-dose daptomycin for bacteremia caused by daptomycin susceptible *Enterococcus faecium* harboring LiaSR substitutions. Clin Infect Dis 2014;59(9):1277–80.
3. Bradley C, Fraise A. Heat and chemical resistance of enterococci. J Hosp Infect 1996;34(3):191–6.
4. Sievert D, Ricks P, Edwards J, et al. Antimicrobial-resistant pathogens associated with healthcare-associated infections: summary of data reported to the National Healthcare Safety Network at the Centers for Disease Control and Prevention, 2009-2010. Infect Control Hosp Epidemiol 2013;34(1):1–14.
5. Galloway-Peña J, Roh JH, Latorre M, et al. Genomic and SNP analyses demonstrate a distant separation of the hospital and community-associated clades of *Enterococcus faecium*. PLoS One 2012;7(1):e30187.
6. Lebreton F, van Schaik W, McGuire AM, et al. Emergence of epidemic multidrug-resistant *Enterococcus faecium* from animal and commensal strains. MBio 2013;4:e00534–613.
7. Hegstad K, Mikalsen T, Coque TM, et al. Mobile genetic elements and their contribution to the emergence of antimicrobial resistant *Enterococcus faecalis* and *Enterococcus faecium*. Clin Microbiol Infect 2010;16(6):541–54.
8. Palmer K, Gilmore M. Multidrug-resistant enterococci lack CRISPR-cas. MBio 2010;1(4):e00227–310.
9. Horvath P, Barrangou R. CRISPR/Cas, the immune system of bacteria and archaea. Science 2010;327(5962):167–70.
10. Murray BE. The life and times of the Enterococcus. Clin Microbiol Rev 1990;3:46–65.
11. Grayson ML, Eliopoulos GM, Wennersten CB, et al. Increasing resistance to beta-lactam antibiotics among clinical isolates of *Enterococcus faecium*: a 22-year review at one institution. Antimicrob Agents Chemother 1991;35(11):2180–4.
12. Galloway-Peña JR, Nallapareddy SR, Arias CA, et al. Analysis of clonality and antibiotic resistance among early clinical isolates of *Enterococcus faecium* in the United States. J Infect Dis 2009;200(10):1566–73.
13. Sifaoui F, Arthur M, Rice L, et al. Role of penicillin-binding protein 5 in expression of ampicillin resistance and peptidoglycan structure in *Enterococcus faecium*. Antimicrob Agents Chemother 2001;45:2594–7.
14. Galloway-Pena JR, Rice LB, Murray BE. Analysis of PBP5 of early U.S. isolates of *Enterococcus faecium*: sequence variation alone does not explain

increasing ampicillin resistance over time. Antimicrob Agents Chemother 2011; 55:3272–7.

15. Reynolds PE. Structure, biochemistry and mechanism of action of glycopeptide antibiotics. Eur J Clin Microbiol Infect Dis 1989;8(11):943–50.
16. Arias CA, Courvalin P, Reynolds PE. vanC cluster of vancomycin-resistant *Enterococcus gallinarum* BM4174. Antimicrob Agents Chemother 2000;44:1660–6.
17. Courvalin P. Vancomycin resistance in gram-positive cocci. Clin Infect Dis 2006; 42:S25–34.
18. Carias LL, Rudin SD, Donskey CJ, et al. Genetic linkage and cotransfer of a novel, vanB-containing transposon (Tn5382) and a low-affinity penicillin-binding protein 5 gene in a clinical vancomycin-resistant *Enterococcus faecium* isolate. J Bacteriol 1998;180(17):4426–34.
19. Xu X, Lin D, Yan G, et al. *vanM*, a new glycopeptide resistance gene cluster found in *Enterococcus faecium*. Antimicrob Agents Chemother 2010;54:4643–7.
20. Guardabassi L, Agersø Y. Genes homologous to glycopeptide resistance vanA are widespread in soil microbial communities. FEMS Microbiol Lett 2006;259: 221–5.
21. Uttley AH, Collins CH, Naidoo J, et al. Vancomycin-resistant enterococci. Lancet 1988;1(8575–6):57–8.
22. Top J, Willems R, Bonten M. Emergence of CC17 *Enterococcus faecium*: from commensal to hospital adapted pathogen. FEMS Immunol Med Microbiol 2008;52(3):297–308.
23. Sydnor ER, Perl TM. Hospital epidemiology and infection control in acute-care settings. Clin Microbiol Rev 2011;24(1):141–73.
24. Drees M, Snydman DR, Schmid CH, et al. Prior environmental contamination increases the risk of acquisition of vancomycin-resistant enterococci. Clin Infect Dis 2008;46(5):678–85.
25. Snyder GM, D'Agata EM. Novel antimicrobial-resistant bacteria among patients requiring chronic hemodialysis. Curr Opin Nephrol Hypertens 2012;21(2):211–5.
26. Paterson DL, Muto CA, Ndirangu M, et al. Acquisition of rectal colonization by vancomycin-resistant Enterococcus among intensive care unit patients treated with piperacillin-tazobactam versus those receiving cefepime-containing antibiotic regimens. Antimicrob Agents Chemother 2008;52(2):465–9.
27. Brandl K, Plitas G, Mihu CN, et al. Vancomycin-resistant enterococci exploit antibiotic-induced innate immune deficits. Nature 2008;455(7214):804–7.
28. Cash H, Whitham C, Behrendt C, et al. Symbiotic bacteria direct expression of an intestinal bactericidal lectin. Science 2006;313(5790):1126–30.
29. Ubeda C, Taur Y, Jenq R, et al. Vancomycin-resistant Enterococcus domination of intestinal microbiota is enabled by antibiotic treatment in mice and precedes bloodstream invasion in humans. J Clin Invest 2010;120(12):4332–41.
30. Somarajan SR, Roh JH, Singh KV, et al. CcpA is important for growth and virulence of *Enterococcus faecium*. Infect Immun 2014;82(9):3580–7.
31. Singh KV, Nallapareddy SR, Sillanpää J, et al. Importance of the collagen adhesin ace in pathogenesis and protection against *Enterococcus faecalis* experimental endocarditis. PLoS Pathog 2010;6(1):e1000716.
32. Nallapareddy S, Singh K, Okhuysen P, et al. A functional collagen adhesin gene, acm, in clinical isolates of *Enterococcus faecium* correlates with the recent success of this emerging nosocomial pathogen. Infect Immun 2008;76:4110–9.
33. Montealegre MC, La Rosa SL, Roh JH, et al. The *Enterococcus faecalis* EbpA pilus protein: attenuation of expression, biofilm formation, and adherence to fibrinogen start with the rare initiation codon ATT. MBio 2015;6(3):e00467–515.

34. Nielsen H, Flores-Mireles A, Kau A, et al. Pilin and sortase residues critical for endocarditis- and biofilm-associated pilus biogenesis in *Enterococcus faecalis*. J Bacteriol 2013;195(19):4484–95.
35. Sillanpää J, Chang C, Singh K, et al. Contribution of individual Ebp Pilus subunits of *Enterococcus faecalis* OG1RF to pilus biogenesis, biofilm formation and urinary tract infection. PLoS One 2013;8(7):e68813.
36. Sillanpää J, Nallapareddy S, Singh K, et al. Characterizationof the ebp(fm) pilus encoding operon of *Enterococcus faecium* and its role in biofilm formation and virulence in a murine model of urinary tract infection. Virulence 2010;1(4):236–46.
37. Chuang-Smith O, Wells C, Henry-Stanley M, et al. Acceleration of *Enterococcus faecalis* biofilm formation by aggregation substance expression in an ex vivo model of cardiac valve colonization. PLoS One 2010;5(12):e15798.
38. Schlievert PM, Gahr PJ, Assimacopoulos AP, et al. Aggregation and binding substances enhance pathogenicity in rabbit models of *Enterococcus faecalis* endocarditis. Infect Immun 1998;66(1):218–23.
39. Heikens E, Bonten M, Willems R. Enterococcal surface protein Esp is important for biofilm formation of *Enterococcus faecium* E1162. J Bacteriol 2007;189:8233–40.
40. Heikens E, Singh KV, Jacques-Palaz KD, et al. Contribution of the enterococcal surface protein Esp to pathogenesis of *Enterococcus faecium* endocarditis. Microbes Infect 2011;13(14–15):1185–90.
41. Brinster S, Furlan S, Serror P. C-terminal WxL domain mediates cell wall binding in *Enterococcus faecalis* and other gram-positive bacteria. J Bacteriol 2007;189(4):1244–53.
42. Brinster S, Posteraro B, Bierne H, et al. Enterococcal leucine-rich repeat-containing protein involved in virulence and host inflammatory response. Infect Immun 2007;75(9):4463–71.
43. Galloway-Peña J, Liang X, Singh K, et al. The identification and functional characterization of WxL proteins from *Enterococcus faecium* reveal surface proteins involved in extracellular matrix interactions. J Bacteriol 2015;197(5):882–92.
44. Fabretti F, Theilacker C, Baldassarri L, et al. Alanine esters of enterococcal lipoteichoic acid play a role in biofilm formation and resistance to antimicrobial peptides. Infect Immun 2006;74(7):4164–71.
45. Thurlow L, Thomas V, Hancock L. Capsular polysaccharide production in *Enterococcus faecalis* and contribution of CpsF to capsule serospecificity. J Bacteriol 2009;191(20):6203–10.
46. Teng F, Jacques-Palaz K, Weinstock M, et al. Evidence that the enterococcal polysaccharide antigen gene (epa) cluster is widespread in *Enterococcus faecalis* and influences resistance to phagocytic killing of *E. faecalis*. Infect Immun 2002;70:2010–5.
47. Xu Y, Jiang L, Murray BE, et al. *Enterococcus faecalis* antigens in human infections. Infect Immun 1997;65(10):4207–15.
48. Singh KV, Lewis RJ, Murray BE. Importance of the epa locus of *Enterococcus faecalis* OG1RF in a mouse model of ascending urinary tract infection. J Infect Dis 2009;200(3):417–20.
49. Theilacker C, Sanchez-Carballo P, Toma I, et al. Glycolipids are involved in biofilm accumulation and prolonged bacteraemia in *Enterococcus faecalis*. Mol Microbiol 2009;71(4):1055–69.
50. Coque TM, Patterson JE, Steckelberg JM, et al. Incidence of hemolysin, gelatinase, and aggregation substance among enterococci isolated from patients

with endocarditis and other infections and from feces of hospitalized and community-based persons. J Infect Dis 1995;171(5):1223–9.
51. Van Tyne D, Martin M, Gilmore M. Structure, function, and biology of the *Enterococcus faecalis* cytolysin. Toxins (Basel) 2013;5(5):895–911.
52. Huycke M, Spiegel C, Gilmore M. Bacteremia caused by hemolytic, high-level gentamicin-resistant *Enterococcus faecalis*. Antimicrob Agents Chemother 1991; 35(8):1626–34.
53. Vergis E, Shankar N, Chow J, et al. Association between the presence of enterococcal virulence factors gelatinase, hemolysin, and enterococcal surface protein and mortality among patients with bacteremia due to *Enterococcus faecalis*. Clin Infect Dis 2002;35(5):570–5.
54. Qin X, Singh K, Weinstock G, et al. Effects of *Enterococcus faecalis fsr* genes on production of gelatinase and a serine protease and virulence. Infect Immun 2000;68(5):2579–86.
55. Thomas VC, Hiromasa Y, Harms N, et al. A fratricidal mechanism is responsible for eDNA release and contributes to biofilm development of *Enterococcus faecalis*. Mol Microbiol 2009;72(4):1022–36.
56. Thurlow LR, Thomas VC, Narayanan S, et al. Gelatinase contributes to the pathogenesis of endocarditis caused by *Enterococcus faecalis*. Infect Immun 2010; 78(11):4936–43.
57. Singh KV, Nallapareddy SR, Nannini EC, et al. Fsr-independent production of protease(s) may explain the lack of attenuation of an *Enterococcus faecalis fsr* mutant versus a *gelE-sprE* mutant in induction of endocarditis. Infect Immun 2005;73(8):4888–94.
58. Arias CA, Murray BE. The rise of the Enterococcus: beyond vancomycin resistance. Nat Rev Microbiol 2012;10(4):266–78.
59. Miller WR, Munita JM, Arias CA. Mechanisms of antibiotic resistance in enterococci. Expert Rev Anti Infect Ther 2014;12(10):1221–36.
60. Hollenbeck BL, Rice LB. Intrinsic and acquired resistance mechanisms in enterococcus. Virulence 2012;3(5):421–33.
61. Steenbergen JN, Alder J, Thorne GM, et al. Daptomycin: a lipopeptide antibiotic for the treatment of serious Gram-positive infections. J Antimicrob Chemother 2005;55:283–8.
62. Zanetti M. Cathelicidins, multifunctional peptides of the innate immunity. J Leukoc Biol 2004;75(1):39–48.
63. Silverman JA, Perlmutter NG, Shapiro HM. Correlation of daptomycin bactericidal activity and membrane depolarization in *Staphylococcus aureus*. Antimicrob Agents Chemother 2003;47(8):2538–44.
64. Zhang T, Muraih JK, Tishbi N, et al. Cardiolipin prevents membrane translocation and permeabilization by daptomycin. J Biol Chem 2014;289(17):11584–91.
65. Tran TT, Panesso D, Mishra NN, et al. Daptomycin-resistant *Enterococcus faecalis* diverts the antibiotic molecule from the division septum and remodels cell membrane phospholipids. MBio 2013;4:e00281–313.
66. Arias CA, Panesso D, McGrath DM, et al. Genetic basis for *in vivo* daptomycin resistance in Enterococci. N Engl J Med 2011;365:892–900.
67. Palmer KL, Daniel A, Hardy C, et al. Genetic basis for daptomycin resistance in Enterococci. Antimicrob Agents Chemother 2011;55:3345–56.
68. Jones T, Yeaman MR, Sakoulas G, et al. Failures in clinical treatment of *Staphylococcus aureus* infection with daptomycin are associated with alterations in surface charge, membrane phospholipid asymmetry, and drug binding. Antimicrob Agents Chemother 2008;52:269–78.

69. Jordan S, Junker A, Helmann J, et al. Regulation of LiaRS-dependent gene expression in *Bacillus subtilis*: identification of inhibitor proteins, regulator binding sites, and target genes of a conserved cell envelope stress-sensing two-component system. J Bacteriol 2006;188(14):5153–66.
70. Davlieva M, Shi Y, Leonard PG, et al. A variable DNA recognition site organization establishes the LiaR-mediated cell envelope stress response of enterococci to daptomycin. Nucleic Acids Res 2015;43(9):4758–73.
71. Munita JM, Tran TT, Diaz L, et al. A liaF codon deletion abolishes daptomycin bactericidal activity against vancomycin-resistant *Enterococcus faecalis*. Antimicrob Agents Chemother 2013;57:2831–3.
72. Munita J, Panesso D, Diaz L, et al. Correlation between mutations in liaFSR of *Enterococcus faecium* and MIC of daptomycin: revisiting daptomycin breakpoints. Antimicrob Agents Chemother 2012;56:4354–9.
73. Diaz L, Tran TT, Munita JM, et al. Whole-genome analyses of *Enterococcus faecium* isolates with diverse daptomycin MICs. Antimicrob Agents Chemother 2014;58:4527–34.
74. Fraher MH, Corcoran GD, Creagh S, et al. Daptomycin-resistant *Enterococcus faecium* in a patient with no prior exposure to daptomycin. J Hosp Infect 2007;65:376–8.
75. Lesho EP, Wortmann GW, Craft D, et al. De novo daptomycin nonsusceptibility in a clinical isolate. J Clin Microbiol 2006;44(2):673.
76. Dubrac S, Bisicchia P, Devine KM, et al. A matter of life and death: cell wall homeostasis and the WalKR (YycGF) essential signal transduction pathway. Mol Microbiol 2008;70:1307–22.
77. Türck M, Bierbaum G. Purification and activity testing of the full-length YycFGHI proteins of *Staphylococcus aureus*. PLoS One 2012;7(1):e30403.
78. Moglich A, Ayers RA, Moffat K. Structure and signaling mechanism of Per-ARNT-Sim domains. Structure 2009;17:1282–94.
79. Tran TT, Panesso D, Gao H, et al. Whole-genome analysis of a daptomycin-susceptible *Enterococcus faecium* strain and its daptomycin-resistant variant arising during therapy. Antimicrob Agents Chemother 2013;57(1):261–8.
80. Miller C, Kong J, Tran TT, et al. Adaptation of *Enterococcus faecalis* to daptomycin reveals an ordered progression to resistance. Antimicrob Agents Chemother 2013;57:5373–83.
81. Davlieva M, Zhang W, Arias CA, et al. Biochemical characterization of cardiolipin synthase mutations associated with daptomycin resistance in enterococci. Antimicrob Agents Chemother 2013;57(1):289–96.
82. Shinabarger D, Marotti K, Murray R, et al. Mechanism of action of oxazolidinones: effects of linezolid and eperezolid on translation reactions. Antimicrob Agents Chemother 1997;41:2132–6.
83. Leach K, Swaney S, Colca J, et al. The site of action of oxazolidinone antibiotics in living bacteria and in human mitochondria. Mol Cell 2007;26:393–402.
84. Shaw KJ, Poppe S, Schaadt R, et al. *In vitro* activity of TR-700, the antibacterial moiety of the prodrug TR-701, against linezolid-resistant strains. Antimicrob Agents Chemother 2008;52(12):4442–7.
85. Marshall S, Donskey C, Hutton-Thomas R, et al. Gene dosage and linezolid resistance in *Enterococcus faecium* and *Enterococcus faecalis*. Antimicrob Agents Chemother 2002;46:3334–6.
86. Bourgeois-Nicolaos N, Massias L, Couson B, et al. Dose dependence of emergence of resistance to linezolid in *Enterococcus faecalis in vivo*. J Infect Dis 2007;195:1480–8.

87. Boumghar-Bourtchaï L, Dhalluin A, Malbruny B, et al. Influence of recombination on development of mutational resistance to linezolid in *Enterococcus faecalis* JH2-2. Antimicrob Agents Chemother 2009;53(9):4007–9.
88. Locke JB, Hilgers M, Shaw KJ. Mutations in ribosomal protein L3 are associated with oxazolidinone resistance in staphylococci of clinical origin. Antimicrob Agents Chemother 2009;53(12):5275–8.
89. Chen H, Wu W, Ni M, et al. Linezolid-resistant clinical isolates of enterococci and *Staphylococcus cohnii* from a multicentre study in China: molecular epidemiology and resistance mechanisms. Int J Antimicrob Agents 2013;42(4):317–21.
90. Billal D, Feng J, Leprohon P, et al. Whole genome analysis of linezolid resistance in *Streptococcus pneumoniae* reveals resistance and compensatory mutations. BMC Genomics 2011;12:512.
91. Mendes R, Deshpande L, Costello A, et al. Molecular epidemiology of *Staphylococcus epidermidis* clinical isolates from U.S. hospitals. Antimicrob Agents Chemother 2012;56(9):4656–61.
92. Tewhey R, Gu B, Kelesidis T, et al. Mechanisms of linezolid resistance among coagulase-negative Staphylococci determined by whole-genome sequencing. MBio 2014;5(3):e00894–914.
93. Mendes R, Deshpande L, Castanheira M, et al. First report of cfr-mediated resistance to linezolid in human staphylococcal clinical isolates recovered in the United States. Antimicrob Agents Chemother 2008;52:2244–6.
94. Diaz L, Kiratisin P, Mendes R, et al. Transferable plasmid-mediated resistance to linezolid due to cfr in a human clinical isolate *of Enterococcus faecalis*. Antimicrob Agents Chemother 2012;56:3917–22.
95. Toh S, Xiong L, Arias C, et al. Acquisition of a natural resistance gene renders a clinical strain of methicillin-resistant *Staphylococcus aureus* resistant to the synthetic antibiotic linezolid. Mol Microbiol 2007;64:1506–14.
96. Rybak JM, Marx K, Martin CA. Early experience with tedizolid: clinical efficacy, pharmacodynamics, and resistance. Pharmacotherapy 2014;34(11):1198–208.
97. Wang Y, Lv Y, Cai J, et al. A novel gene, *optrA*, that confers transferable resistance to oxazolidinones and phenicols and its presence *in Enterococcus faecalis* and *Enterococcus faecium* of human and animal origin. J Antimicrob Chemother 2015;70(8):2182–90.
98. Higgins DL, Chang R, Debabov DV, et al. Telavancin, a multifunctional lipoglycopeptide, disrupts both cell wall synthesis and cell membrane integrity in methicillinresistant *Staphylococcus aureus*. Antimicrob Agents Chemother 2005; 49(3):1127–34.
99. Belley A, McKay G, Arhin F, et al. Oritavancin disrupts membrane integrity of *Staphylococcus aureus* and vancomycin-resistant Enterococci to effect rapid bacterial killing. Antimicrob Agents Chemother 2010;54(12):5369–71.
100. Zhanel G, Calic D, Schweizer F, et al. New lipoglycopeptides: a comparative review of dalbavancin, oritavancin and telavancin. Drugs 2010;70(7):859–86.
101. Kim S, Cegelski L, Stueber D, et al. Oritavancin exhibits dual mode of action to inhibit cell-wall biosynthesis in *Staphylococcus aureus*. J Mol Biol 2008;377(1): 281–93.
102. Zhanel G, Schweizer F, Karlowsky JA. Oritavancin: mechanism of action. Clin Infect Dis 2012;54(Suppl 3):S214–9.
103. Arthur M, Depardieu F, Reynolds P, et al. Moderate-level resistance to glycopeptide LY333328 mediated by genes of the *vanA* and *vanB* clusters in enterococci. Antimicrob Agents Chemother 1999;43(8):1875–80.

104. Canu A, Leclercq R. Overcoming bacterial resistance by dual target inhibition: the case of streptogramins. Curr Drug Targets Infect Disord 2001;1:215–25.
105. Singh K, Weinstock G, Murray B. An *Enterococcus faecalis* ABC homologue (Lsa) is required for the resistance of this species to clindamycin and quinupristin-dalfopristin. Antimicrob Agents Chemother 2002;46:1845–50.
106. Werner G, Klare I, Witte W. Molecular analysis of streptogramin resistance in enterococci. Int J Med Microbiol 2002;292:81–94.
107. Korczynska M, Mukhtar T, Wright G, et al. Structural basis for streptogramin B resistance in *Staphylococcus aureus* by virginiamycin B lyase. Proc Natl Acad Sci U S A 2007;104:10388–93.
108. Hershberger E, Donabedian S, Konstantinou K, et al. Quinupristin-dalfopristin resistance in gram-positive bacteria: mechanism of resistance and epidemiology. Clin Infect Dis 2004;38(1):92–8.
109. Fantin B, Leclercq R, Garry L, et al. Influence of inducible cross-resistance to macrolides, lincosamides, and streptogramin B-type antibiotics in *Enterococcus faecium* on activity of quinupristin-dalfopristin *in vitro* and in rabbits with experimental endocarditis. Antimicrob Agents Chemother 1997;41(5):931–5.
110. Isnard C, Malbruny B, Leclercq R, et al. Genetic basis for *in vitro* and *in vivo* resistance to lincosamides, streptogramins A, and pleuromutilins (LSAP phenotype) in *Enterococcus faecium*. Antimicrob Agents Chemother 2013;57:4463–9.
111. Bauer G, Berens C, Projan S, et al. Comparison of tetracycline and tigecycline binding to ribosomes mapped by dimethylsulphate and drug-directed Fe2+ cleavage of 16S rRNA. J Antimicrob Chemother 2004;53:592–9.
112. Fluit A, Florijn A, Verhoef J, et al. Presence of tetracycline resistance determinants and susceptibility to tigecycline and minocycline. Antimicrob Agents Chemother 2005;49:1636–8.
113. Werner G, Gfrörer S, Fleige C, et al. Tigecycline-resistant *Enterococcus faecalis* strain isolated from a German intensive care unit patient. J Antimicrob Chemother 2008;61:1182–3.
114. Cordina C, Hill R, Deshpande A, et al. Tigecycline-resistant *Enterococcus faecalis* associated with omeprazole use in a surgical patient. J Antimicrob Chemother 2012;67:1806–7.
115. Freitas AR, Novais C, Correia R, et al. Non-susceptibility to tigecycline in enterococci from hospitalised patients, food products and community sources. Int J Antimicrob Agents 2011;38(2):174–6.
116. Cattoir V, Isnard C, Cosquer T, et al. Genomic analysis of reduced susceptibility to tigecycline in *Enterococcus faecium*. Antimicrob Agents Chemother 2015;59(1):239–44.
117. Beabout K, Hammerstrom T, Perez A, et al. The ribosomal S10 protein is a general target for decreased tigecycline susceptibility. Antimicrob Agents Chemother 2015;59:5561–6.
118. Herzstein J, Ryan JL, Mangi RJ, et al. Optimal therapy for enterococcal endocarditis. Am J Med 1984;76(2):186–91.
119. Munita JM, Murray BE, Arias CA. Daptomycin for the treatment of bacteraemia due to vancomycin-resistant enterococci. Int J Antimicrob Agents 2014;44(5):387–95.
120. Whang DW, Miller LG, Partain NM, et al. Systematic review and meta-analysis of linezolid and daptomycin for treatment of vancomycin-resistant enterococcal bloodstream infections. Antimicrob Agents Chemother 2013;57(10):5013–8.

121. Balli EP, Venetis CA, Miyakis S. Systematic review and meta-analysis of linezolid versus daptomycin for treatment of vancomycin-resistant enterococcal bacteremia. Antimicrob Agents Chemother 2014;58(2):734–9.
122. Chuang YC, Wang JT, Lin HY, et al. Daptomycin versus linezolid for treatment of vancomycin-resistant enterococcal bacteremia: systematic review and meta-analysis. BMC Infect Dis 2014;14:687.
123. Britt NS, Potter EM, Patel N, et al. Comparison of the effectiveness and safety of linezolid and daptomycin in vancomycin-resistant enterococcal bloodstream infection: a national cohort study of veterans affairs patients. Clin Infect Dis 2015;61:871–8.
124. Akins RL, Rybak MJ. Bactericidal activities of two daptomycin regimens against clinical strains of glycopeptide intermediate-resistant *Staphylococcus aureus*, vancomycin-resistant *Enterococcus faecium*, and methicillin-resistant *Staphylococcus aureus* isolates in an *in vitro* pharmacodynamic model with simulated endocardial vegetations. Antimicrob Agents Chemother 2001;45(2):454–9.
125. Hall AD, Steed ME, Arias CA, et al. Evaluation of standard- and high-dose daptomycin versus linezolid against vancomycin-resistant Enterococcus isolates in an *in vitro* pharmacokinetic/pharmacodynamic model with simulated endocardial vegetations. Antimicrob Agents Chemother 2012;56(6):3174–80.
126. Fernández-Hidalgo N, Almirante B, Gavaldà J, et al. Ampicillin plus ceftriaxone is as effective as ampicillin plus gentamicin for treating *Enterococcus faecalis* infective endocarditis. Clin Infect Dis 2013;56:1261–8.
127. Mainardi JL, Gutmann L, Acar JF, et al. Synergistic effect of amoxicillin and cefotaxime against *Enterococcus faecalis*. Antimicrob Agents Chemother 1995; 39(9):1984–7.
128. Brandt CM, Rouse MS, Laue NW, et al. Effective treatment of multidrug-resistant enterococcal experimental endocarditis with combinations of cell wall-active agents. J Infect Dis 1996;173(4):909–13.
129. Antony SJ, Ladner J, Stratton CW, et al. High-level aminoglycoside-resistant enterococcus causing endocarditis successfully treated with a combination of ampicillin, imipenem and vancomycin. Scand J Infect Dis 1997;29(6):628–30.
130. Dhand A, Bayer A, Pogliano J, et al. Use of antistaphylococcal beta-lactams to increase daptomycin activity in eradicating persistent bacteremia due to methicillin-resistant *Staphylococcus aureus*: role of enhanced daptomycin binding. Clin Infect Dis 2011;53(2):158–63.
131. Sakoulas G, Bayer AS, Pogliano J, et al. Ampicillin enhances daptomycin- and cationic host defense peptide-mediated killing of ampicillin- and vancomycin-resistant *Enterococcus faecium*. Antimicrob Agents Chemother 2012;56(2): 838–44.
132. Sakoulas G, Rose W, Nonejuie P, et al. Ceftaroline restores daptomycin activity against daptomycin-nonsusceptible vancomycin-resistant *Enterococcus faecium*. Antimicrob Agents Chemother 2014;58(3):1494–500.
133. Hall Snyder A, Werth BJ, Barber KE, et al. Evaluation of the novel combination of daptomycin plus ceftriaxone against vancomycin-resistant enterococci in an *in vitro* pharmacokinetic/pharmacodynamic simulated endocardial vegetation model. J Antimicrob Chemother 2014;69(8):2148–54.
134. Smith JR, Barber KE, Raut A, et al. β-Lactams enhance daptomycin activity against vancomycin-resistant *Enterococcus faecalis* and *Enterococcus faecium* in *in vitro* pharmacokinetic/pharmacodynamic models. Antimicrob Agents Chemother 2015;59(5):2842–8.

135. Hindler JA, Wong-Beringer A, Charlton CL, et al. *In vitro* activity of daptomycin in combination with β-lactams, gentamicin, rifampin, and tigecycline against daptomycin-nonsusceptible enterococci. Antimicrob Agents Chemother 2015; 59(7):4279–88.
136. Entenza JM, Giddey M, Vouillamoz J, et al. *In vitro* prevention of the emergence of daptomycin resistance in *Staphylococcus aureus* and enterococci following combination with amoxicillin/clavulanic acid or ampicillin. Int J Antimicrob Agents 2010;35(5):451–6.
137. Silvestri C, Cirioni O, Arzeni D, et al. *In vitro* activity and *in vivo* efficacy of tigecycline alone and in combination with daptomycin and rifampin against Gram-positive cocci isolated from surgical wound infection. Eur J Clin Microbiol Infect Dis 2012;31(8):1759–64.
138. Munita JM, Arias CA, Murray BE. Enterococcal endocarditis: can we win the war? Curr Infect Dis Rep 2012;14(4):339–49.
139. Arias CA, Torres HA, Singh KV, et al. Failure of daptomycin monotherapy for endocarditis caused by an *Enterococcus faecium* strain with vancomycin-resistant and vancomycin-susceptible subpopulations and evidence of in vivo loss of the vanA gene cluster. Clin Infect Dis 2007;45(10):1343–6.
140. Caron F, Kitzis MD, Gutmann L, et al. Daptomycin or teicoplanin in combination with gentamicin for treatment of experimental endocarditis due to a highly glycopeptide-resistant isolate of *Enterococcus faecium*. Antimicrob Agents Chemother 1992;36(12):2611–6.
141. Pankey G, Ashcraft D, Patel N. *In vitro* synergy of daptomycin plus rifampin against *Enterococcus faecium* resistant to both linezolid and vancomycin. Antimicrob Agents Chemother 2005;49(12):5166–8.
142. Luther MK, Arvanitis M, Mylonakis E, et al. Activity of daptomycin or linezolid in combination with rifampin or gentamicin against biofilm-forming *Enterococcus faecalis* or *E. faecium* in an *in vitro* pharmacodynamic model using simulated endocardial vegetations and an *in vivo* survival assay using *Galleria mellonella* larvae. Antimicrob Agents Chemother 2014;58(8):4612–20.
143. Cui L, Isii T, Fukuda M, et al. An RpoB mutation confers dual heteroresistance to daptomycin and vancomycin in *Staphylococcus aureus*. Antimicrob Agents Chemother 2010;54(12):5222–33.
144. Descourouez JL, Jorgenson MR, Wergin JE, et al. Fosfomycin synergy *in vitro* with amoxicillin, daptomycin, and linezolid against vancomycin-resistant *Enterococcus faecium* from renal transplant patients with infected urinary stents. Antimicrob Agents Chemother 2013;57(3):1518–20.
145. Sweeney MT, Zurenko GE. *In vitro* activities of linezolid combined with other antimicrobial agents against Staphylococci, Enterococci, Pneumococci, and selected gram-negative organisms. Antimicrob Agents Chemother 2003;47(6):1902–6.
146. Allen GP, Cha R, Rybak MJ. *In vitro* activities of quinupristin-dalfopristin and cefepime, alone and in combination with various antimicrobials, against multidrug-resistant staphylococci and enterococci in an *in vitro* pharmacodynamic model. Antimicrob Agents Chemother 2002;46(8):2606–12.
147. Linden PK, Moellering RC Jr, Wood CA, et al. Treatment of vancomycin-resistant *Enterococcus faecium* infections with quinupristin/dalfopristin. Clin Infect Dis 2001;33(11):1816–23.
148. Raad I, Hachem R, Hanna H, et al. Treatment of vancomycin-resistant enterococcal infections in the immunocompromised host: quinupristin-dalfopristin in combination with minocycline. Antimicrob Agents Chemother 2001;45(11): 3202–4.

149. Pérez Salmerón J, Martínez García F, Roldán Conesa D, et al. Comparative study of treatment with quinupristin-dalfopristin alone or in combination with gentamicin, teicoplanin, imipenem or levofloxacin in experimental endocarditis due to a multidrug-resistant *Enterococcus faecium*. Rev Esp Quimioter 2006; 19(3):258–66.
150. Eliopoulos GM, Wennersten CB. Antimicrobial activity of quinupristin-dalfopristin combined with other antibiotics against vancomycin-resistant enterococci. Antimicrob Agents Chemother 2002;46(5):1319–24.

New β-Lactamase Inhibitors in the Clinic

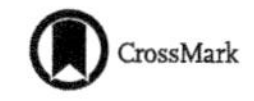

Krisztina M. Papp-Wallace, PhD[a,b], Robert A. Bonomo, MD[a,b,c,d,e,*]

KEYWORDS

- β- Lactamases • Inhibitor • Diazabicyclooctanones • Boronic acids • Sulfones
- Monobactams • Carbapenems • Metallo-beta-lactamases

KEY POINTS

- Obstacles in the development of beta-lactamase inhibitors.
- Diazabicyclooctanones, an ever expanding novel beta-lactamase inhibitor class.
- Boronic acids, non-hydrolyzable beta-lactamase inhibitors.
- Beta-lactams as beta-lactamase inhibitors.

WHAT TRANSPIRED? THE FALL OF THE CURRENT CLINICALLY AVAILABLE β-LACTAM-β-LACTAMASE INHIBITOR COMBINATIONS

In gram-negative pathogens, the production of β-lactamases, which hydrolyze β-lactam antibiotics, is a foremost threat in modern medicine.[1–3] β-Lactam-β-lactamase inhibitor combinations (ie, amoxillin-clavulanic acid, ampicillin-sulbactam, cefoperazone-sulbactam, piperacillin-tazobactam, and ticarcillin-clavulanic acid)

Funding: Research reported in this publication was supported in part by funds and/or facilities provided by the Cleveland Department of Veterans Affairs to K.M. Papp-Wallace and R.A. Bonomo, the Veterans Affairs Career Development Program to K.M. Papp-Wallace, the Veterans Affairs Merit Review Program Award 1I01BX002872 to K.M. Papp-Wallace and the Veterans Affairs Merit Review Program Award 1I01BX001974 to R.A. Bonomo and the Geriatric Research Education and Clinical Center VISN 10 to R.A. Bonomo. R.A. Bonomo is also supported by the Harrington Foundation, and The National Institute of Allergy and Infectious Diseases of the National Institutes of Health under Award Numbers R01 AI100560 and R01 AI063517 to R.A. Bonomo. The content is solely the responsibility of the authors and does not necessarily represent the official views of the National Institutes of Health.
[a] Research Service, Louis Stokes Cleveland Department of Veterans Affairs Medical Center, 10701 East Boulevard, Cleveland, OH 44106, USA; [b] Department of Medicine, Case Western Reserve University, 10900 Euclid Avenue, Cleveland, OH 44106, USA; [c] Department of Biochemistry, Case Western Reserve University, 10900 Euclid Avenue, Cleveland, OH 44106, USA; [d] Department of Pharmacology, Case Western Reserve University, 10900 Euclid Avenue, Cleveland, OH 44106, USA; [e] Department of Molecular Biology and Microbiology, Case Western Reserve University, 10900 Euclid Avenue, Cleveland, OH 44106, USA
* Corresponding author. Research Service, Louis Stokes Cleveland Department of Veterans Affairs Medical Center, 10701 East Boulevard, Cleveland, OH 44106.
E-mail address: robert.bonomo@va.gov

Infect Dis Clin N Am 30 (2016) 441–464
http://dx.doi.org/10.1016/j.idc.2016.02.007 id.theclinics.com
0891-5520/16/$ – see front matter

were first introduced into the clinic in the 1980s and 1990s (**Fig. 1**). The premise was simple: the β-lactamase inhibitor targeted the β-lactamase inactivating it, so that the partner β-lactam could inactivate the penicillin binding protein (PBP) target, eventually resulting in bacterial cell death. When introduced, these compounds were highly effective because they mimicked the β-lactam core. However, resistance to these inhibitors (ie, clavulanic acid, tazobactam, and sulbactam) is highly prevalent in the clinic because of 3 mechanisms. First, from the beginning, clavulanic acid, sulbactam, and tazobactam targeted only class A serine β-lactamases, thus 3 structurally and functionally distinct groups of β-lactamases: metallo-β-lactamases (MBLs) of class B, AmpCs serine β-lactamases belonging to class C, and OXAs serine β-lactamases of class D, were resistant to inhibition. Second, variants of previously susceptible class A β-lactamases (eg, TEM-1 and SHV-1) evolved single amino acid substitutions (eg, S130G, K234R) that resulted in these inhibitors failing to inactivate these enzymes.[3] These variant β-lactamases were considered inhibitor-resistant and are classically more resistant to clavulanic acid than the sulfone inhibitors, sulbactam and tazobactam. Last, new class A β-lactamases, such as KPC-2, evolved (circa 1996) with the ability to hydrolyze clavulanic acid, sulbactam, and tazobactam.[4] Thus, these first-generation β-lactam-β-lactamase inhibitor combinations are unable to inactivate most β-lactamases expressed by multi-drug-resistant (MDR) clinical isolates today.

MAJOR OBSTACLES IN β-LACTAMASE INHIBITOR DEVELOPMENT

The development of novel inhibitors is an arduous task because the mechanisms by which β-lactamases are resistant to clavulanic acid, tazobactam and/or sulbactam, are different even within the same class of β-lactamase. The mechanistic characterization of the greater than 1600 β-lactamases identified to date is critical to understanding how to evade their action (http://www.lahey.org/Studies/). In addition,

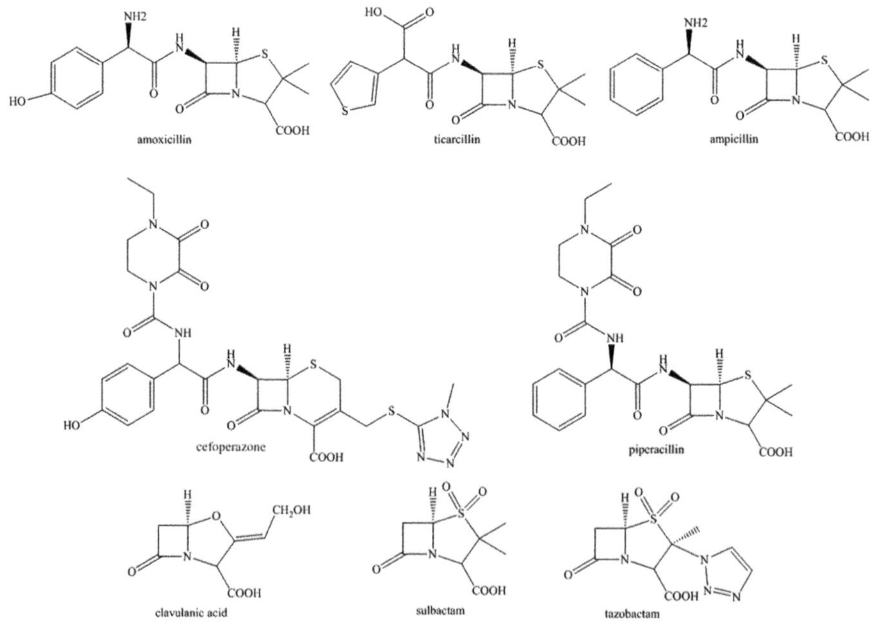

amoxicillin ticarcillin ampicillin cefoperazone piperacillin clavulanic acid sulbactam tazobactam

Fig. 1. β-Lactamase inhibitors of the past and their β-lactam partners.

most MDR Gram-negatives possess more than one of these β-lactamases. A large gap exists that needs to be filled by identifying novel β-lactamase inhibitors or modified β-lactams that can inhibit this ever-growing population of diverse enzymes. MBLs and OXA β-lactamases pose the most difficult challenge. MBLs possess a Zn^{2+}-mediated noncovalent mechanism, whereas the OXA class is extremely heterogeneous with over 500 different variants at the time this article was written. In addition, the β-lactam hydrolytic mechanism of OXAs is fundamentally different and not like the other serine-based mechanisms. As a result, a single "magic bullet" β-lactam-β-lactamase inhibitor combination that targets all clinically important β-lactamases (eg, KPC-2, OXA-24/40, AmpC, and NDM-1) seems unlikely. This debated question is addressed and the novel β-lactam-β-lactamase inhibitor combinations are discussed in this article.

CHANGING THE β-LACTAM PARTNER: CEFTOLOZANE-TAZOBACTAM

One technique to combat strains that carry multiple different classes of β-lactamases is to switch the β-lactam partner of a clinically available inhibitor. Cubist (now owned by Merck) used this approach with tazobactam when they paired tazobactam with the novel cephalosporin, ceftolozane (**Fig. 2** and **Table 1**). Ceftolozane-tazobactam was approved in December 2014 by the US Food and Drug Administration (FDA) for the treatment of complicated intra-abdominal infections (cIAIs) and complicated urinary tract infections (cUTIs). Ceftolozane-tazobactam will also be tested in clinical trials for ventilator-associated pneumonia, cystic fibrosis patients, and for diabetic lower limb infections (**Table 1**). What makes this combination successful? Ceftolozane is more stable against the AmpC β-lactamase than the predecessor β-lactam partners of tazobactam. AmpC possesses a low catalytic efficiency (k_{cat}/K_m) for ceftolozane.[5] Thus, ceftolozane inhibits PBPs and inhibitor-resistant TEMs and SHVs as well as AmpC (unlike tazobactam), allowing tazobactam to target class A serine β-lactamases (eg, TEM-1) and extended-spectrum beta-lactamases (ESBLs) (eg, CTX-M-15). In addition, ceftolozane works against some class D oxacillinases (eg, OXA-1).[6] Thus, the ceftolozane-tazobactam combination is able to target class A, C, and some class D β-lactamases; the major exception is carbapenemases. Ceftolozane or ceftolozane-tazobactam was demonstrated to be similarly effective or superior to other β-lactams in a variety (eg, lung, urinary tract, burn wound, sepsis, and thigh) of animal infection models using *Pseudomonas aeruginosa*, *Escherichia coli*, or *Klebsiella pneumoniae*[6]; therefore, its utility in the clinic may be expanded for other

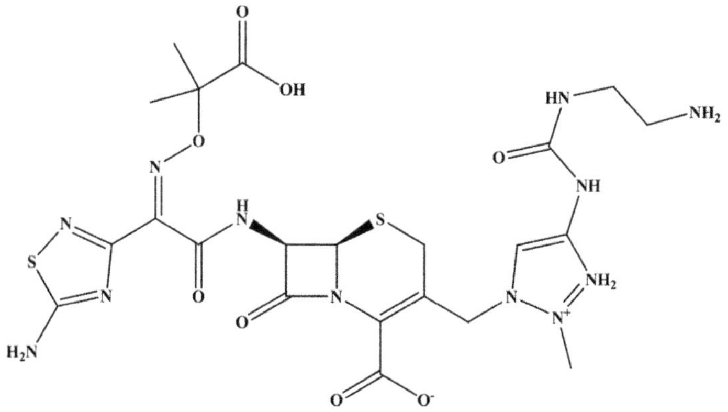

Fig. 2. Chemical structure of ceftolozane.

Table 1
New β-lactam-β-lactamase inhibitor combinations in the clinic or in development

Combination	Company	Type of β-Lactamase Inhibitor	Development Phase	US Clinical Trial Numbers (Status)
Ceftolozane-tazobactam	Merck/Cubist Pharmaceuticals	Sulfone	FDA approved (2014)	NCT01147640 (completed); NCT01853982 (terminated); NCT02266706, NCT02070757, and NCT02387372 (recruiting); NCT02508753 (completed); NCT02421120 (recruiting); NCT02620774 (not open yet)
Ceftazidime-avibactam	AstraZeneca Pharmaceuticals, Forest-Cerexa, Actavis-Allergan	DBO	FDA approved (2014)	NCT01395420, NCT01430910, NCT01290900, NCT01644643, NCT01291602, NCT00752219, NCT00690378, NCT01599806, NCT01595438, NCT01893346, NCT01499290, NCT01500239, NCT01920399, NCT01534247, and NCT01789528 (completed); NCT01726023 (completed); and NCT01808092 (completed); NCT02475733 and NCT02497781 (recruiting)
Ceftaroline-avibactam	AstraZeneca Pharmaceuticals, Forest-Cerexa, Actavis-Allergan	DBO	Phase 2	NCT01624246, NCT01281462, NCT01290900, and NCT01789528 (completed)
Aztreonam-avibactam	AstraZeneca Pharmaceuticals, Forest-Cerexa, Actavis-Allergan	DBO	Phase 1	NCT01689207 (completed); NCT02655419 (not open yet)
Imipenem-relebactam	Merck Sharp & Dohme Corporation	DBO	Phase 2	NCT01275170 and NCT01506271 (completed); and NCT01505634 (completed); NCT02452047 and NCT02493764 (recruiting)
RG6080 (formerly OP0595)	Meiji Seika Pharma Co, Ltd, Roche, and Fedora	DBO	Phase 1	NCT02134834 (completed)
Meropenem-RPX7009	Rempex Pharmaceuticals (The Medicines Company)	Boronate	Phase 3	NCT01897779, NCT02020434, and NCT02073812 (completed); and NTC02168946 and NCT02166476 (recruiting); NCT01751269 (completed); NCT02687906 (not open yet)
Biapenem-RPX7009	Rempex Pharmaceuticals (The Medicines Company)	Boronate	Phase 1	NCT01772836 (completed)
S-649266	Shionogi	Cephalosporin	Phase 2	NCT02321800 (recruiting); NCT02714595 (not open yet)

infections. In addition, clinical trials are recruiting pediatric patients to test ceftolozane-tazobactam (**Table 1**).

Laboratory-mediated selection of resistance (minimum inhibitory concentration [MIC] range of 4–8 mg/L) to ceftolozane-tazobactam was slower to occur than that with ceftazidime, meropenem, and ciprofloxacin in *P aeruginosa* PAO1; resistance was attributed to global pleiotrophic changes.[7] Higher levels of ceftolozane-tazobactam resistance (MIC range of 32–128 mg/L) were obtained only with a Δ*mutS* strain of PAO1; in these resistant strains, mutations were identified in bla_{ampC} and the bla_{ampC} regulatory pathway. Since the writing of this article, additional amino acid substitutions in the AmpC from *Pseudomonas* were found to confer resistance to ceftolozane-tazobactam.[8]

DIAZABICYCLOOCTANONES, THE "FUTURE" OF β-LACTAMASE INHIBITOR MEDICINAL CHEMISTRY

DBOs are synthetic non-β-lactam-based β-lactamase inhibitors that were discovered in the early 2000s. Over a period of 15 years, this class of compounds has expanded almost exponentially with most modifications occurring at the C2 side chain (**Fig. 3**). Most studies published to date indicate that DBOs possess class A and class C activity with minor class D activity. More recently, the DBOs, FPI-1465 and RG6080 (formerly, OP0595), showcased at the 2013 and 2014 Interscience Conference on Antimicrobial Agents and Chemotherapy (ICAAC) meetings, and WCK 5153 and WO2013/030735, claim activity against PBPs as well. Many pharmaceutical companies (eg, Actavis-Allergan [formerly Forest-Cerexa], AstraZeneca, Fedora Pharmaceuticals, Meiji Seika Pharmaceuticals, Merck [formerly Cubist], Naeja Pharmaceuticals, Roche, and Wockhardt) are developing DBO derivatives (see **Fig. 3**).

AVIBACTAM, THE "PIONEER" DIAZABICYCLOOCTANONE IN THE CLINIC

In December 2014, avibactam was the first DBO to be approved by the FDA in combination with ceftazidime for the treatment of cUTIs and cIAIs; currently the combination is being tested in the pediatric population (see **Fig. 3** and **Table 1**). Thus, the microbiological, pharmacologic, and biochemical characteristics of avibactam are the most known and are discussed in more detail than the other DBOs. Depending on the partner β-lactam (eg, ceftazidime, ceftaroline, aztreonam, cefepime, or imipenem), β-lactam-avibactam combinations have the potential to be highly effective against many MDR gram-negative pathogens, including Enterobacteriaceae and *P aeruginosa*, producing class A, B, C, and some D β-lactamases.[1] Avibactam has been studied primarily with 2 partner cephalosporins, ceftazidime and ceftaroline; these combinations target Gram-negatives expressing class A, C, and some D β-lactamases (see **Fig. 3** and **Table 1**). However, partnership with aztreonam would expand the spectrum of activity to include class B MBLs, because aztreonam is not hydrolyzed by MBLs (see **Fig. 5** and **Table 1**). Imipenem-avibactam and cefepime-avibactam or aztreonam-avibactam and ceftaroline-avibactam are effective against *E coli* and *K pneumoniae* carrying $bla_{OXA\text{-}48}$, respectively, but not *Acinetobacter baumannii* producing bla_{OXA}s.[9–12] Avibactam is restores susceptibility to ceftazidime when tested against clinical isolates of Enterobacteriaceae possessing porin and outer membrane permeability defects.[13]

Avibactam forms a stable carbamyl-adduct with serine β-lactamases that is reversible through recyclization of the 5-membered urea ring.[14] Thus far, decarbamylation-hydrolysis of avibactam was only observed after 24 hours with class A β-lactamase, KPC-2.[15] Formation of the carbamyl-enzyme complex, represented by the kinetic

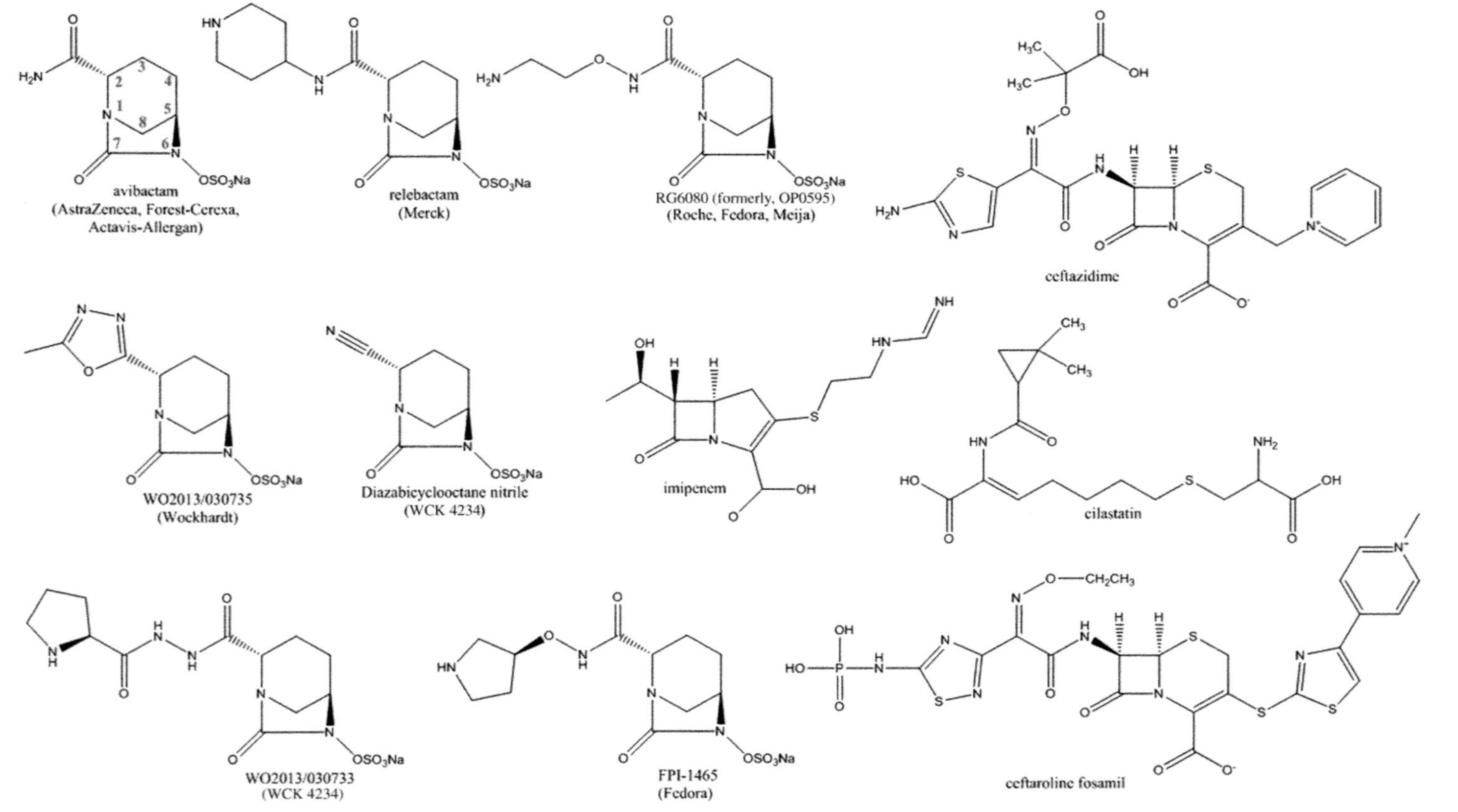

Fig. 3. DBOs and DBO β-lactam partners.

value, k_2/K and recyclization-decarbamylation to reform active avibactam, denoted by a k_{off} value differs for the various classes of serine β-lactamases. These kinetic parameters translate directly to efficacy within bacterial cells; thus, an ideal DBO is one that possesses a high k_2/K value and low k_{off} value. The tested class A and C β-lactamases (with the exception of the class A β-lactamase BlaC from *Mycobacterium tuberculosis*) acylate rapidly with high k_2/K values (range: 10^4 to 10^6 $M^{-1}s^{-1}$) and recyclize slowly with low k_{off} values (range: 10^{-3} to 10^{-4} s^{-1}).[15,16] Conversely, BlaC and class D β-lactamases are slow to acylate with low k_2/K values in the range of 10^1 to 10^3 $M^{-1}s^{-1}$, but once acylated, recyclization is very slow with k_{off} values of 10^{-5} to 10^{-6} s^{-1}. X-ray crystallography as well as molecular modeling revealed that avibactam adopts very similar active site conformations in class A, C, and D β-lactamases.[16–20]

Recent crystal structures and biochemical analysis with avibactam and OXA-24/40 and OXA-48 were conducted and provided some insights into why select class D β-lactamases are inhibited, whereas others are not.[17,19] OXA-24/40's k_2/K value is much lower than OXA-48's, whereas the k_{off} values are very similar. The crystal structures revealed that the binding pocket for avibactam in class D β-lactamases is more hydrophobic with fewer polar residues present, thus potentially affecting binding and acylation. In addition, OXA-24/40 possesses additional hydrophobic moieties (eg, hydrophobic bridge between Y112 and M223), whereas OXA-48 possesses polar residues (eg, T213, R214, and D101) that could aid in Michaelis-complex formation with avibactam. Slow recyclization was suggested to occur because of a decarboxylated Lys84/73.[17,19]

RESISTANCE TO β-LACTAM-AVIBACTAM COMBINATIONS

Selection via passaging of *E coli* producing *bla*CTX-M-15 and *E cloacae* with de-repressed *bla*$_{AmpC}$ on ceftaroline-avibactam identified strains with elevated ceftaroline-avibactam MICs; however, most of the mutations were unstable.[21] *E coli* producing CTX-M-15 Lys237Gln variant conferred resistance with the cost of ESBL activity. Selected-resistant *E cloacae* possessed Ω loop deletions within AmpC as well as porin loss. A similar approach was conducted using *P aeruginosa* with de-repressed *bla*$_{AmpC}$ with ceftazidime-avibactam.[22] Ceftazidime-avibactam–resistant variants possessed MICs from 64 to 256 mg/L as a result of deletions in the Ω loop of the AmpC. Mechanistic analyses revealed that the AmpC variants were less susceptible to avibactam inactivation and possessed improved ceftazidime kinetics.

Resistance to ceftazidime-avibactam was observed in a panel of clinical isolates of *P aeruginosa*.[23] The mechanism of resistance was dissected by sequencing *bla*$_{AmpC}$, the genes in the *bla*$_{AmpC}$ regulon, *pbp*s, and *oprD*, measuring efflux pump expression, and combination antibiotic therapy with ceftazidime-avibactam. Using these methods, membrane permeability and drug efflux were found to be the most important factor influencing ceftazidime-avibactam resistance in these isolates. Resistance to ceftazidime-avibactam was overcome with ceftazidime-avibactam/fosfomycin; this combination targets PBPs, β-lactamases, and MurA, and UDP-*N*-acetylglucosamine-3-enolpyruvyltransferase, which is involved in peptidoglycan synthesis.

In a panel of clinical isolates of *E coli* producing *bla*$_{NDM-1}$, resistance to aztreonam-avibactam was detected.[24] Aztreonam was still able to inhibit the β-lactamases; however, a 4-amino-acid insertion was identified in PBP3.

Variant β-lactamases with single amino acid substitutions in residues that typically result in inhibitor resistance (ie, 69, 130, 234, 220/244, and 276) and ceftazidime-resistance (ie, 164, 167, 169, and 179) in clinical isolates were tested in SHV-1 and KPC-2 β-lactamase isogenic *E coli* strain backgrounds with β-lactam-avibactam combinations.[25–27] The S130G, K234R, and R220M (KPC-2)/R244S (SHV-1) substitutions in the SHV-1 and KPC-2 backgrounds resulted in elevated MICs to ampicillin-avibactam when expressed in *E coli*.[25,27] The S130G variants of SHV-1 and KPC-2 were found to have severely compromised k_2/K values ($\sim$1 $M^{-1}s^{-1}$), thus avibactam failed to inactivate these variants. S130 is an important residue for avibactam acylation. The resistance mechanisms of the K234R and R220M/R244S variants remain to be defined. The R164A, R164P, D179A, D179Q, and D179N substitutions in KPC-2 resulted in increased ceftazidime-avibactam MICs.[26] Loss of susceptibility to ceftazidime-avibactam is thought to be due to enhanced ceftazidime kinetics of the variants because avibactam was still able to inactivate the R164A and D179N variants. In another study, selection of Enterobacteriaceae producing blaKPC for resistance to ceftazidime-avibactam resulted in the identification of KPC variants with D179Y amino acid substitutions.[28] Resistance to a β-lactam-β-lactamase inhibitor combination due to resistance to the partner β-lactam is a very intriguing observation. The choice of a β-lactam partner is critical, as described above with ceftolozane-tazobactam.

During the writing of this manuscript, the first clinical observation of ceftazidime-avibactam resistance was reported.[29] The resistance was observed in Klebsiella pneumoniae expressing blaKPC-3 and mechanism of resistance is unclear.

DIAZABICYCLOOCTANONES, RELEBACTAM AND OP0595, ON THE HORIZON

Relebactam partnered with imipenem-cilastatin demonstrates a similar spectrum of activity as avibactam, thus lacking activity against MBLs and most OXAs (see **Fig. 3** and **Table 1**).[30–32] RG6080 (formerly OP0595) not only is an inhibitor of class A and C β-lactamases but also inhibits PBP-2 of Enterobacteriaceae (see **Fig. 3** and **Table 1**).[33,34] Thus, RG6080 is unique compared with avibactam and relebactam, because it does not need a β-lactam partner for antimicrobial activity. In addition, there is evidence that RG6080 acts to enhance the activity of β-lactams.[35]

DIAZABICYCLOOCTANONES IN PRECLINICAL DEVELOPMENT

FPI-1465 when combined with aztreonam and ceftazidime possesses activity against Enterobacteriaceae containing ESBLs and class A, B, and D carbapenemases (see **Fig. 3**; **Table 2**).[36,37] In addition, FPI-1465 is also active against PBPs (ie, PBP2) from *E coli* and *P aeruginosa*.[38]

Wockhardt, Ltd has 3 DBOs in the pipeline: WCK 4234, WO2013/030735, and WCK 5153 (see **Fig. 3** and **Table 2**).[39] The WCK 4234 combined with meropenem demonstrates activity against oxacillinase-producing strains of *A baumannii*.[39] WO2013/030735 and WCK 5153 possess antibacterial activity against *P aeruginosa* and *E coli*.

During the publication process of this article, Merck (formerly Cubist) published work with another DBO, CB-618.[40] CB-618 tested in combination with meropenem displays activity against clinical isolates of Enterobacteriaceae expressing the KPC-2, KPC-3, FOX-5, OXA-48, SHV-11, SHV-27, and/or TEM-1 beta-lactamases.

BORONIC ACID β-LACTAMASE INHIBITORS ARE MAKING GREAT STRIDES

In the late 1970s, boronic acids were recognized as inhibitors of serine β-lactamases in vitro.[41] Boron forms a reversible bond with the β-lactamase.[42] Boronic acids serve as competitive inhibitors and were not shown to be hydrolyzed by any β-lactamase to date. Historically, despite good affinities for many class A and C serine β-lactamases, boronic acids failed to make it into clinical development, but the tides are changing.

A novel cyclic boronic acid–based β-lactamase inhibitor, RPX7009, is in phase 3 clinical trials in combination with meropenem (RPX2014) under the name Carbavance; in addition, clinical trials in pediatric patients are in the works (**Fig. 4**; see **Table 1**).[43] Initially, development began with biapenem (RPX2003) (see **Fig. 4** and **Table 1**). Biapenem-RPX7009 and meropenem-RPX7009 are most effective against Enterobacteriaceae producing class A carbapenemases and demonstrated against class A ESBLs and AmpC; impermeability had a negative impact on the activity of carbapenem-RPX7009 combinations.[44,45] In addition, biapenem-RPX7009 was not effective against Enterobacteriaceae expressing MBLs or OXA-48.[44]

RPX7009 did not potentiate the activity of carbapenems against nonfermenters *P aeruginosa* and *A baumannii*.[45] RPX7009 also did not increase the activity of biapenem against anaerobes.[46] A neutropenic lung model of infection in mice with *K pneumoniae* producing bla_{KPC-2} revealed that RPX-7009 reduced colony forming units (CFUs) by 2 logs in combination with biapenem and meropenem compared with the carbapenem alone.[43]

BORONIC ACIDS IN PRECLINICAL DEVELOPMENT

In addition, several boronic acid inhibitors in preclinical development showed promise because they reduced MICs or were successful in animal models of infection. Benzo(b)thiophene-2-boronic acids combined with ceftazidime are effective against Enterobacteriaceae and *P aeruginosa* (see **Fig. 4** and **Table 2**).[47] S02030, a novel boronic acid possessing thiophene and triazole carboxylate side chains demonstrates activity against Enterobacteriaceae carrying blaKPCs with a k2/K value (1.2 ± 0.2 × 10(4) M(-1) s(-1)) comparable to avibactam (**Fig. 4** and **Table 2**).[48] TheraBor Pharmaceuticals and the Regents of the University of California developed and patented (patent WO2013/056079) several sulfonamide boronates (eg, CR161) that were shown to reduce ceftazidime MICs against Enterobacteriaceae and *P aeruginosa* (see **Fig. 4** and **Table 2**).[16,49] Moreover, when mice were infected intraperitoneally with *E coli* overexpressing AmpC, after 120 hours, the mice treated with CR161 combined with cefotaxime possessed a 65% survival compared with cefotaxime alone at 15%. VenatoRx Pharmaceuticals also patented a series of cyclic boronic acids, 3,4-dihydro-2H-benzo[e][1,2]oxaborinine-8-carboxylic acids (US 8,912,169 B2), and a set of novel α-aminoboronic acids (US 20100120715 A1) (see **Fig. 4** and **Table 2**). Select cyclic boronates combined with either ceftazidime or meropenem demonstrated activity against *E cloacae*, *K pneumoniae* with bla_{KPC-3}, *P aeruginosa* with bla_{VIM-2}, and *K pneumoniae* with bla_{KPC-2} and bla_{VIM-4} and inhibited SHV-5, KPC-2, VIM-2, AmpC, and OXA-1 with concentration of inhibitor at which 50% inhibition of substrate hydrolysis is observed (IC_{50}) values <1 μM. Select α-aminoboronic acids combined with ceftazidime possessed activity against *E coli* with bla_{SHV-5}, *K pneumoniae* with $bla_{CTX-M-15}$, *E cloacae* with bla_{P99}, and *K pneumoniae* with bla_{KPC-2} and inhibited SHV-5, CTX-M-15, P99, and KPC-2, with IC_{50} values <0.1 μM. Rempex, a subsidiary of The Medicines Company, also patented another group of cyclic boronic acids, 3,4-dihydro-2H-benzo[e][1,2]oxaborinine-8-carboxylic acids (see **Fig. 4** and **Table 2**) (WO2014/107536 A1). Select compounds in this class have K_i values of less than 1 μM against SHV-12, TEM-10, CTX-M-14, KPC-2, P99, CMY-2, OXA-48, VIM-1, and NDM-1, and when combined with carbapenems, demonstrated MICs less than 1 mg/L for Enterobacteriaceae producing bla_{NDM-1}, bla_{VIM-1}, and bla_{KPC-2} and even *A baumannii* expressing bla_{NDM-1}.

Table 2
Promising new β-lactams or β-lactamase inhibitors in preclinical development

β-Lactamase Inhibitor Name	Partner β-Lactam	Company	Type of β-Lactamase Inhibitor
FPI-1465	Aztreonam or ceftazidime	Fedora	DBO (also inhibits PBP activity)
WCK 4234	Meropenem	Wockhardt, Ltd	DBO
WO2013/030735	Not necessary?	Wockhardt, Ltd	DBO (also inhibits PBP activity)
WCK 5153	Not necessary?	Wockhardt, Ltd	DBO (also inhibits PBP activity)
Benzo(b)thiophene-2-boronic acid	Ceftazidime	Therabor and Regents of the University of California	Boronate
Sulfonamide boronates (CR161, compound 4, and compound 9)	Ceftazidime or cefotaxime	Therabor and Regents of the University of California	Boronate
S02030	Cefepime	Case Western Reserve University and Università degli Studi di Modena e Reggio Emilia	Boronate
3,4-dihydro-2H-benzo[e][1,2] oxaborinine-8-carboxylic acids	Ceftazidime or meropenem	VenatoRx Pharmaceuticals	Boronate
α-Aminoboronic acids	Ceftazidime	VenatoRx Pharmaceuticals	Boronate
3,4-Dihydro-2H-benzo[e][1,2] oxaborinine-8-carboxylic acids	Carbapenem	Rempex Pharmaceuticals (The Medicines Company)	Boronate
AA101	Cefepime	Allecra Therapeutics	Sulfone

Sulfone derivatives	Meropenem or imipenem	Orchid Pharmaceuticals	Sulfone
Sulfone derivatives	Meropenem or imipenem	Dr John D. Buynak (Southern Methodist University)	Sulfone
Clavam derivatives	Ceftazidime	Nabriva Therapeutics	Clavam
MG96077	Imipenem	Mirati Therapeutics	Phosphonate
BAL30072	Meropenem or no β-lactam required	Basilea Pharmaceuticals	Siderophore monobactam
BAL30376 (BAL19764, BAL29880, & clavulanic acid)	No β-lactam required	Basilea Pharmaceuticals	Siderophore monobactam, bridged monobactam, and a clavam
MK-8712	Imipenem	Merck Sharp & Dohme Corporation	Bridged monobactam
Siderophore monobactams	Aztreonam or meropenem	Pfizer	Siderophore monobactam
Syn2190	Ceftazidime	Taiho Pharmaceuticals Co	Siderophore monobactam
3′-Thiobenzoyl cephalosporins	Meropenem	University of Waterloo, Wilfrid Laurier University	β-Lactam
FSI-1686 and FSI-1671	No β-lactam required	FOB Synthesis Inc	β-Lactam
BTZs	Imipenem	Universidad de la República, Montevideo, Uruguay	Bisthiazolidine
ME1071	Ceftazidime or biapenem	Meiji Seika Kaisha Ltd	Maleic acid derivative

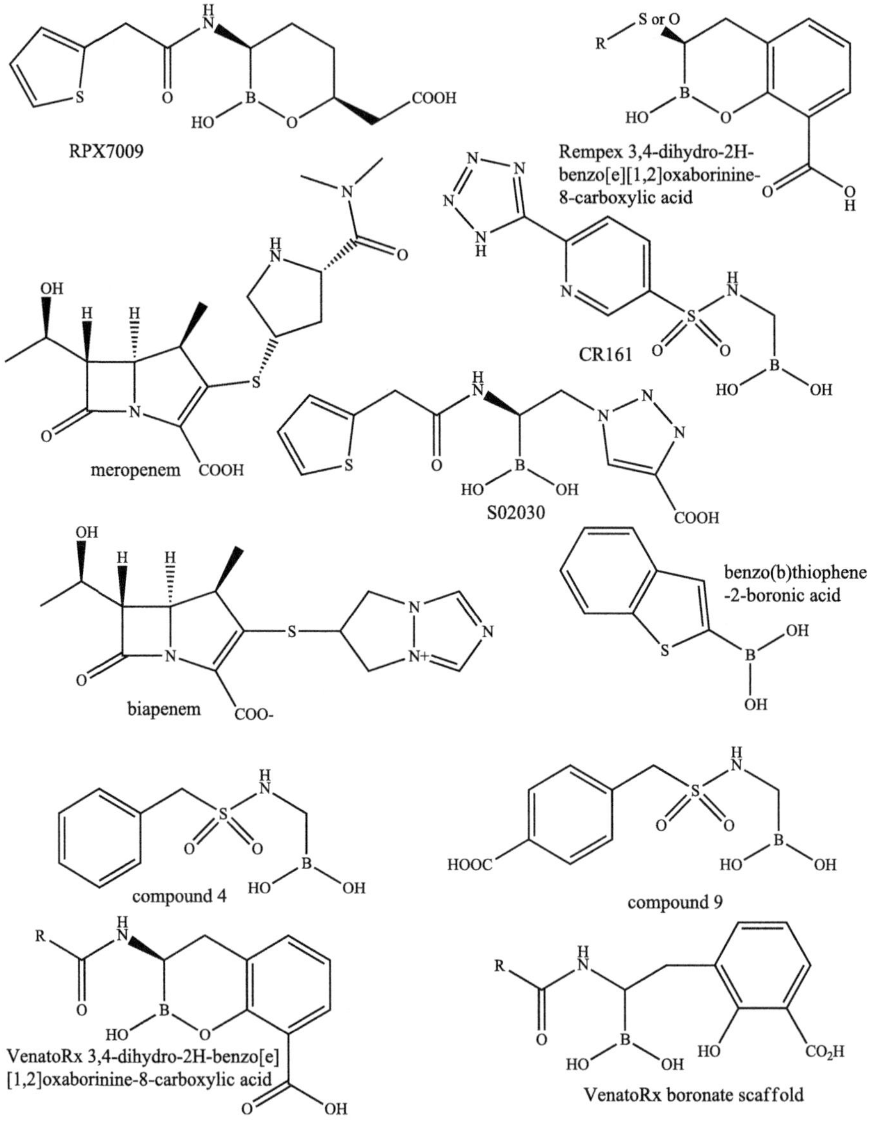

Fig. 4. Chemical structures of the carbavance (meropenem-RPX7009) combination, biapenem, and other boronates.

NOVEL SULFONES AND CLAVAMS IN PRECLINICAL DEVELOPMENT

Allecra Therapeutics is developing a novel sulfone, AAI101, in combination with cefepime; cefepime-AAI101 demonstrated activity against some Enterobacteriaceae with ESBLs or carbapenemases (**Fig. 5**; see **Table 2**).[50] In a neutropenic thigh mouse infection model, the cefepime-AAI101 combination reduced bacterial CFUs by more than 0.5 log CFU for 12 of the 20 strains tested; cefepime alone only worked in 3 of 20 strains. Orchid Pharmaceuticals synthesized a series of sulfone derivatives with no

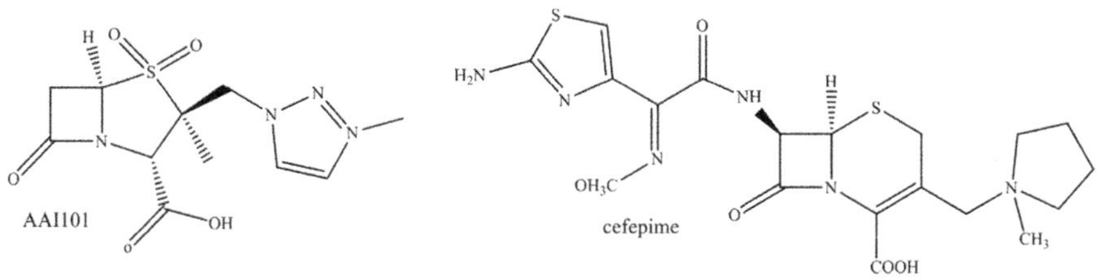

Fig. 5. Chemical structures of AAI101 and cefepime.

R1 side chain and different R2 side chains, and some lowered meropenem and imipenem MICs from 32 to 64 mg/L to 1 to 2 mg/L against *K pneumoniae* with bla_{KPC-2} (WO/2012/070071) when tested in combination (see **Table 2**). These sulfones were also tested in combination with imipenem or meropenem against other Enterobacteriaceae with bla_{KPC-2} or bla_{KPC-3}, and MICs decreased from 2 to 4 mg/L to 0.25 to 0.5 mg/L for some compounds. Another set of novel sulfones was developed by Dr John D. Buynak, and one of these compounds lowered meropenem and imipenem MICs for carbapenem-susceptible *A baumannii* producing $bla_{OXA-24/40}$ from 32 mg/L to 1 mg/L when tested in combination (see **Table 2**).[51] Nabriva Therapeutics created clavam spinoffs that possessed activity against *K pneumoniae* and *Citrobacter freundii* with MICs decreasing for ceftazidime from 26 mg/L to 0.2 mg/L and 3.2 mg/L, respectively, with a clavam derivative (see **Table 2**).

PHOSPHONATES IN PRECLINICAL DEVELOPMENT

Like with the boronates, literature shows that phosphonates are good inhibitors of class A and C and even some B and D β-lactamases kinetically.[52–54] Mirati Therapeutics conducted preclinical studies on a phosphonate, MG96077, which is a novel broad-spectrum, non-β-lactam β-lactamase inhibitor (**Fig. 6**; see **Table 2**).[39,55] Imipenem combined with MG96077 decreased greater than 90% of the MICs for imipenem-resistant *P aeruginosa* and *K pneumoniae* to 4 mg/L. In a mouse spleen infection model with imipenem-resistant *P aeruginosa*, imipenem-MG96077 caused a 4 to 6 log reduction in CFUs and increased mouse survival.

MONOBACTAMS ARE PROMISING β-LACTAMASE INHIBITORS OR EVADE β-LACTAMASE ACTIVITY

Already available in the clinic, the monobactam, aztreonam, is a β-lactam that can also circumvent certain β-lactamases (**Fig. 7**). Aztreonam inhibits certain AmpC β-lactamases and binds poorly to MBLs.[56–58]

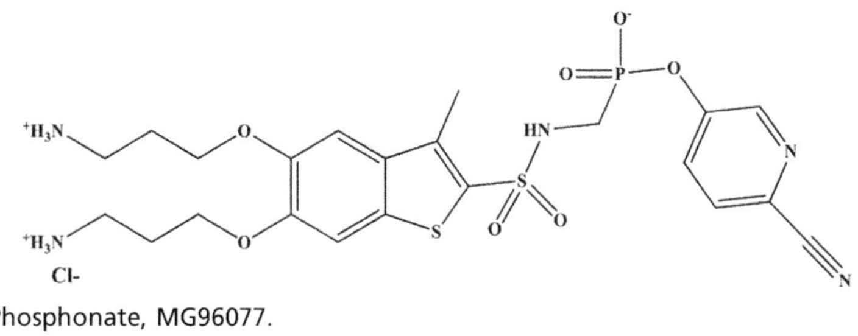

Fig. 6. Phosphonate, MG96077.

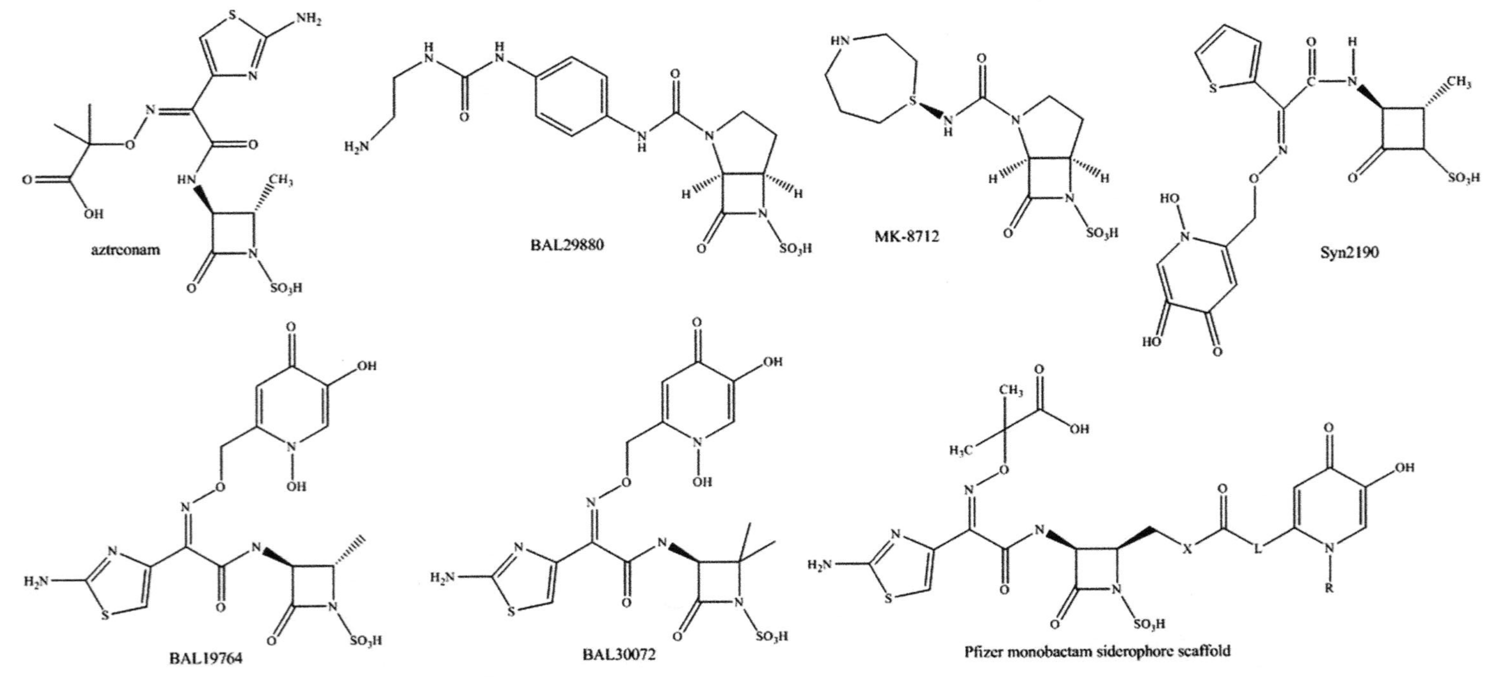

Fig. 7. Chemical structures of monobactams and bridged monobactams.

MONOBACTAMS AND DERIVATIVES IN PRECLINICAL DEVELOPMENT

The monobactam scaffold is encouraging for future MBL inhibitors as well as inhibitors of AmpCs, and Basilea Pharmaceuticals, Merck, Pfizer, and Taiho Pharmaceutical Co are working on these agents.

For Basilea, expansion of the monobactam class has resulted in several new monobactams (eg, BAL30072 and BAL19764) and a novel class of bridged monobactams (eg, BAL29880) that serve as β-lactamase inhibitors. BAL30072 contains a 1,5-dihydroxy-4-pyridone group that is a siderophore moiety that allows for transport of the compound into the bacterial cell via the TonB iron transport system (see **Fig. 7** and **Table 2**). BAL30072 possessed bactericidal activity against *Acinetobacter* spp, which include those with some bla_{OXA}s, *P aeruginosa*, *Burkholderia* spp, Enterobacteriaceae with class A carbapenemases, and against strains that produced bla_{MBL}s.[59–62] BAL30072 demonstrated efficacy in rat soft tissue infection by *A baumanniii* as well as a mouse septicemia model when combined with meropenem against *Serratia marcescens* producing bla_{SME-1} (a class A carbapenemase), *P aeruginosa*, and *A baumannii*.[61,63]

BAL30376 combines BAL19764, another siderophore monobactam, with the bridged monobactam BAL29880 and clavulanic acid (see **Fig. 7** and **Table 2**).[64,65] BAL30376 was effective against most clinical Enterobacteriaceae isolates producing bla_{AmpC}s and bla_{ESBL}s, *P aeruginosa*, *A baumannii* producing bla_{OXA-23}, or the southeast region clonal lineage and some *Stenotrophomonas maltophilia*. BAL30376 was not effective against Enterobacteriaceae expressing bla_{MBLs}, bla_{KPC}, or bla_{OXA-48}, or those with impermeability, *P aeruginosa* or *B cepacia* complex isolated from cystic fibrosis patients, *P aeruginosa* expressing bla_{MBL}s, and other *A baumannii*. In addition, in a mouse septicemia model of infection, BAL30376 demonstrated efficacy against selected isolates of *A baumannii*, *E cloacae*, and *P aeruginosa*.[65]

Merck is conducting preclinical testing with a bridged monobactam, MK-8712 (see **Fig. 7** and **Table 2**).[66] MK-8712 combined with imipenem reduced MICs against *P aeruginosa* strain CL5701from 32 mg/L to 4 mg/L. MK-8712 was also a potent inhibitor of AmpC of *P aeruginosa* with an IC_{50} value of 1 μM. MK-8712 combined with imipenem-cilastatin resulted in a 4.6 log fold reduction in CFU in a mouse spleen model of infection compared with imipenem-cilastatin alone.[67]

Pfizer developed a series of siderophore monobactams, similar to BAL30072; however, the siderophore moiety is on the R2 side chain (see **Fig. 7** and **Table 2**).[68] Several of these compounds worked in combination with aztreonam or meropenem to lower MIC values to the susceptible range against *P aeruginosa* and also possessed efficacy in a mouse pneumonia model of infection. The siderophore monobactams were modified to increase the length of the R2 side chain with linkers resulting in expansion of activity against *K pneumoniae*, *E coli*, and *A baumannii*, including *P aeruginosa* carrying a bla_{MBL}; these compounds target the PBPs and evade MBL activity.[69]

Similar to Merck, Taiho Pharmaceutical Co is working on a siderophore monobactam, Syn2190, that inhibited AmpC β-lactamases and reduced ceftazidime MICs to the susceptible range against Enterobacteriaceae and *P aeruginosa* expressing bla_{AmpC} (see **Fig. 7** and **Table 2**).[70] In addition, Syn2190 combined with ceftazidime or cefpirome demonstrated activity in mouse systemic and urinary tract infection models using *P aeruginosa*. However, Syn2190 induced expression of bla_{AmpC}.

A NEW SIDEROPHORE CEPHALOSPORIN IN CLINICAL DEVELOPMENT

S-649266, a novel catechol-substituted siderophore cephalosporin, is in phase II clinical trials (see **Table 1** and **Fig. 8**).[71] This compound demonstrated potent in vitro activity against a diverse panel of gram-negative bacteria[39] S-649266 was not hydrolyzed by KPC-2, P99, or OXA-23; minimal hydrolysis with k_{cat}/K_m values in the 10^3–10^4 $M^{-1}s^{-1}$ for MBLs, IMP-1, VIM-2, L1, and CTX-M-15 was observed.[72] S-649266 demonstrated activity against *P aeruginosa*, *S maltophilia*, *K pneumoniae*, and *A baumannii* with MIC_{90} values <2 mg/L.[73] Furthermore, against MDR strains of Enterobacteriaceae, *P aeruginosa*, and *A baumannii*, the MIC_{90} values were less than 4 mg/L.[73] In a rat lung infection model, S-649266 was shown to have efficacy against *P aeruginosa* and *A baumannii*, including MDR strains.[74] In addition, several different mouse models of infections (ie, systemic, lung, urinary tract, and subcutaneous infection) using various Gram-negatives were used to assess the efficacy of S-649266; the compound was effective against *K pneumoniae* producing bla_{KPC-2}.[75]

NOVEL 3′-THIOBENZOYL CEPHALOSPORINS IN PRECLINICAL DEVELOPMENT

3′-Thiobenzoyl cephalosporins demonstrated inhibitory activity against class A, B, C, and D β-lactamases with IC_{50} values in the range of 1.4 μM to 140 μM (**Fig. 8** and see **Table 2**) (US 20120329770 A1). In addition, when combined with meropenem, selected compounds possessed activity against *P aeruginosa*, *S maltophilia*, and *Chryseobacterium meningosepticum*.

NOVEL CARBAPENEMS IN PRECLINICAL DEVELOPMENT: FSI-1671 AND FSI-1686

Two novel carbapenems, FSI-1671 and FSI-1686, were shown to possess activity against MDR *A baumannii*, Enterobacteriaceae, and some *P aeruginosa* (**Fig. 9**; see **Table 2**).[76] Mice were intraperitoneally infected by carbapenem-resistant *A baumannii*, *K pneumoniae*, and *P aeruginosa* and treated with FSI-1671, FSI-1686, meropenem, doripenem, colistin, or tigecycline.[77] Both novel carbapenems demonstrated good potency (lower ED_{50} [50% effective dose] values) against carbapenem-resistant *A baumannii*, *K pneumoniae*, and *P aeruginosa* compared with the other carbapenems

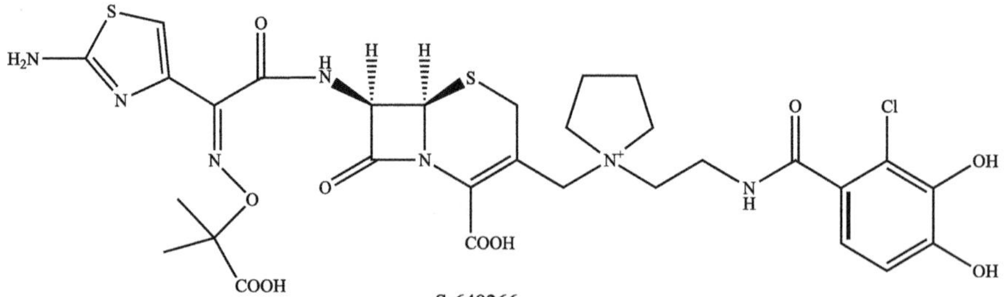

S-649266

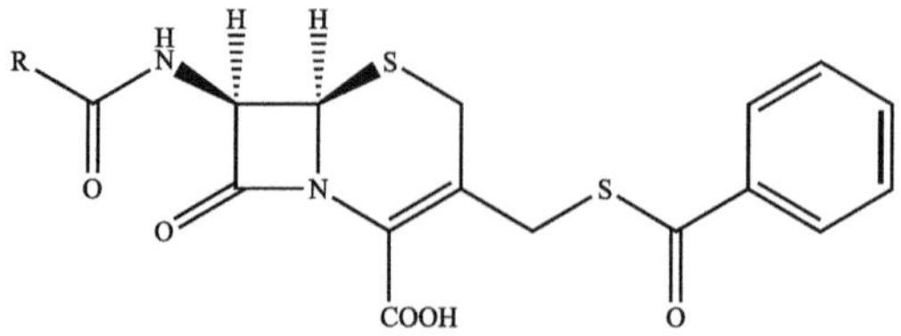

3'-thiobenzoyl cephalosporins.

Fig. 8. Chemical structure of 3′-thiobenzoyl cephalosporins.

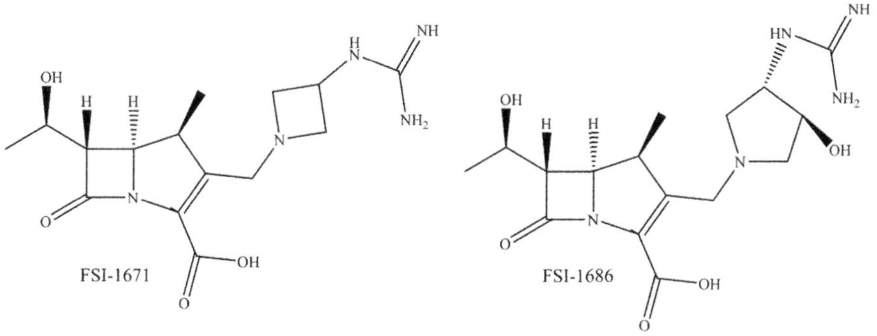

Fig. 9. Chemical structures of FSI-1671 and FSI-1686.

tested. The β-lactamase inhibitory properties of these compounds were not assessed, but all other clinically available carbapenems are dual agents inhibiting PBPs and some β-lactamases.

METALLO-β-LACTAMASE-SPECIFIC INHIBITORS IN PRECLINICAL DEVELOPMENT: BISTHIAZOLIDINES AND ME1071

Four bisthiazolidine (BTZ) inhibitors were tested against VIM-2 and VIM-24 and possessed K_i values between 3.7 and 14 μM (**Fig. 10**; see **Table 2**).[78] Most importantly, the BTZs restored imipenem susceptibility of clinical isolates, *P aeruginosa* producing bla_{VIM-2} and *K pneumoniae* carrying bla_{VIM-24}. In addition, BTZs demonstrate activity against NDM-1 with K_i values from 7 to 19 μM and are effective against *A. baumannii, K. pneumoniae, and P. rettgeri* expressing bla_{NDM-1} when combined with imipenem (ACS Infect. Dis., 2015, 1 (11), pp 544–54).

ME1071 is a maleic acid derivative, and when combined with ceftazidime, increased susceptibility to ceftazidime against *P aeruginosa* expressing bla_{IMP} and bla_{VIM}, although never for 100% of the isolates tested (see **Fig. 10** and **Table 2**).[79] Biapenem-ME1071 combination decreased MICs for Enterobacteriaceae with bla_{IMP} and bla_{VIM}, but not bla_{NDM}.[80] ME1071 in combination with biapenem was effective in a mouse model for ventilator-associated pneumonia by *P aeruginosa* producing bla_{MBL}.[81]

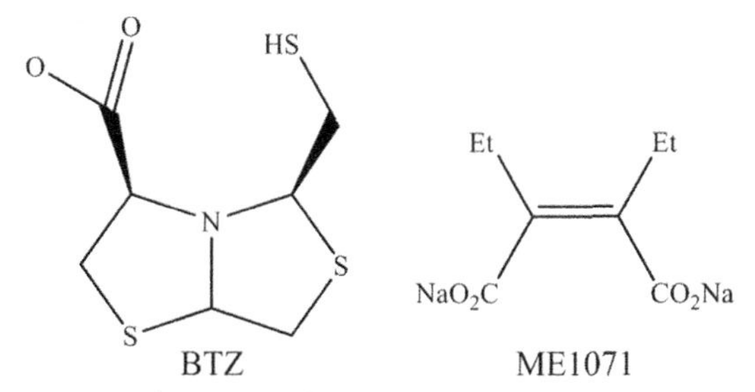

Fig. 10. Chemical structure of MBL-specific inhibitors the BTZ, (3R,5R,7aS)-5-(sulfanylmethyl) tetrahydro[1,3] thiazol[4,3-b][1,3]thiazole-3-carboxylic acid and ME1071.

SUMMARY

When one thinks about designing drugs to treat infections caused by MDR bacteria, there are 2 approaches to keep in mind. One strategy involves designing "niche" drugs to target specific bacteria with certain resistance mechanisms. These "niche" agents would be highly useful especially for uncommon or hard-to-treat infections (eg, *S maltophilia* or MDR *A baumannii* or Gram-negatives producing bla_{MBL}s). However, using drugs that only target a specific pathogen will force clinicians to rely heavily on accurate and rapid molecular diagnostics. The second tactic is designing drugs that possess a very broad spectrum and can be given as empirical therapy. With this second scenario, "time is no longer the enemy," and molecular diagnostics are not nearly as important. However, the risk of the bacteria evolving resistance to the novel agents is higher the more these agents are used in the clinic. If other older agents would work equally well, why accelerate the decline in utility of a novel agent?

Taking these ideas into consideration and looking back at this article, how do these approaches fit with the novel β-lactam-β-lactamase inhibitor combinations described? Clavulanic acid and the sulfones seem to be classified between a "niche" and a broad-spectrum agent category because their spectrum is somewhat limited given the MDR organisms observed today. Moreover, because they were first introduced more than 30 years ago, further derivatization of these compounds has not resulted in any novel inhibitors reaching clinical development. There were slight gains such as increased penetration and the ability to target other classes of β-lactamase. However, based on this history, the novel inhibitors may be a better route.

The DBOs in the preclinical development target PBPs. Is this PBP activity enough to propel this class forward as a broad-spectrum agent? With that in mind, could a novel DBO be a potential "magic bullet" to target all Gram-negatives producing β-lactamases? Will β-lactamases ever evolve to hydrolyze DBOs? Probably, as KPC-2 hydrolyzes avibactam albeit at a very slow rate.

Boronates have historically possessed activity against class A and C β-lactamases. Now, boronates were expanded to inhibit class A and B carbapenemases and some class D β-lactamases with 3,4-dihydro-2H-benzo[e][1,2]oxaborinine-8-carboxylic acids showing the most promise. Can they be expanded to target OXA carbapenemases? Could a novel carbapenem-3,4-dihydro-2H-benzo[e][1,2]oxaborinine-8-carboxylic acid combination be a potential "magic bullet" to inhibit all Gram-negatives producing β-lactamases? Will β-lactamases evolve to hydrolyze them? Hydrolysis seems less likely because, to date, hydrolysis of boronic acids has not been documented. However, β-lactamases could still evolve to resist inhibition by boronates.

The other compounds discussed here possess more limited spectra compared with the DBOs and boronates that are in preclinical development. Some inhibitors would be categorized as "niche" agents, such as the BTZs and ME1071. Where does this leave us now, and what is the best path forward? Clinical agents need to be developed that treat the resistant pathogens that exist now. It should be kept in mind that other resistance mechanisms (eg, loss of porins, expression of efflux pumps, and other permeability barriers) are still going to be a challenge. Also, the evolution of resistance in both PBPs and β-lactamases to these novel β-lactams and β-lactamase inhibitor should be studied to understand their mechanisms of action in order to come up with strategies to circumvent resistance, when it eventually appears. The war against resistant pathogens will most likely not have a definitive end. However, luckily, several new agents are in the arsenal that momentarily will keep pace with the challenging pathogens in the clinic today.

REFERENCES

1. Drawz SM, Papp-Wallace KM, Bonomo RA. New β-lactamase inhibitors: a therapeutic renaissance in an MDR world. Antimicrob Agents Chemother 2014;58:1835–46.
2. Clinical and Laboratory Standards Institute. Performance standards for antimicrobial susceptibility testing; Twenty-fifth Informational supplement M100-S25. Wayne (PA): CLSI; 2015.
3. Drawz SM, Bonomo RA. Three decades of β-lactamase inhibitors. Clin Microbiol Rev 2010;23:160–201.
4. Papp-Wallace KM, Bethel CR, Distler AM, et al. Inhibitor resistance in the KPC-2 β-lactamase, a preeminent property of this class A β-lactamase. Antimicrob Agents Chemother 2010;54:890–7.
5. Takeda S, Ishii Y, Hatano K, et al. Stability of FR264205 against AmpC β-lactamase of Pseudomonas aeruginosa. Int J Antimicrob Agents 2007;30:443–5.
6. Zhanel GG, Chung P, Adam H, et al. Ceftolozane/tazobactam: a novel cephalosporin/β-lactamase inhibitor combination with activity against multidrug-resistant gram-negative bacilli. Drugs 2014;74:31–51.
7. Cabot G, Bruchmann S, Mulet X, et al. Pseudomonas aeruginosa ceftolozane-tazobactam resistance development requires multiple mutations leading to overexpression and structural modification of AmpC. Antimicrob Agents Chemother 2014;58:3091–9.
8. Berrazeg M, Jeannot K, Ntsogo Enguéné VY, et al. Mutations in β-Lactamase AmpC Increase Resistance of Pseudomonas aeruginosa Isolates to Antipseudomonal Cephalosporins. Antimicrob Agents Chemother 2015;59(10):6248–55.
9. Aktas Z, Kayacan C, Oncul O. In vitro activity of avibactam (NXL104) in combination with β-lactams against Gram-negative bacteria, including OXA-48 β-lactamase-producing Klebsiella pneumoniae. Int J Antimicrob Agents 2012;39:86–9.
10. Livermore DM, Mushtaq S, Warner M, et al. Activities of NXL104 combinations with ceftazidime and aztreonam against carbapenemase-producing Enterobacteriaceae. Antimicrob Agents Chemother 2011;55:390–4.
11. Mushtaq S, Warner M, Livermore DM. In vitro activity of ceftazidime+NXL104 against Pseudomonas aeruginosa and other non-fermenters. J Antimicrob Chemother 2010;65:2376–81.
12. Mushtaq S, Warner M, Williams G, et al. Activity of chequerboard combinations of ceftaroline and NXL104 versus β-lactamase-producing Enterobacteriaceae. J Antimicrob Chemother 2010;65:1428–32.
13. Pagès JM, Peslier S, Keating TA, et al. Role of the Outer Membrane and Porins in Susceptibility of β-Lactamase-Producing Enterobacteriaceae to Ceftazidime-Avibactam. Antimicrob Agents Chemother 2015;60(3):1349–59.
14. Ehmann DE, Jahic H, Ross PL, et al. Avibactam is a covalent, reversible, non-β-lactam β-lactamase inhibitor. Proc Natl Acad Sci U S A 2012;109:11663–8.
15. Ehmann DE, Jahic H, Ross PL, et al. Kinetics of avibactam inhibition against class A, C, and D β-lactamases. J Biol Chem 2013;288:27960–71.
16. Xu H, Hazra S, Blanchard JS. NXL104 irreversibly inhibits the β-lactamase from Mycobacterium tuberculosis. Biochemistry 2012;51:4551–7.
17. Lahiri SD, Mangani S, Jahic H, et al. Molecular basis of selective inhibition and slow reversibility of avibactam against class D carbapenemases: a structure-guided study of OXA-24 and OXA-48. ACS Chem Biol 2015;10:591–600.
18. Lahiri SD, Mangani S, Durand-Reville T, et al. Structural insight into potent broad-spectrum inhibition with reversible recyclization mechanism: avibactam

in complex with CTX-M-15 and Pseudomonas aeruginosa AmpC β-lactamases. Antimicrob Agents Chemother 2013;57:2496–505.
19. King DT, King AM, Lal SM, et al. Molecular mechanism of avibactam-mediated β-lactamase inhibition. ACS Infect Dis 2015;1:175–84.
20. Krishnan NP, Nguyen NQ, Papp-Wallace KM, et al. Inhibition of Klebsiella β-Lactamases (SHV-1 and KPC-2) by Avibactam: A Structural Study. PLoS One 2015; 10(9):e0136813.
21. Livermore DM, Mushtaq S, Barker K, et al. Characterization of β-lactamase and porin mutants of Enterobacteriaceae selected with ceftaroline + avibactam (NXL104). J Antimicrob Chemother 2012;67:1354–8.
22. Lahiri SD, Walkup GK, Whiteaker JD, et al. Selection and molecular characterization of ceftazidime/avibactam-resistant mutants in Pseudomonas aeruginosa strains containing derepressed AmpC. J Antimicrob Chemother 2015;70:1650–8.
23. Winkler ML, Papp-Wallace KM, Hujer AM, et al. Unexpected challenges in treating multidrug-resistant Gram-negative bacteria: resistance to ceftazidime-avibactam in archived isolates of Pseudomonas aeruginosa. Antimicrob Agents Chemother 2015;59:1020–9.
24. Alm RA, Johnstone MR, Lahiri SD. Characterization of Escherichia coli NDM isolates with decreased susceptibility to aztreonam/avibactam: role of a novel insertion in PBP3. J Antimicrob Chemother 2015;70:1420–8.
25. Papp-Wallace KM, Winkler ML, Taracila MA, et al. Variants of the KPC-2 β-lactamase which are resistant to inhibition by avibactam. Antimicrob Agents Chemother 2015;59(7):3710–7.
26. Winkler ML, Papp-Wallace KM, Bonomo RA. Activity of ceftazidime/avibactam against isogenic strains of Escherichia coli containing KPC and SHV β-lactamases with single amino acid substitutions in the Ω-loop. J Antimicrob Chemother 2015;70(8):2279–86.
27. Winkler ML, Papp-Wallace KM, Taracila MA, et al. Avibactam and inhibitor resistant SHV β-lactamases. Antimicrob Agents Chemother 2015;59(7):3700–9.
28. Livermore DM, Warner M, Jamrozy D, et al. In vitro selection of ceftazidime-avibactam resistance in Enterobacteriaceae with KPC-3 carbapenemase. Antimicrob Agents Chemother 2015;59(9):5324–30.
29. Humphries RM, Yang S, Hemarajata P, et al. First Report of Ceftazidime-Avibactam Resistance in a KPC-3-Expressing Klebsiella pneumoniae Isolate. Antimicrob Agents Chemother 2015;59(10):6605–7.
30. Hirsch EB, Ledesma KR, Chang KT, et al. In vitro activity of MK-7655, a novel β-lactamase inhibitor, in combination with imipenem against carbapenem-resistant Gram-negative bacteria. Antimicrob Agents Chemother 2012;56:3753–7.
31. Livermore DM, Warner M, Mushtaq S. Activity of MK-7655 combined with imipenem against Enterobacteriaceae and Pseudomonas aeruginosa. J Antimicrob Chemother 2013;68(10):2286–90.
32. Young K, Hackel M, Lascols C, et al. Response to imipenem plus MK-7655, a novel β-lactamase inhibitor, among 212 recent clinical isolates of *P. aeruginosa*, Abstr 1620, abstr IDSA Week 2012. San Diego (CA), October 17–21, 2012.
33. Morinaka A, Tsutsumi Y, Yamada M, et al. F-946: OP0595, a novel serine-β-lactamase inhibitor: mode of action as β-lactamase inhibitor, antibiotic agent and β-lactam enhancer. Abstr 54th Interscience Conference on Antimicrobial Agents and Chemotherapy. Washington, DC, September 5–9, 2014.
34. Ishii Y, Tsutsumi Y, Yoshizumi A, et al. F-953: OP0595, a novel serine-β-lactamase inhibitor: enzymatic studies of OP0595 against serine-β-lactamases. Abstr 54th

Interscience Conference on Antimicrobial Agents and Chemotherapy. Washington, DC, September 5–9, 2014.
35. Morinaka A, Tsutsumi Y, Yamada M, et al. OP0595, a new diazabicyclooctane: mode of action as a serine β-lactamase inhibitor, antibiotic and β-lactam 'enhancer'. J Antimicrob Chemother 2015;70(10):2779–86.
36. Mendes RE, Rhomberg P, Becker H, et al. F-1188: Activity of β-lactam agents tested in combination with novel β-lactamase inhibitor compounds against Enterobacteriaceae producing extended-spectrum β-lactamases. Abstr 53rd International Interscience Conference on Antimicrobial Agents Chemotherapy. Denver (CO), September 10–13, 2013.
37. Mendes RE, Rhomberg PR, Becker HK, et al. F-1189: β-lactam activity tested in combination with β-lactamase inhibitor candidates against Enterobacteriaceae producing class A, B and D carbapenemases. Abstr 53rd Interscience Conference on Antimicrobial Agents and Chemotherapy. Denver (CO), September 10–13, 2013.
38. Salama SM, Brouillette E, Malouin F, et al. F-1191: mechanistic studies of FPI-1465 a novel β-lactamase inhibitor. Abstr 54th Interscience Conference on Antimicrobial Agents and Chemotherapy. Washington, DC, September 5–9, 2014.
39. Qin W, Panunzio M, Biondi S. β-Lactam antibiotics renaissance. Antibiotics 2014; 3:193–215.
40. VanScoy BD, Trang M, McCauley J, et al. Pharmacokinetics-Pharmacodynamics of a Novel Beta-Lactamase Inhibitor, CB-618, in Combination with Meropenem in an. In Vitro Infection Model. Antimicrob Agents Chemother 2016. [Epub ahead of print].
41. Kiener PA, Waley SG. Reversible inhibitors of penicillinases. Biochem J 1978;169: 197–204.
42. Beesley T, Gascoyne N, Knott-Hunziker V, et al. The inhibition of class C β-lactamases by boronic acids. Biochem J 1983;209:229–33.
43. Hecker SJ, Reddy KR, Totrov M, et al. Discovery of a cyclic boronic acid β-lactamase inhibitor (RPX7009) with utility vs class A serine carbapenemases. J Med Chem 2015;58:3682–92.
44. Livermore DM, Mushtaq S. Activity of biapenem (RPX2003) combined with the boronate β-lactamase inhibitor RPX7009 against carbapenem-resistant enterobacteriaceae. J Antimicrob Chemother 2013;68:1825–31.
45. Lapuebla A, Abdallah M, Olafisoye O, et al. Activity of meropenem combined with RPX7009, a novel β-lactamase inhibitor, against Gram-negative clinical isolates in New York City. Antimicrob Agents Chemother 2015;59(8):4856–60.
46. Goldstein EJ, Citron DM, Tyrrell KL, et al. In vitro activity of biapenem plus RPX7009, a carbapenem combined with a serine β-lactamase inhibitor, against anaerobic bacteria. Antimicrob Agents Chemother 2013;57:2620–30.
47. Powers RA, Blazquez J, Weston GS, et al. The complexed structure and antimicrobial activity of a non-β-lactam inhibitor of AmpC β-lactamase. Protein Sci 1999; 8:2330–7.
48. Rojas LJ, Taracila MA, Papp-Wallace KM, et al. Boronic Acid Transition State Inhibitors Active against KPC and Other Class A β-Lactamases: Structure-Activity Relationships as a Guide to Inhibitor Design. Antimicrob Agents Chemother 2016;60(3):1751–9.
49. Eidam O, Romagnoli C, Caselli E, et al. Design, synthesis, crystal structures, and antimicrobial activity of sulfonamide boronic acids as β-lactamase inhibitors. J Med Chem 2010;53:7852–63.

50. Crandon JL, Nicolau DP. In vivo activities of simulated human doses of cefepime and cefepime-AAI101 against multidrug-resistant Gram-negative Enterobacteriaceae. Antimicrob Agents Chemother 2015;59:2688–94.
51. Bou G, Santillana E, Sheri A, et al. Design, synthesis, and crystal structures of 6-alkylidene-2'-substituted penicillanic acid sulfones as potent inhibitors of Acinetobacter baumannii OXA-24 carbapenemase. J Am Chem Soc 2010;132:13320–31.
52. Majumdar S, Pratt RF. Inhibition of class A and C β-lactamases by diaroyl phosphates. Biochemistry 2009;48:8285–92.
53. Adediran SA, Nukaga M, Baurin S, et al. Inhibition of class D β-lactamases by acyl phosphates and phosphonates. Antimicrob Agents Chemother 2005;49:4410–2.
54. Lassaux P, Hamel M, Gulea M, et al. Mercaptophosphonate compounds as broad-spectrum inhibitors of the metallo-β-lactamases. J Med Chem 2010;53:4862–76.
55. Martell LA, Rahil G, Vaisburg A, et al. C1–1373: novel β-lactamase inhibitor potentiates and extends the antibacterial activity of imipenem against β-lactam-resistant P. aeruginosa and K. pneumoniae. Abstr 49th Interscience Conference on Antimicrobial Agents and Chemotherapy. San Francisco (CA), September 12–15, 2009.
56. Poeylaut-Palena AA, Tomatis PE, Karsisiotis AI, et al. A minimalistic approach to identify substrate binding features in B1 metallo-β-lactamases. Bioorg Med Chem Lett 2007;17:5171–4.
57. Sakurai Y, Yoshida Y, Saitoh K, et al. Characteristics of aztreonam as a substrate, inhibitor and inducer for β-lactamases. J Antibiot (Tokyo) 1990;43:403–10.
58. Papp-Wallace KM, Mallo S, Bethel CR, et al. A kinetic analysis of the inhibition of FOX-4 β-lactamase, a plasmid-mediated AmpC cephalosporinase, by monocyclic β-lactams and carbapenems. J Antimicrob Chemother 2014;69:682–90.
59. Page MG, Dantier C, Desarbre E. In vitro properties of BAL30072, a novel siderophore sulfactam with activity against multiresistant Gram-negative bacilli. Antimicrob Agents Chemother 2010;54:2291–302.
60. Mushtaq S, Warner M, Livermore D. Activity of the siderophore monobactam BAL30072 against multiresistant non-fermenters. J Antimicrob Chemother 2010;65:266–70.
61. Russo TA, Page MG, Beanan JM, et al. In vivo and in vitro activity of the siderophore monosulfactam BAL30072 against Acinetobacter baumannii. J Antimicrob Chemother 2011;66:867–73.
62. Mima T, Kvitko BH, Rholl DA, et al. In vitro activity of BAL30072 against Burkholderia pseudomallei. Int J Antimicrob Agents 2011;38:157–9.
63. Hofer B, Dantier C, Gebhardt K, et al. Combined effects of the siderophore monosulfactam BAL30072 and carbapenems on multidrug-resistant Gram-negative bacilli. J Antimicrob Chemother 2013;68:1120–9.
64. Livermore DM, Mushtaq S, Warner M. Activity of BAL30376 (monobactam BAL19764 + BAL29880 + clavulanate) versus Gram-negative bacteria with characterized resistance mechanisms. J Antimicrob Chemother 2010;65:2382–95.
65. Page MG, Dantier C, Desarbre E, et al. In vitro and in vivo properties of BAL30376, a β-lactam and dual β-lactamase inhibitor combination with enhanced activity against Gram-negative bacilli that express multiple β-lactamases. Antimicrob Agents Chemother 2011;55:1510–9.
66. Chen H, Blizzard TA, Kim S, et al. Side chain SAR of bicyclic β-lactamase inhibitors (BLIs). 2. N-Alkylated and open chain analogs of MK-8712. Bioorg Med Chem Lett 2011;21:4267–70.

67. Blizzard TA, Chen H, Kim S, et al. Side chain SAR of bicyclic β-lactamase inhibitors (BLIs). 1. Discovery of a class C BLI for combination with imipinem. Bioorg Med Chem Lett 2010;20:918–21.
68. Mitton-Fry MJ, Arcari JT, Brown MF, et al. Novel monobactams utilizing a siderophore uptake mechanism for the treatment of Gram-negative infections. Bioorg Med Chem Lett 2012;22:5989–94.
69. Brown MF, Mitton-Fry MJ, Arcari JT, et al. Pyridone-conjugated monobactam antibiotics with Gram-negative activity. J Med Chem 2013;56:5541–52.
70. Nishida K, Kunugita C, Uji T, et al. In vitro and in vivo activities of Syn2190, a novel β-lactamase inhibitor. Antimicrob Agents Chemother 1999;43:1895–900.
71. Ito A, Kohira N, Bouchillon SK, et al. In vitro antimicrobial activity of S-649266, a catechol-substituted siderophore cephalosporin, when tested against non-fermenting Gram-negative bacteria. J Antimicrob Chemother 2016;71(3):670–7.
72. Ishii Y, Horiyama T, Nakamura R, et al. F-1557: S-649266, a novel siderophore cephalosporin: III. Stability against clinically relevant β-lactamases. Abstr 53rd Interscience Conference on Antimicrobial Agents and Chemotherapy. Washington, DC, September 5–9, 2014.
73. Ito A, Yoshizawa H, Nakamura R, et al. F-1562: S-649266, a novel siderophore cephalosporin: I. In vitro activity against Gram-negative bacteria including multidrug-resistant strains. Abstr 53rd Interscience Conference on Antimicrobial Agents and Chemotherapy. Washington, DC, September 5–9, 2014.
74. Horiyama T, Singley CM, Nakamura R, et al. F-1556: S-649266, a novel siderophore cephalosporin: VIII. Efficacy against Pseudomonas aeruginosa and Acinetobacter baumannii in rat lung infection model with humanized exposure profile of 2 gram dose with 1 hour and 3 hours infusion. Abstr 53rd Interscience Conference on Antimicrobial Agents and Chemotherapy. Washington, DC, September 5–9, 2014.
75. Nakamura R, Toba S, Tsuji M, et al. F-1558: S-649266, a novel siderophore cephalosporin: IV. In vivo efficacy in various murine infection models. Abstr 53rd Interscience Conference on Antimicrobial Agents and Chemotherapy. Washington, DC, September 5–9, 2014.
76. Joo HY, Kim DI, Kowalik E, et al. F1-1202: FSI–1671, a novel anti-Acinetobacter carbapenem: in vivo efficacy against carbapenem-resistance Gram-negative bacterial infection. Abstr 53rd Interscience Conference on Antimicrobial Agents and Chemotherapy. Denver (CO), September 10–13, 2013.
77. Joo HY, Kim DI, Kowalik E, et al. F1–143: efficacy of FSI-1686 in animal model of carbapenem-resistance Gram-negative bacterial infection. Abstr 51st Interscience Conference on Antimicrobial Agents and Chemotherapy. Chicago (IL), September 17–20, 2011.
78. Mojica MF, Mahler SG, Bethel CR, et al. Exploring the role of residue 228 in substrate and inhibitor recognition by VIM metallo-β-lactamases. Biochemistry 2015; 54:3183–96.
79. Ishii Y, Eto M, Mano Y, et al. In vitro potentiation of carbapenems with ME1071, a novel metallo-β-lactamase inhibitor, against metallo-β-lactamase- producing Pseudomonas aeruginosa clinical isolates. Antimicrob Agents Chemother 2010; 54:3625–9.
80. Livermore DM, Mushtaq S, Morinaka A, et al. Activity of carbapenems with ME1071 (disodium 2,3-diethylmaleate) against Enterobacteriaceae and Acinetobacter spp. with carbapenemases, including NDM enzymes. J Antimicrob Chemother 2013;68:153–8.

81. Yamada K, Yanagihara K, Kaku N, et al. In vivo efficacy of biapenem with ME1071, a novel metallo-β-lactamase (MBL) inhibitor, in a murine model mimicking ventilator-associated pneumonia caused by MBL-producing Pseudomonas aeruginosa. Int J Antimicrob Agents 2013;42:238–43.

Antibiotic-Resistant Infections and Treatment Challenges in the Immunocompromised Host

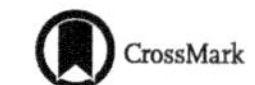

Donald M. Dumford III, MD[a,b,*], Marion Skalweit, MD[c,d]

KEYWORDS

• MDRO • Immunocompromise • HIV/AIDS • Organ transplant recipients • Infection

KEY POINTS

- Rates of infection with multidrug resistant organisms (MDRO) are increasing among immunocompromised persons, as greater numbers of MDRO are observed throughout the population.
- Antibiotic prophylaxis and empiric antibiotic therapy influences the selection of these MDRO; susceptibility patterns vary among regions and even within hospitals.
- The astute clinician is aware of his or her regional unique antibiogram.
- MDRO can be associated with worse outcomes among immunocompromised persons, and empiric antibiotic choices must be selected with the local antibiogram in mind.
- Studies are needed among immunocompromised persons to evaluate these novel approaches to improve outcomes.

INTRODUCTION

This article reviews antibiotic resistance and treatment of bacterial infections in the growing number of patients who are immunocompromised: solid organ transplant (SOT) recipients, the neutropenic host, and persons with human immunodeficiency virus (HIV) and AIDS. A literature review of the role of antibiotic resistance in infections in patients with primary and secondary immunodeficiencies, and associated infections, as well as fungal and viral resistance, is beyond the scope of this article and is not included. Specific mechanisms of resistance in both gram-negative and

[a] Akron General Medical Center, 1 Akron General Way, Akron, OH 44302, USA; [b] Northeast Ohio Medical University, 4209 St. Rt. 44, PO Box 95, Rootstown, Ohio 44272, USA; [c] Louis Stokes Cleveland Department of Veterans Affairs, 10701 East Blvd 111(W), Cleveland, OH 44106, USA; [d] Case Western Reserve University School of Medicine, 2109 Adelbert Road, Cleveland, OH 44106, USA
* Corresponding author. Akron General Medical Center, 1 Akron General Avenue (formerly 400 Wabash Avenue), Akron, OH 44307.
E-mail address: donald.dumford@akrongeneral.org

Infect Dis Clin N Am 30 (2016) 465–489
http://dx.doi.org/10.1016/j.idc.2016.02.008
id.theclinics.com

gram-positive bacteria, as well as newer treatment options are addressed elsewhere, and are only briefly discussed in the context of the immunocompromised host.

THE IMMUNE SYSTEM AND HOST SUSCEPTIBILITY TO BACTERIAL PATHOGENS

A complete review of immunology is beyond the scope of this paper. The interested reader is referred to a number of excellent textbooks.[1,2] As a brief introduction, focusing on specific immune defects and related infections, the immune system is divided into components that represent innate and adaptive immunity to bacterial pathogens. Innate immunity includes mucosal barriers and the skin, the complement system as well as cellular components, such as dendritic cells and neutrophils and phagocytic cells in circulation and in tissues (eg, Langerhans cells, Kuppfer cells, alveolar macrophages). Defects in innate immunity can be primary (congenital) or secondary (eg, related to other diseases or as adverse reactions to medications) and lead to specific susceptibility to bacterial pathogens. The adaptive immune response (B and T lymphocytes) includes both humoral and cell-mediated immune mechanisms. Some immunodeficiency states involve a combination of both defects in innate and adaptive immunity, for example, cytotoxic chemotherapy and the neutropenic host, common variable immunodeficiency, or AIDS. In recent years, the human microbiome has been considered as an additional immune defense whose disruption can contribute to susceptibility to specific pathogens, for example, *Clostridium difficile* infection, requiring unique treatments like fecal microbiota transplant.[3]

SOLID ORGAN TRANSPLANTATION

Since its inception, SOT have saved many lives. In an analysis of United Network for Organ Sharing data from 1987 to 2012, Rana and colleagues[4] found that 2,270,859 life-years were saved with a mean of 4.3 life-years per organ transplant. SOT are associated with significant morbidity and mortality after transplant with infections being significant cause of complications of SOT. In an analysis of 156 deceased single organ transplant recipients who underwent autopsy, infections were found to be the most common cause of mortality, accounting for 41% of deaths (64/156) and typically occurred within the first year of transplantation.[5] Mortality owing to infection varied by organ transplant type. In the heart transplant group, 21% of deaths were attributable to infection compared with 59.4% in the liver transplant group, 58.6% in the kidney transplant group, and 63.1% in the lung transplant group.[5] Of the 64 cases of infection-related mortality, bacterial infections accounted for the majority, with 43 (67.1%) being bacterial in origin.[5] A high mortality rate owing to infection in the first year posttransplant is not necessarily surprising given high incidence of infection during this time period compared with later time periods posttransplant. For example, Al-Hasan and colleagues[6] showed a drastically higher incidence of gram-negative bloodstream infection (BSIs) in the first month posttransplant at 210 in 1000 patient-years compared with 2 to 12 months and greater than 1 year posttransplant with incidence of 25.7 and 8.2 per 1000 patient-years during those time periods respectively. Even in the late posttransplant period (>1 year), the incidence of gram-negative bacteremia in the SOT population was still 10-fold greater than that of the general population.[6] As with other patient populations, infections owing to antibiotic resistant pathogens are a concern, especially with those considered multidrug resistant (MDR). In this review, issues regarding SOT and antimicrobial resistance are addressed, including incidence of antibiotic-resistant pathogens, risk factors for antibiotic-resistant pathogens, mortality associated with antibiotic-resistant pathogens, and risk factors for mortality associated with antibiotic-resistant pathogens in this patient population.

Prevalence of Pathogens in Solid Organ Transplant

Table 1 presents the prevalence of resistant pathogens in studies addressing different types of SOT. More data are available on gram-negative pathogens than on gram-positive pathogens. Data for methicillin-resistant *Staphylococcus aureus* (MRSA) were limited, with only 4 studies reviewed reporting on MRSA.[7–10] The prevalence of MRSA had wide variability being as low as 18%[9] and as high as 80%.[10] Few of these studies looked at *Enterococcus* spp. In those that did, the prevalence of vancomycin-resistant *Enterococcus faecium* (VRE) was low; Bodro and colleagues[7] reporting no *Enterococcus* spp. isolates to be VRE, Kawecki and colleagues[11] reporting 11% VRE, and Song and colleagues[10] reporting only 10%.

Gram-negative infections were represented more often in these studies with resistance being very common. Extended spectrum β-lactamase (ESBL) production was common in enteric pathogens in most studies. Twelve studies had available data on ESBL production in enteric pathogens. One additional study reported cefepime resistance, but did not describe this as an ESBL.[8] With the exception of the studies from Al-Hasan and colleagues,[6] Azap and colleagues,[13] and Riera and colleagues,[9] the incidence of ESBL production in enteric pathogens was at least 40%.[6–9,11,12,14,21,23,25] Two other studies reported the proportion of enteric bacilli that were MDR (14.5% and 54.8%, respectively), but did not specify if these were ESBL producing or not.[26,28] One other study looked at the number of patients who were colonized with ESBL producing pathogens before liver transplantation.[14] In this study, 15.8% of liver transplant patients were found to have fecal carriage with ESBL pathogens before liver transplant. Independent risk factors for colonization in this study were prior antibiotic use and prior spontaneous bacterial peritonitis. In a risk score that these authors developed, prior ESBL infection was included, although it could not be included in the multivariate modeling. All patients with all 3 risk factors had fecal colonization with ESBL pathogens, with the conclusion being that these patients should receive perioperative coverage of ESBL pathogens.[14]

Acinetobacter baumannii frequently was described as MDR, and several studies also analyzed the incidence of carbapenem resistance. Two studies looked at the number of *A baumannii* isolates that were extensively drug resistant (XDR).[18,19] XDR status was common in these 2 studies, with Kim and colleagues reporting rates of 75.7% and Kitazano and colleagues reporting 21.2%. In addition to these studies on XDR *A baumannii*, several other studies investigated carbapenem resistance in *A baumannii* and found it was quite common.[8,15,20,27,28] Carbapenem resistance in *A baumannii* in these studies ranged from 15.3% from Reddy and colleagues[27] to 75% from De Gouvea and colleagues.[8,15]

Six studies investigated *Pseudomonas aeruginosa*.[6,8,20–22,24,30] Carbapenem resistance rates were high ranging from 18%[24] to 87.5%.[8] Additionally, in the study by Mlynarczyk and colleagues,[24] production of metallo-β lactamase was found in 10.5% of isolates. Two other studies described the isolates strictly as MDR with relatively low incidence in one of 10.3%[6] versus 31% in another study.[22]

Risks for Multidrug-resistant Organisms

Across the studies reviewed, a number of factors were found to be risk factors for MDRO pathogens. Several studies showed that specific types of transplants were risk factors with liver transplant significant in 1 study,[22] lung transplantation in another,[20] and kidney transplantation in a third21, however, the other studies did

Table 1
Studies of resistant pathogens in different types of solid organ transplants

Author	Study Subjects	Type of Infection	Data on Antibiotic Resistant Pathogens
Aguiar et al,[12] 2014	997 with liver or kidney transplant	112 with Enterobacteracieae bloodstream infections	52/112 (48%) ESBL-producing
Al-Hasan et al,[6] 2009	3367 patients with SOT	223 with gram-negative bloodstream infections	Incidence of ESBL producing *E coli increased* from 0% in 2000 (first year the screen was available) to 8% in 2008 3/29 *Pseudomonas* isolates MDR Common fluoroquinolone resistance (25.6% of *E coli* and 27.6% of *Pseudomonas aeruginosa* were ciprofloxacin resistant) 50% of *E coli* isolates resistant to trimethoprim–sulfamethoxazole
Azap et al,[13] 2013	398 renal transplant patients	703 urinary isolates 172 with ≥1 UTI	97/407 (12.6%) *E. coli* isolates ESBL positive 59.4% resistant to fluoroquinolones 85.7% resistant to trimethoprim–sulfamethoxazole
Bert et al,[14] 2014	317 liver transplant patients	50 (15.8%) with fecal ESBL colonization	24/50 (48%) ESBL carriers had subsequent ESBL infection vs 18/267 (6.7%) noncarriers
Bodro et al,[7] 2013	276 episodes of bacteremia in 190 SOT	50/190 (19.6%) with resistant-ESKAPE pathogens	rESKAPE per species type: 0/16 *E faecium* 5/13 (38.5%) *S aureus* isolates 10/29 (25.6%) *K pneumonia* 5/11 *Enterobacter* spp. (45.4% ESBL) 8/11 (72.7%) *A baumannii* 26/35 (74.3%) *P aeruginosa*
Camargo et al,[8] 2015	2563 patients with nosocomial bacteremia, 83 of which SOT	42/65 (64.6%) in SOT were antibiotic resistant vs 911/1811 (50.3)	6/14 (42.9%) MRSA 9/11 (81.8%) *Klebsiella* spp. cefepime resistant 4/10 (40%) *E coli* ciprofloxacin resistant 5/8 (62.5%) *Enterobacter* spp. cefepime resistant 3/4 (75%) *Acinetobacter* spp. carbapenem resistant 7/8 (87.5%) *Pseudomonas* meropenem resistant
de Gouvea et al,[15] 2012	800 liver or kidney transplants	49 cases of *A baumannii*	18/49 (36.7%) with carbapenem resistance

Freire et al,[16] 2015	1101 kidney transplants	35 carbapenem-resistant *Klebsiella* infections	31/35 with *bla*$_{kpc}$
Giannella et al,[17] 2014	47 SOT patients with pneumonia	24/31 occurred >6 mo after SOT	MDR in 2/3 (66.7%) at <1 mo, 2/4 (50%) at 1–6 mo, and (37.5%) at >6 mo. In patients with community acquired pneumonia, MDR pathogens caused 2/11 (18%)
Kawecki et al,[11] 2011	295 patients with kidney transplant in first 4 wk after transplant	582 urine cultures yielded 291 isolates	52.5% of Enterobacteriaceae were ESBL positive 11% of *Enterococcus* spp. were VRE
Kim et al,[18] 2011	451 liver transplants	26/451 (5.8%) with *A. baumannii* with a total of 37 isolates	28/37 (75.7%) were XDR with only susceptibility to colistin
Kitazono et al,[19] 2015	33 SOT with *A. baumannii* infections	—	21/33 (63.6%) MDR 7/33 (21.2%) XDR with resistance to all antimicrobials except colistin
Lanini et al,[20] 2015	887 SOT	185 gram-negative infections	49/185 (26.5%) carbapenem resistant: 49% of *Klebsiella* spp., 1.9% *E coli*, 31% *P aeruginosa*, 44% *A. baumannii*, and 10% other Enterobacteriaceae
Linares et al,[21] 2010bib21	1057 transplants	92 patients with 116 *K pneumonia* infections	62/116 (53.4%) ESBL
Linares et al,[22] 2009	902 SOT	191 with bloodstream infection	54% *E coli* ESBL producing 57% *K pneumoniae* ESBL producing 77% *Enterobacter* spp. ESBL producing 31% *Pseudomonas* MDR
Men et al,[23] 2013	350 SOT	78 (22.3%) with gram-negative bacilli infection	33 (42.3%) with ESBL: 16/18 *E coli*, 4/4 *Enterobacter* spp., 13/16 *K pneumoniae*, 32/71 (45.1%) with MBL
Mlynarczyk et al,[24] 2009	311 *Pseudomonas* isolates from 228 patients	—	41/228 (18%) carbapenem resistant 24/228 (10.5%) MBL
Mlynarczyk et al,[25] 2009	257 SOT patients with *S marascens*	—	188/257 (73%) ESBL
Morena et al,[26] 2007	2935 SOT 991 HSCT	730 bloodstream infections	14.5% Enteric bacilli MDR 9.7% nonfermentative 16.2% *S aureus*

(*continued on next page*)

Table 1
(continued)

Author	Study Subjects	Type of Infection	Data on Antibiotic Resistant Pathogens
Reddy et al,[27] 2010	248 patients with *A baumannii*	14 SOT 234 non-SOT	38/248 (15.3%) Carbapenem resistant. More prevalent in liver transplant (6/14 [42.9%) vs non-liver transplant (32/234 [13.7%])
Shi et al,[28] 2009	475 liver transplant	152 (32%) with gram-negative bacillus bacteremia with 190 isolates	107/190 (56.3%0) MDR: 21/32 (62.5%) of *A. baumannii*, 20/35 (57.1%) of *O anthropic*, 23/42 (54.8%) of Enterobacteriaceae; 26/48 (54.2%) *S maltophilia*; 17/33 (51.5%) of *Pseudomonas* species
Shields et al,[29] 2012	XDR *A baumannii* isolated from 69 SOT	28 (40.5%) colonized 41 (59.4%) infected	—
Riera et al,[9] 2015	170 lung transplants	24 VAP	2/11 (18.1%) MRSA 4/19 (21%) Enterobacteriaceae with ESBL 14/28 (50%) *P aeruginosa* MDR
Song et al,[10] 2014	51 liver transplants	53 ESKAPE infections	28/53 (52.8%) resistant-ESKAPE: 1/10 VRE, 8/10 (80%) MRSA, 6/7 *K pneumoniae* ESBL, 1/3 *Enterobacter* spp. ESBL, 10/18 *A baumannii* MDR

Abbreviations: ESBL, extended spectrum β-lactamase; ESKAPE, Enterococcus faecium, Staphylococcus aureus, Klebsiella pneumoniae, Acinetobacter baumannii, Pseudomonas aeruginosa, and Enterobacter species; HSCT, hematopoietic stem cell transplant; MBL, metallo-β lactamase; MDR, multidrug resistant; MRSA, methicillin-resistant Staphylococcus aureus; SOT, solid organ transplant; UTI, urinary tract infection; VRE, vancomycin-resistant Enterococcus faecium; XDR, extremely drug resistant.

not show significance for any specific type of transplant, so there is likely no association. Risk factors that were found to be significant in more than 1 study included prior transplant,[7,16] length of stay before infection,[20,31] advancing age,[16,20] hemodialysis,[15,21] and prior antibiotic.[7,15,19,31] As far as antecedent antibiotics are concerned, XDR *A baumannii* and carbapenem-resistant *A baumannii* were found to be associated with prior carbapenem use.[15,19] Greater acuity of illness was found to be associated with resistant pathogens in several studies with septic shock,[7] admission to the intensive care unit,[31] and respiratory failure[31] being associated in 3 separate studies.

Inappropriate Empiric Antibiotics

Not all studies reported appropriateness of empiric antibiotic regimen for resistant pathogens. In those that did have available data, inappropriate empiric antibiotic regimens were frequently used in patients with MDR pathogens. This was highest in the retrospective case series of ESBL infections in SOT patients by Winters and colleagues,[32] where they found that 85% of empiric regimens for first episode of ESBL infections were inappropriate. Median time to change to appropriate therapy was reported as 3.5 days. Other studies with proportion of empiric antibiotics being appropriate included 21.6% in resistant *Enterococcus faecium*, *Staphylococcus aureus*, *Klebsiella pneumoniae*, *Acinetobacter baumannii*, *Pseudomonas aeruginosa*, and *Enterobacter* species (ESKAPE pathogens) in the study by Bodro and colleagues,[7] 38% in the study looking at incidence of ESBL-producing organisms in patients with *Enterobacteriaceae* bacteremia by Aguiar and colleagues,[12] and 42.3% in the study of MDR *A baumannii* infections by Kim and colleagues.[18]

Interestingly, the study by Aguiar and colleagues[12] showed that use of appropriate empiric antibiotics was associated with increased mortality (6/10 [60%] of deaths vs 7/29 [24%] of survivors; $P = .056$) The authors concluded that this paradox was attributable to selection bias, because these patients typically were sicker with higher Charlson comorbidity index and Pitt bacteremia scores. Additionally, Kalil and colleagues[33] in their comparison of mortality owing to bacteremia in transplant versus nontransplant patients found that transplant patients are less likely to receive appropriate antibiotics (84% vs 98%). Presumably this would be owing to presence of resistance among isolates; however, those data were not included.

Other studies did not find this paradoxic relationship between appropriate antibiotic use and mortality as they found that appropriate antibiotics were protective.[19] In the study by Kim and colleagues,[18] those patients who died were far more likely to have inadequate empiric antibiotics versus those who survived with a hazard ratio (HR) of 4.19; however, this was a study in which 75.7% of isolates were considered panresistant (defined in their study as resistant to all commercially available antibiotics except colistin), so antibiotic selection was very limited. In the study by De Gouvea and colleagues,[15] appropriate antibiotics were found to be associated with a 96% reduction in mortality (odds ratio [OR], 0.04). In the study by Men and colleagues,[23] 75% of patients with inappropriate antibiotics perished compared with 32% of those on correct antibiotics. And, last, Lupei and colleagues[31] found that the 28-day mortality for those on inappropriate antibiotics at 24 hours was 14%, compared with 2% of those on appropriate antibiotics. This last study investigated the risks associated with inadequate antibiotics and found that younger age, longer courses of intravenous antibiotics before transplant, and greater duration of stay before transplant were associated.

Morbidity and Mortality Associated with Multidrug-resistant Organisms

Mortality rates tend to be high in SOT patients with MDRO pathogens compared with nonresistant organism. This was seen in Bodro and colleagues,[7] with 35.3% of patients with ESKAPE pathogens dying compared with 14.4% of patients with non-ESKAPE pathogens.

The risk of mortality does not seem to be related to the immunosuppression owing to antirejection medications and may in fact be protective. Two studies are included that compare mortality in bacteremic patients who have undergone SOT versus those who have not. Camargo and colleagues[8] showed statistically similar rates of mortality between the SOT group (34.5%) and the nontransplant group (40.5%). Patients with stem cell transplant were also included in this analysis and had a statistically significant decrease in mortality (16.7%), but were much more likely to have gram-positive infections with higher proportion of coagulase-negative *Staphylococcus* (CNS). Another study by Kalil and colleagues[33] comparing bacteremic sepsis in transplant and nontransplant patients found that SOT was associated with a decrease risk of death when controlling for other factors. The 28-day mortality in the SOT group was 78% lower (HR, 0.22; $P = .001$) and 57% lower at 90 days (HR, 0.43; $P = .25$).[33] The other factors in the multivariable hazard model included WBC count, platelet count, elevated heart rate, elevated respiratory rate, Sepsis-related Organ Failure Assessment (SOFA) score, and presence of multiorgan system failure.[33]

Mortality Risks

Antimicrobial resistance itself was not typically associated with mortality in these studies, except in the study by Kitazono and colleagues,[19] who found that those with extremely drug-resistant isolates had increased risk of mortality. Mortality was associated more commonly with increased severity of illness, whether it was by a specific system (Charlson comorbidity index,[12] Pitt bacteremia score,[12] SOFA score,[16] Acute Physiology And Chronic Health Evaluation [APACHE] II),[19] or by other objective data, for example, respiratory failure,[7] mechanical ventilation,[15,26] heart failure upon admission,[31] multiorgan system failure,[31] and septic shock.[10,26]

One study looking at XDR *A baumannii* did assess type of therapy and mortality.[29] In the study, all patients on monotherapy died. Of the 11 patients on colistin plus a non-carbapenem antibiotic, 10 died, including 0 of 7 on tigecycline plus colistin. Of the 21 patients on colistin plus a carbapenem, 16 survived although the isolates should have been resistant to the carbapenem. This may further support combination therapy for XDR pathogens.

THE NEUTROPENIC HOST

Early in the treatment of hematologic malignancies in children and young adults, it was recognized that empiric antibiotics directed at bacterial pathogens including Pseudomonas aeruginosa (PSDA) were important in the supportive care of the neutropenic patient.[34] Considerations include host risk stratification using scoring systems such as Multinational Association Of Supportive Care In Cancer,[35] the type of cytotoxic chemotherapy, projected duration of neutropenia, and whether granulocyte colony stimulating factors can be used, and the use of antibiotic prophylaxis (eg, fluoroquinolones, trimethoprim–sulfamethoxazole). Clinical infectious disease syndromes will also dictate which pathogens are of greatest concern: severe mucositis syndromes and oral *Streptococcus* spp.; pneumonia and *P aeruginosa*, *Klebsiella pneumoniae, Streptococcus pneumoniae*, MRSA; skin and skin structure infections, device-related bacteremias and MRSA, *K pneumoniae, A baumannii*; typhilitis-enteric gram-negative rods, *Enterococcus* spp. including VRE; and urinary tract infection–enteric gram-negative bacilli, *P aeruginosa*, MRSA, *Enterococcus* spp. The changing epidemiology of bacterial infections in neutropenic hosts reflects all of the host risks, as well as the emergence of antibiotic resistant pathogens in the hospital and the community.[36,37] More care is being delivered to patients with malignancies in the outpatient setting, and thus the epidemiology reflects that of the community as well as the hospital (eg, CTX-M–producing *E coli*, fluoroquinolone-resistant *Enterobacteriaceae* and *P aeruginosa*, *A baumannii*; community-acquired MRSA (CA-MRSA); and penicillin-resistant *Streptococcus pneumoniae*). Empiric antibiotic therapies must take the changing microbial landscape into consideration. The role of newer agents with antipseudomonal spectrum have not yet been defined: ceftazidime-avibactam[38] and ceftolozane-tazobactam.[39] Alternative gram-positive therapies such asceftaroline, daptomycin, dalbvancin, oritavancin, and tedizolid also offer possible prospects for treatment of infections with MDRO gram-positive organisms.[40]

Prevalence of Multidrug-resistant Organisms in Cancer Patients with Neutropenic Fever

The organisms responsible for bacteremic neutropenic fever have been characterized over many decades of clinical observation and a shift in the type of organisms and antibiotic susceptibility phenotypes has been noted. One of the most comprehensive early studies in 1993 showed that, among 1051 bacteremias in 9 French and 1 Belgian hospital, a total of 1147 isolates were obtained, with 86 blood cultures showing polymicrobial infection.[41] The other pathogens isolated included *Escherichia coli* (10.7%), *Klebsiella–Enterobacter–Serratia* (6.1%), other Enterobacteriaceae (2.2%), *P aeruginosa* (4.8%), other nonfermenters (4.7%), CNS (40.8%), *Staphylococcus aureus* (9.9%), streptococci (5.4%), enterococci (2.2%), anaerobes (3.4%), yeasts (3.5%), and other bacteria (6.9%). Antibiotic prophylaxis was not being used in patients at the time, but in 34.6% of the cases, patients were receiving systemic antibiotics when blood cultures were obtained. The role of antimicrobial resistance in outcomes for these patients was not addressed. It was noted, however, that gram-positive organisms predominated in cancer patients at this time, reflecting a shift in pathogens owing to the adoption of empiric antipseudomonal coverage.[34]

In more contemporary surveys that overlapped some with this very early period, Mebis and colleagues[42] and Ortega and colleagues[43] looked at all bloodstream isolates from neutropenic fever patients from 1994 to 2008, and 1991 to 2012. In both large series, gram-positive organisms (namely, CNS) predominated, but a shift in susceptibility to oxacillin-resistant CNS was observed.[42] Among *S aureus* isolates, the majority remained methicillin susceptible with 214 methicillin-sensitive *S aureus* (5.9%) and 48 (1.3%) MRSA.[42] During this time, it became standard practice to administer oral fluoroquinolones to patients who were neutropenic, and in the Mebis study, to use cefepime/amikacin for empiric therapy of febrile neutropenic patients. An increase of gram-negative isolates, namely *E coli*, was foreshadowed in the latter period (2006–2012).[43] High rates of fluoroquinolone resistance were noted (66% gram-negative pathogens[42] and 73% *E coli* isolates[43]). A reduced susceptibility of *P aeruginosa* strains to meropenem and cefepime was also noted. Twenty-nine isolates (7.2%) were observed in the period of study.[42] Resistance to cefotaxime, presumably because of the production of ESBLs, was noted in 26% of the *E coli* isolates.[43] Similar findings were reported in Australia from 2001 to 2010.[44]

However, in a large retrospective study conducted in France between 2003 and 2010,[45] examining 723 bacterial bloodstream isolates researchers began to notice a definite predominance of gram-negative bacteria. Among 723 isolates, they found gram-negative bacilli (70.8%) and gram-positive cocci (18.7%). The rate of MRSA was 6.45% and of coagulase-negative staphylococci, 61.2%. No resistance to glycopeptides was detected. In *E coli*, as in the *Klebsiella–Enterobacter–Serratia* group, a

27% resistance to fluoroquinolones was observed. Concerning *P aeruginosa*, the phenotypes were distributed over penicillinase (23.4%) and cephalosporinase (13.1% were resistant to ceftazidime). The impermeability rate of imipenem was 9.3%. Increasing rates of gram-negative bacteria from less than 20% in 1996 to 80% in 2009 with a parallel decrease in gram-positive cocci (~80% in 1996 and ~5% in 2009) were noted. *E coli* isolates increased 2-fold, *Klebsiella pneumoniae* isolates 3-fold, and there was a 2.5-fold increase in nonfermenters with increases in fluoroquinolone resistance to 25% of *E coli*. Four percent of *E coli* were ESBL producers. There was a concomitant 50% decrease in MRSA observed, but no VRE were isolated. In a more recent study, in Barcelona, Spain, Gudiol and colleagues[46] compared 272 episodes of BSIs in adult neutropenic patients with cancer prospectively collected from January 1991 to December 1996 (first period), when quinolone prophylaxis was used, with 283 episodes recorded from January 2006 to March 2010 (second period), when antibacterial prophylaxis was stopped. Patients in the second period were significantly older and were more likely to have graft-versus-host disease and a urinary catheter in place, whereas the presence of a central venous catheter, parenteral nutrition, corticosteroids, and antifungal and quinolone prophylaxis were more frequent in the first period. More patients in the first period had mucositis and soft tissue infection as the origin of BSIs, but an endogenous source was more common during the second. Gram-positive BSI was more frequent in the first period (64% vs 41%; $P < .001$), mainly owing to coagulase-negative staphylococci and viridans group streptococci. Increases in MRSA BSI from 17% to 28.6% and enterococcal BSI (6% to 23%) were noted. In the second period, gram-negative BSI increased (28% vs 49%; $P < .001$), mostly owing to an increase in *K pneumoniae* isolates (7%–21%). Quinolone susceptibilities were recovered, but multidrug-resistant gram-negative BSI increased (from 3% to 11%; $P = .04$), including ESBL and AmpC hyperproducers, MDR *P aeruginosa* and *A baumannii*, and *Streptococcus maltophila*. Blennow and colleagues[47] also reported on the increase in gram-negatives over this period.

Since that time, many authors throughout the world have reported on the shift to more resistant gram-negative bacteria, and the possible role of prophylactic fluoroquinolones in the selection of fluoroquinolone resistant bacteria, and ESBL producers, especially among Enterobacteriaceae (reviewed by[37,48–62]) Because of this, Zhang and colleagues[63] looked at the issue of whether empiric oral fluoroquinolone is appropriate in low-risk neutropenic patients in China who presented with fever and BSI: 38 patients were studied and 74% had bloodstream isolates with *E coli*, with 46% resistance to fluoroquinolones. Other isolates included 2 *K pneumoniae* (1 resistant to fluoroquinolones). In a Swiss pediatric neutropenic fever cohort,[64] although gram-positive organisms predominated overall, it was noted that in centers that did not use fluoroquinolone prophylaxis, more *P aeruginosa* isolates were found; more fluoroquinolone-resistant gram-negative bacteria were found in centers where fluoroquinolone prophylaxis was used frequently. In university hospitals in Italy, high rates of *P aeruginosa* BSIs (20% of all BSI) were observed in febrile neutropenic patients, with 33% to 70% MDR PSDA isolates reported.[61,62,65,66] Other centers have reported increasing rates of MDR *A baumannii* and other ESKAPE pathogens,[6,50,51,57,65] including carbapenem-resistant *K pneumoniae* (35%).[61] Garza-Ramos and colleagues[67] also described a high prevalence of ESBL and GES carbapenemases in carbapenem-resistant *P aeruginosa* in their hospitals. In their study, they observed 124 imipenem-resistant *P aeruginosa* with 36.2% producing carbapenemases of IMP, VIM, and GES types. ESBL GES-19 and carbapenemase GES-20 β-lactamases were most prevalent (84%).

Gram-positive infections continue to predominate in some settings, such as pediatric cancer hospitals,[64,68,69] and was reported in 1 adult cancer hospital in Sweden.[70] These BSI in febrile neutropenic patients are predominantly caused by CNS and viridans streptococci, with relatively low rates of *S aureus* (including MRSA) and enterococci (including VRE). Some studies noted an increase in the number of *S pneumoniae* isolates, especially those resistant to ceftazidime, among febrile neutropenic patients, prompting an inquiry into the rates of pneumococcal vaccination.[71,72] Gudiol and colleagues[72] reported an increase in the number of vancomycin susceptible *E faecium* isolates with high-level resistance to ampicillin and fluoroquinolones, related to the use of antibiotic prophylaxis in these patients. These authors expressed concerns that this was a harbinger of future VRE as vancomycin use increases in such patients.

Risks for Multidrug-resistant Organisms in the Febrile Neutropenic Patient

Bassetti and Righi[73] reviewed risk factors for development of MDRO infections in oncology patients, including patients with neutropenic fever. Colonization, previous infection, previous exposure to broad spectrum antibiotics, and/or prophylaxis with fluoroquinolones were associated with these types of infections, as well as advanced disease with severe presentation and prolonged hospitalization, as well as the presence medical devices and instrumentation.[74,75]

A number of additional studies have found similar associations between MDRO infections and febrile neutropenia. In a retrospective study of 747 bacteremias in a 4-year period in Barcelona, Spain,[76] antibiotic exposures before neutropenic fever increased the odds of an MDRO being isolated by 3.57-fold (95% CI, 1.63–7.80); presence of a urinary catheter (OR, 2.41; 95% CI, 1.01–5.74). In this series, 13.7% of the gram-negative bacteria isolated were multidrug resistant. In a separate study, these authors found that carbapenem use was associated with increased rates of ampicillin resistant, vancomycin susceptible *E faecium* bacteremias.[77] In a Melbourne pediatric oncology hospital, antibiotic-resistant gram-negative BSI were associated with high-intensity chemotherapy (OR, 3.7; 95% CI, 1.2–11.4), hospital-acquired bacteremia (OR, 4.3; 95% CI, 2.0–9.6), and isolation of antibiotic-resistant gram-negative bacteria from any site within the preceding 12 months (OR, 9.9; 95% CI, 3.8–25.5).[53] Kim and colleagus[78] showed that a hospital stay of longer than 2 weeks during the 3 months preceding bacteremia (adjusted OR, 5.887; 95% CI, 1.572–22.041) and the use of broad-spectrum cephalosporins in the 4 weeks before bacteremia (adjusted OR, 6.186; 95% CI, 1.616–23.683) were significantly related to the acquisition of ESBL producing *Enterobacteriaceae*. However, the 30-day mortality rates for ESBL bacteremia and non-ESBL bacteremia were not significantly different (15 vs 5%; $P = .199$). A matched case-control study (1:2) in hospitals in New York City, including both pediatric and adult oncology patients in intensive care between February 2007 and January 2010, found that immunocompromised state (OR, 1.55; $P = .047$) and exposure to amikacin (OR, 13.81; $P < .001$), levofloxacin (OR, 2.05; $P = .005$), or trimethoprim–sulfamethoxazole (OR, 3.42; $P = .009$) were factors associated with XDR gram-negative bacilli health care–associated infections.[79] A retrospective chart review of 192 adults with cancer in China who had *Enterobacter* bacteremia evaluated risk factors and treatment outcomes associated with extended-spectrum cephalosporin resistance. Recent use of a third-generation cephalosporins, older age, tumor progression at last evaluation, recent surgery, and nosocomial acquisition were all associated with extended spectrum cephalosporin resistant *Enterobacter* bacteremia.[80]

Investigators in Mexico city evaluated the impact of fecal colonization with extended-spectrum β-lactamase-producing *E coli* for BSI, clinical outcome, and costs in patients with hematologic malignancies and severe neutropenia.[51] Colonization with ESBL *E coli* increased the risk of BSI by the same strain (relative risk, 3.4; 95% CI, 1.5–7.8; $P = .001$), shorter time to death (74 ± 62 vs 95 ± 83 days; $P < .001$), longer hospital stay (64 ± 39 vs 48 ± 32 days; $P = .01$), and higher infection-related costs ($6528 ± $4348 vs $4722 ± $3173; $P = .01$). There was no difference in overall mortality between the groups. The authors concluded that stool colonization by ESBL *E coli* was associated with increased risk of BSI by this strain, longer hospital stay, and higher related costs. However, Nesher and colleagues[81] at MD Anderson found in a 2-year retrospective review of all patients who received allogeneic hematopoietic stem cell transplants that the incidence of fecal colonization with *P aeruginosa*, including MDR strains, was low, and that the rate of infections with these bacteria was also low. The incidence of MDR *P aeruginosa* in the entire cohort was only 2.2% (18/794); 12 had positive surveillance stool cultures and 7 of these patients later developed MDR *P aeruginosa* infections. Older patients and patients with acute myelogenous leukemia were more likely to be colonized, and to develop subsequent infection. No infection-related deaths were observed during the first 30 days after infection. In this study, the positive predictive value of the PSDA plus surveillance stool culture was only 23% for infection. Notably, 83% of the patients were on fluoroquinolones in the 30 days after hematopoietic cell transplantation. Patients who were not colonized had a low chance of developing *P aeruginosa* infection. Most patients who developed infection did not have fecal colonization, suggesting a different source of infection.

Inappropriate Empiric Antibiotics

Given the profound immunosuppression associated with neutropenia in cancer patients, reliance on early diagnosis and appropriate antibiotic selection would seem to be even more critical in this subset of infectious disease patients. In a recent review,[62] antimicrobial resistance and/or the inadequacy of empirical antibiotic treatment have been frequently linked to a worse outcome in cancer patients with BSIs caused by gram-negative isolates.

In 1 study,[82] immunocompetent patients with BSIs caused by ESBL-producing organisms who received inappropriate antibiotics (defined as receipt of treatment with an active antibiotic >72 hours after collection of the first positive blood culture) had an overall mortality of 38.2% over a 21-day period. In their multivariate analysis, these authors found that inadequate initial antimicrobial therapy (OR, 6.28; 95% CI, 3.18–12.42; $P < .001$) and unidentified primary infection site (OR = 2.69; 95% CI = 1.38–5.27; $P = .004$) were factors associated with mortality. The patients who received inappropriate empiric antibiotics (89/186 [47.8%]) were 3 times more likely to die compared with the adequately treated group (59.5% vs 18.5%; OR = 2.38; 95% CI = 1.76–3.22; $P < .001$). In a large study looking at hospitalized cancer patients, Bodro and colleagues[49] showed that, in patients with bacteremia with ESKAPE organisms, inappropriate empiric antibiotics were given more frequently (55.6% vs 21.5%, $P < .001$), were associated with more persistence of bacteremia (25% vs 9.7%; $P < .05$), septic metastases (8% vs 4%; $P < .05$), and early case fatality (23% vs 11%; $P < .05$). In a subgroup analysis of data from 54 patients with an absolute neutrophil count of less than 500/mm^3 in a larger study of *P aeruginosa* BSI in 234 cancer patients[83] (n = 54), the patients who had appropriate empirical or targeted combination therapy showed better outcomes than those who underwent monotherapy or inappropriate therapy ($P < .05$). In a smaller study looking at MDR *P aeruginosa* bacteremias in neutropenic fever patients, 6 of 22 patients received inappropriate antibiotics or developed resistance during therapy, and demonstrated an increased mortality of 83.3% versus 27% in those who received appropriate antibiotics.[65] A retrospective study looking at *K pneumoniae* BSI in southern Europe[84] demonstrated a high rate of resistance in the hospitals studied: of 217

BSIs, 92 (42%) involved KPC-positive *K pneumoniae*, 49 (23%) ESBL-positive, and 1 (0.5%) metallo-β lactamase–positive isolates. Appropriate empiric antibiotics were administered in 74% of infections caused by non-ESBL non-KPC strains, versus 33% of ESBL and 23% of KPC cases ($P < .0001$). In a multivariate analysis accounting for disease severity, inappropriate antibiotic therapy demonstrated close to a 2-fold higher rate of death (adjusted HR, 1.9; 95% CI, 1.1–3.4; $P = .02$). Even in lower risk patients, Zhang and colleagues[63] showed that inappropriate antibiotics in 22 of 38 patients led to higher rates of clinical deterioration (29%) and further infection (29%), but did not impact mortality in these low-risk neutropenic patients.

One study examined BSI-related mortality in 400 patients who underwent hematopoietic stem cell transplants, before and after engraftment, and found a difference in the rates of inappropriate antibiotic administration between the preengraftment and postengraftment periods.[72] In the preengraftment period, 17% of patients had a delay of more than 48 hours in receipt of appropriate antibiotics, versus 27% in the postengraftment group. This resulted in a greater number of admissions to the intensive care unit (7% vs 25%) and a higher case fatality rate (4% vs 25%).[72] However, overall mortality in the cohort was not increased, and these authors did not find an association with inappropriate antibiotics when looking at overall mortality. This may be related to the fact that 50% of the patients on inappropriate antibiotics had central line–associated BSIs and central venous catheter lines were removed.

These authors also looked prospectively at the administration of inappropriate antibiotics to cancer patients with enterococcal BSIs, and found that patients with *E faecium* were more likely to receive inappropriate antibiotics than patients with *Enterobacter faecalis* (44% vs 24%), but found no difference in overall mortality (30% *E faecium*, 26% *E faecalis*).[77] Similarly, in settings where CNS accounts for the majority of MDR organisms, mortality is not increased as a result.[51]

Morbidity and Mortality Associated with Multidrug-resistant Organisms

As noted, the presence of MDRO and the receipt of inappropriate antibiotic therapy early in the course of an infection are linked with increased mortality in neutropenic and other cancer patients, but there is a relationship between the specific type of infection and mortality, with greater mortality for MDR gram-negative pathogens in most studies.[44,62,65,82] BSI with a multidrug-resistant organism (OR, 3.61; 95% CI, 1.40–9.32; $P = .008$) was an independent predictor of mortality at 7 days after a positive blood culture.[44]

In a pediatric setting, overall mortality was not affected by the presence of antibiotic resistant gram-negative pathogens[53]; however, these authors did show that antibiotic-resistant gram-negative infections were associated with longer median hospital length of stay (23.5 vs 14.0 days; $P = .0007$), longer median intensive care unit length of stay (3.8 vs 1.6 days; $P = .02$), and a higher rate of invasive ventilation (15% vs 5.2%; $P = .03$). In addition, mortality rates were not increased in association with drug resistance in the setting of gram-positive infections[68,77] or in low-risk neutropenic patients.[63]

Mortality Risks and Multidrug-resistant Organisms

Antimicrobial resistance and/or the inadequacy of empirical antibiotic treatment have been frequently linked with a worse outcome in cancer patients with BSIs caused by gram-negative isolates.[62] BSI with a multidrug-resistant organism (OR, 3.61; 95% CI, 1.40–9.32; $P = .008$) was an independent predictor of mortality at 7 days after a positive blood culture.[44] In a large study of the effect of antibiotic resistance on outcomes in intensive care patients, including immunocompromised and neutropenic patients, multiple factors in both case and control subjects significantly predicted increased mortality at different time intervals after hospital-acquired infection diagnosis.[79] At 7 days, liver disease (HR, 5.52), immunocompromised state (HR, 3.41), and BSI (HR, 2.55) predicted mortality; at 15 days, age (HR, 1.02 per year increase), liver disease (HR, 3.34), and immunocompromised state (HR, 2.03) predicted mortality. Mortality at 30 days was predicted by age (HR, 1.02 per 1-year increase), liver disease (HR, 3.34), immunocompromised state (HR, 2.03), and hospitalization in a medical intensive care unit (HR, 1.85). Infections caused by XDR gram-negative pathogens were associated with potentially modifiable factors. Moghnieh and colleagues[56] performed a retrospective study of 75 episodes of bacteremia occurring in febrile neutropenic patients admitted to a hematology-oncology unit from 2009 to 2012. Increased mortality was associated with MDRO BSI (22.7% died with extended spectrum cephalosporin resistance vs susceptible 3.8%; MDR bacteremia resulted in death in 4/7 [57%] versus 3/68 4.4% in non-MDR bacteremia patients). Risks associated with MDRO included carbapenem or piperacillin-tazobactam exposure greater than 4 days before the bacteremia. Two studies did not show an association between MDRO and mortality; in these studies, mortality in neutropenic fever patients with BSI were associated with a septic shock presentation, and polymicrobial sepsis.[43,59] Factors associated with lower mortality were isolation of CNS [OR, 0.38; 95% CI, 0.20–0.73, $P = .004$] and empirical therapy with amikacin (OR, 0.50; 95% CI, 0.29–0.88; $P = .016$)[43]; appropriate combination therapy also increased survival in patients with febrile neutropenia.[83] Carbapenems have been associated with a trend toward increased survival[85] in patients with neutropenic fever and ESBL-producing *E coli* and *K pneumoniae* BSI.

P aeruginosa and MDR *P aeruginosa*,[61,65,83] ESBL-producing *E coli*, especially CTX-M–producing and ST131[86]; *K pneumoniae*[61,84] and *Enterobacter aerogenes*,[80] KPC and metallo-β lactamase–producing *K pneumoniae*,[84] and *A baumannii*[61] were all associated with increased overall mortality in cancer patients with neutropenic fever, adjusting for other risks, such as degree of neutropenia, advanced or relapsed disease, APACHE score, age, and septic shock, typically associated with worse outcomes in immunocompromised patients. Discontinuation of prophylaxis with fluoroquinolones in some settings did not affect the overall mortality, only shifted the etiology from gram-positive bacteria to gram-negative bacteria.[46]

HUMAN IMMUNODEFICIENCY VIRUS INFECTION AND AIDS

HIV/AIDS is a common cause of immune suppression. The increased incidence of infection compared with non-HIV patients has been well documented. In an Ugandan cohort including HIV-positive and -negative subjects, the incidence of septicemia for HIV-infected patients was 32.4 per 1000 person-years versus 2.6 per 1000 person-years for uninfected subjects.[87] In a study looking at the incidence of CA-MRSA, those with HIV had a 17.7-fold higher incidence of infection compared with uninfected subjects (40.3 cases/1000 person-years vs 2.3 infections/1000 person-years).[88] A separate study found the rate of CA-MRSA to be 6-fold higher than the general population (9.96 per 1000 person-years vs 1.57 per 1000 person-years).[89] In a separate retrospective study of a large United States health care network, it was found that 11% of HIV-infected individuals had an MRSA infection versus 1.4% of uninfected individuals.[90] Not surprisingly, the incidence of infection increased as CD4 count decreases. The Ugandan cohort investigating incidence of septicemia reported a 7-fold higher incidence in those with CD4 below 200 versus those with CD4 of greater than 500 (78 per 1000 person-years vs 11 per 1000 person-years).[87]

The purpose of this final section is to review the impact of antibacterial resistance on nonmycobacterial infections in persons living with HIV/AIDS.

Incidence and Risks for Methicillin-resistant Staphylococcus aureus Colonization and Infection in Human Immunodeficiency Virus-infected Individuals

There is a large body of literature investigating MRSA colonization and infection in persons living with HIV. Colonization with *S aureus* is common in the HIV population.[91–93] Colonization with *S aureus* ranged from 23.1%[93] up to 76.7%.[91] The prevalence of *S aureus* colonization has been shown to be higher in HIV-infected than uninfected individuals. In an Indian case-control study, the prevalence of *S aureus* colonization in HIV-infected individuals was nearly 4 times that of non-HIV individuals (44% vs 12%).[94] Although *S aureus* colonization is common, the prevalence of MRSA colonization among the *S aureus* isolates is variable. The study by Giuliani and colleagues[93] showed that although 23.1% of their HIV-infected men who have sex with men cohort was colonized with *S aureus*, none of them were colonized with MRSA. Other studies that showed relatively low prevalence of MRSA colonization included the study by Kotpal and colleagues[94] in which only 6% of subjects were colonized, and the study by Crum-Cianflone and coworkers,[92] in which only 4% of subjects were colonized. Other studies showed higher rates of MRSA colonization in HIV-infected individuals of 11% from Popovich and colleagues,[89] 13.3% from Chacko and colleagues,[91] 15.4% from Farley and colleagues,[95] and 13% to 15% between baseline and 12 months.[96] The variability may come from the number of sites tested; Farley and colleagues[95] found that 40% of their MRSA-colonized individuals had negative nares tests. One study compared the rate of colonization in HIV-infected versus noninfected subjects and found that MRSA colonization was significantly higher in the HIV-infected (11% vs 4.2%).[97] Numerous factors associated with colonization were found. Socioeconomic factors associated with increased risk of MRSA colonization included lower income,[95] previous arrest,[95] African American race,[92] history of substance abuse,[95] and "alternative" housing (defined as either homelessness or residence in shelter, halfway house, substance abuse center, public housing, subsidized housing, supported living, nursing home, or mental health facility).[97] In the same study, there was also a trend toward geographic location as a risk for colonization in 1 study, but this was not found to be significant. In fact, the investigators found that, after controlling for incarceration, residence, and geography, HIV status was no longer significantly associated with MRSA colonization. This study found that Hispanic ethnicity was a protective factor. Medical factors associated with colonization included prior MRSA infection and recent sexually transmitted infection,[92] current or prior abscess, and recent hospitalization.[95] The use of antiretroviral therapy was found to be protective in this study as well.

As several studies discussed previously show, the rate of MRSA infection in HIV-infected individuals is high. In 1 study, it was shown to be the cause of 0.5% of hospitalizations among HIV patients.[98] Additionally, 2 studies that looked at *S aureus* bacteremia found that MRSA accounted for 43.5%[99] and 66% of episodes of bacteremia, respectively.[100] In looking at the causative strains, it has been found that the USA 300 strain is very common. It accounted for 54% of cases of *S aureus* bacteremia in the study by Furuno and colleagues[100] In other studies, the USA 300 strain accounted for 64%,[96] 80%,[97] and 86% of infections, respectively.[95]

Risks for MRSA infection were similar to those for colonization. Socioeconomic factors included African American race,[99] residence in alternative housing, and residence in high-risk zip codes.[89]

Personal habits associated with MRSA infection included intravenous drug use,[99] methamphetamine use, having a sex partner with skin infection, routine hands-on contact with customers at work, frequent fingernail biting, and routine use of a public hot tub or sauna.[101] In this study, use of a condom during every sexual encounter was found to be associated with a 90% decrease in MRSA infection.

Medical risks included end-stage renal disease,[99] lower CD4 count,[88,91,99,102] invasive procedures in the previous year,[98] history of syphilis,[88] history of MRSA infection[96] hospital admission (with 1 study finding that admission >10 days was a risk,[91] and another finding that every 5 days of a hospital stay increased risk for MRSA infection by 14%[98]). Prior β-lactam use was found to be a risk in 2 different studies.[88,102] The OR for MRSA infection increased from 2.76 for 1 β-lactam prescription in the past year to 36.42 for 4 or more β-lactam prescriptions in the past year.[88] Additionally, MRSA colonization in the groin was found to have an adjusted relative risk of 4.8 in 1 study.[101] Use of trimethoprim–sulfamethoxazole for prophylaxis of opportunistic infection was found to be protective with an 80% reduction in risk[101] Although this association was interesting, the impact on resistance for those on prophylaxis is significant, because a study on HIV-infected children showed that 91% of the *S aureus* isolates that were isolated were trimethoprim–sulfamethoxazole resistant.[103] Few of the studies investing MRSA in HIV-infected individuals assessed the morbidity and mortality associated with it. In 1 study looking at *S aureus* bacteremia, the overall mortality rate was found to be 8% with CA-MRSA associated with an increase in mortality (OR, 2.93).[100] In other studies, however, MRSA patients did not have an increased risk of mortality. The study by Everett and colleagues[104] found that MRSA patients "experienced a combined outcome of ICU admission, intubation, and/or chest tube 58% of the time, compared with 30% of the time for methicillin-sensitive *S aureus* patients, but not increased mortality." Additionally, the study by Tumbarello and colleagues[102] showed that MRSA was not associated with higher mortality. Additional studies comparing CA-MRSA with hospital-acquired MRSA in HIV patients would be needed to determine if the CA-MRSA has increased mortality in this population compared with other strains.

Antibiotic Resistance in Streptococcus pneumoniae in Patients with Human Immunodeficiency Virus Infection

S pneumoniae manifests differently in HIV-infected individuals versus noninfected individuals; HIV-infected individuals are more likely to develop pneumonia rather than meningitis.[105] This older study also found that there was no difference in resistance between HIV-infected and noninfected individuals. Other studies showed that antibiotic resistance was found to be high in HIV-infected patients with *S pneumoniae* infections, although a comparison was not made with noninfected individuals. Trimethoprim–sulfamethoxazole resistance was high in all studies[87,103,106–109] ranging from 41% to 100%. β-Lactam resistance was less common, but still prevalent. In the reviewed studies, one showed that all isolates were susceptible to amoxicillin.[106] Two other studies found penicillin resistance in one-third of cases.[87] The highest reported incidence of resistance to penicillin was 44% in a French study.[107]

Antibiotic Resistance in Enterococcus spp. Among Human Immunodeficiency Virus-infected Patients

Data on VRE among HIV-infected individuals are sparse. One case-control study found that VRE colonization occurred in 8 of 103 patients (7.8%). HIV-infected individuals demonstrated a trend toward higher rates of colonization than non–HIV-infected controls (3.1%), but this was not statistically significant.[110] In this study, the HIV-infected patients were also more likely to be colonized with an amoxicillin/ampicillin resistant isolate. In another study, none of the 89 HIV-infected individuals were colonized with VRE.[111]

Does Trimethoprim–Sulfamethoxazole Prophylaxis Cause Resistance?

Several studies have looked at colonization by trimethoprim-sulfamethoxazole–resistant organisms among HIV-infected individuals. One study found that trimethoprim–sulfamethoxazole resistance was 97.7% after 2 weeks of prophylaxis, compared with 70.1% for those not on prophylaxis.[112] In Tanzania, patients on prophylaxis had increase in trimethoprim–sulfamethoxazole resistance from 64.9 to 86.2 after 1 week of prophylaxis.[113] Another study found that 90.6% of HIV-infected children were colonized with trimethoprim-sulfamethoxazole–resistant Enterobacteriaceae.[103] Approximately 70% of this cohort was using trimethoprim–sulfamethoxazole prophylaxis. Use of trimethoprim–sulfamethoxazole was associated with trimethoprim–sulfamethoxazole resistance (86% vs 91%) and dicloxacillin resistance (70% vs 87%), but not cefotaxime resistance (54 v 50%).

Other Antibiotic Resistance Among Gram-negative Pathogens, Including Extended Spectrum β-Lacatamase, Among Human Immunodeficiency Virus-infected Patients

In a study among HIV-infected individuals with symptomatic urinary tract infection in South India, 29 of 36 *E coli* urine isolates (80.6%) were resistant to multiple drugs.[114] Resistance to trimethoprim–sulfamethoxazole was observed in 30 (83.3%) of these urinary isolates. Seven isolates (19.4%) in this study were resistant to all antibiotics except imipenem. In other studies, fluoroquinolone resistance was found to be high. One group looked at 79 cases of Shigella dysentery, of which 54 occurred in HIV-infected individuals.[115] Sixty-six percent of the HIV-infected individuals had fluoroquinolone-resistant isolates versus 24% of the non–HIV-infected individuals. Another study investigating ESBL uropathogens found that fluoroquinolone resistance occurred in 77.6% of isolates from HIV-infected individuals versus 26.2% non–HIV-infected individuals.[116]

Data on ESBL pathogens among HIV-infected individuals is also sparse, but the limited data do show ESBL pathogens to be common in this population. One study found that HIV-infected individuals with uropathogenic *E coli* were more likely to have ESBL and AmpC coproducers than non–HIV-infected individuals (71.1% vs 35.7%), although ESBL producers (without AmpC) were more common among non–HIV-infected individuals (16.7% vs 3.9%).[116] In a South African study, 13 of 25 HIV-infected children with Enterobacteriaceae causing bacteremia were found to be infected with ESBL isolates.[103] In the same study, nasopharyngeal colonization was investigated and found that of the 32 children with nasal colonization by Enterobacteriaceae, 16 (50%) were ESBL isolates.

SUMMARY

Rates of infection with MDR organisms are increasing among immunocompromised persons, as greater numbers of MDRO are observed throughout the population. Antibiotic prophylaxis and empiric antibiotic therapy influences the selection of these MDRO; susceptibility patterns vary among regions and even within hospitals. The astute clinician is aware of his or her regional unique antibiogram. MDRO, especially gram-negative pathogens, can be associated with worse outcomes among immunocompromised persons, and empiric antibiotic choices must be selected with the local antibiogram in mind if appropriate life-saving antibiotics are to be administered in a timely fashion. The role of rapid diagnostics and newer agents for MDRO is addressed elsewhere; studies are needed among immunocompromised persons to evaluate these novel approaches to improve outcomes.

REFERENCES

1. Paul WE. Fundamental immunology. 7th edition. Philadelphia: Wolters Kluwer; 2014.
2. Owen J. Kuby immunology. 7th edition. New York: W. H. Freeman; 2013.
3. Drekonja D, Reich J, Gezahegn S, et al. Fecal microbiota transplantation for Clostridium difficile infection: a systematic review. Ann Intern Med 2015;162:630–8.
4. Rana A, Gruessner A, Agopian VG, et al. Survival benefit of solid-organ transplant in the United States. JAMA Surg 2015;150:252–9.
5. Sanroman Budino B, Vazquez Martul E, Pertega Diaz S, et al. Autopsy-determined causes of death in solid organ transplant recipients. Transplant Proc 2004;36:787–9.
6. Al-Hasan MN, Razonable RR, Eckel-Passow JE, et al. Incidence rate and outcome of Gram-negative bloodstream infection in solid organ transplant recipients. Am J Transplant 2009;9:835–43.
7. Bodro M, Sabe N, Tubau F, et al. Risk factors and outcomes of bacteremia caused by drug-resistant ESKAPE pathogens in solid-organ transplant recipients. Transplantation 2013;96:843–9.
8. Camargo LF, Marra AR, Pignatari AC, et al. Nosocomial bloodstream infections in a nationwide study: comparison between solid organ transplant patients and the general population. Transpl Infect Dis 2015;17:308–13.
9. Riera J, Caralt B, Lopez I, et al, Vall d'Hebron Lung Transplant Study Group. Ventilator-associated respiratory infection following lung transplantation. Eur Respir J 2015;45:726–37.
10. Song SH, Li XX, Wan QQ, et al. Risk factors for mortality in liver transplant recipients with ESKAPE infection. Transplant Proc 2014;46:3560–3.
11. Kawecki D, Kwiatkowski A, Sawicka-Grzelak A, et al. Urinary tract infections in the early posttransplant period after kidney transplantation: etiologic agents and their susceptibility. Transplant Proc 2011;43:2991–3.
12. Aguiar EB, Maciel LC, Halpern M, et al. Outcome of bacteremia caused by extended-spectrum beta-lactamase-producing Enterobacteriaceae after solid organ transplantation. Transplant Proc 2014;46:1753–6.
13. Azap O, Togan T, Yesilkaya A, et al. Antimicrobial susceptibilities of uropathogen Escherichia coli in renal transplant recipients: dramatic increase in ciprofloxacin resistance. Transplant Proc 2013;45:956–7.
14. Bert F, Larroque B, Dondero F, et al. Risk factors associated with preoperative fecal carriage of extended-spectrum beta-lactamase-producing Enterobacteriaceae in liver transplant recipients. Transpl Infect Dis 2014;16:84–9.
15. de Gouvea EF, Martins IS, Halpern M, et al. The influence of carbapenem resistance on mortality in solid organ transplant recipients with Acinetobacter baumannii infection. BMC Infect Dis 2012;12:351.
16. Freire MP, Abdala E, Moura ML, et al. Risk factors and outcome of infections with Klebsiella pneumoniae carbapenemase-producing K. pneumoniae in kidney transplant recipients. Infection 2015;43:315–23.
17. Giannella M, Munoz P, Alarcon JM, et al, PISOT Study Group. Pneumonia in solid organ transplant recipients: a prospective multicenter study. Transpl Infect Dis 2014;16:232–41.
18. Kim YJ, Yoon JH, Kim SI, et al. High mortality associated with Acinetobacter species infection in liver transplant patients. Transplant Proc 2011;43:2397–9.
19. Kitazono H, Rog D, Grim SA, et al. Acinetobacter baumannii infection in solid organ transplant recipients. Clin Transplant 2015;29:227–32.

20. Lanini S, Costa AN, Puro V, et al, Donor-Recipient Infection Collaborative Study Group. Incidence of carbapenem-resistant gram negatives in Italian transplant recipients: a nationwide surveillance study. PLoS One 2015;10:e0123706.
21. Linares L, Cervera C, Hoyo I, et al. Klebsiella pneumoniae infection in solid organ transplant recipients: epidemiology and antibiotic resistance. Transplant Proc 2010;42:2941–3.
22. Linares L, Garcia-Goez JF, Cervera C, et al. Early bacteremia after solid organ transplantation. Transplant Proc 2009;41:2262–4.
23. Men TY, Wang JN, Li H, et al. Prevalence of multidrug-resistant gram-negative bacilli producing extended-spectrum beta-lactamases (ESBLs) and ESBL genes in solid organ transplant recipients. Transpl Infect Dis 2013;15:14–21.
24. Mlynarczyk G, Sawicka-Grzelak A, Szymanek K, et al. Resistance to carbapenems among Pseudomonas aeruginosa isolated from patients of transplant wards. Transplant Proc 2009;41:3258–60.
25. Mlynarczyk A, Szymanek K, Sawicka-Grzelak A, et al. CTX-M and TEM as predominant types of extended spectrum beta-lactamases among Serratia marcescens isolated from solid organ recipients. Transplant Proc 2009;41:3253–5.
26. Moreno A, Cervera C, Gavalda J, et al. Bloodstream infections among transplant recipients: results of a nationwide surveillance in Spain. Am J Transplant 2007;7:2579–86.
27. Reddy P, Zembower TR, Ison MG, et al. Carbapenem-resistant Acinetobacter baumannii infections after organ transplantation. Transpl Infect Dis 2010;12:87–93.
28. Shi SH, Kong HS, Xu J, et al. Multidrug resistant gram-negative bacilli as predominant bacteremic pathogens in liver transplant recipients. Transpl Infect Dis 2009;11:405–12.
29. Shields RK, Clancy CJ, Gillis LM, et al. Epidemiology, clinical characteristics and outcomes of extensively drug-resistant Acinetobacter baumannii infections among solid organ transplant recipients. PLoS One 2012;7:e52349.
30. Bodro M, Sabe N, Tubau F, et al. Extensively drug-resistant Pseudomonas aeruginosa bacteremia in solid organ transplant recipients. Transplantation 2015;99:616–22.
31. Lupei MI, Mann HJ, Beilman GJ, et al. Inadequate antibiotic therapy in solid organ transplant recipients is associated with a higher mortality rate. Surg Infect (Larchmt) 2010;11:33–9.
32. Winters HA, Parbhoo RK, Schafer JJ, et al. Extended-spectrum beta-lactamase-producing bacterial infections in adult solid organ transplant recipients. Ann Pharmacother 2011;45:309–16.
33. Kalil AC, Syed A, Rupp ME, et al. Is bacteremic sepsis associated with higher mortality in transplant recipients than in nontransplant patients? A matched case-control propensity-adjusted study. Clin Infect Dis 2015;60:216–22.
34. Pizzo PA, Hathorn JW, Hiemenz J, et al. A randomized trial comparing ceftazidime alone with combination antibiotic therapy in cancer patients with fever and neutropenia. N Engl J Med 1986;315:552–8.
35. Freifeld AG, Bow EJ, Sepkowitz KA, et al, Infectious Diseases Society of America. Clinical practice guideline for the use of antimicrobial agents in neutropenic patients with cancer: 2010 update by the Infectious Diseases Society of America. Clin Infect Dis 2011;52:e56–93.
36. Mikulska M. How to Manage Infections Caused by Antibiotic Resistant Gram-negative Bacteria - EBMT Educational Meeting from the Severe Aplastic

Anaemia and Infectious Diseases Working Parties, Naples, Italy, 2014. Curr Drug Targets 2015. [Epub ahead of print].

37. Mikulska M, Viscoli C, Orasch C, et al, Fourth European Conference on Infections in Leukemia Group (ECIL-4), a joint venture of EBMT, EORTC, ICHS, ELN and ESGICH/ESCMID. Aetiology and resistance in bacteraemias among adult and paediatric haematology and cancer patients. J Infect 2014;68: 321–31.
38. Zhanel GG, Lawson CD, Adam H, et al. Ceftazidime-avibactam: a novel cephalosporin/beta-lactamase inhibitor combination. Drugs 2013;73:159–77.
39. Zhanel GG, Chung P, Adam H, et al. Ceftolozane/tazobactam: a novel cephalosporin/beta-lactamase inhibitor combination with activity against multidrug-resistant gram-negative bacilli. Drugs 2014;74:31–51.
40. Tsoulas C, Nathwani D. Review of meta-analyses of vancomycin compared with new treatments for Gram-positive skin and soft-tissue infections: are we any clearer? Int J Antimicrob Agents 2015;46:1–7.
41. Coullioud D, Van der Auwera P, Viot M, et al. Prospective multicentric study of the etiology of 1051 bacteremic episodes in 782 cancer patients. CEMIC (French-Belgian Study Club of Infectious Diseases in Cancer). Support Care Cancer 1993;1:34–46.
42. Mebis J, Jansens H, Minalu G, et al. Long-term epidemiology of bacterial susceptibility profiles in adults suffering from febrile neutropenia with hematologic malignancy after antibiotic change. Infect Drug Resist 2010;3:53–61.
43. Ortega M, Almela M, Soriano A, et al. Bloodstream infections among human immunodeficiency virus-infected adult patients: epidemiology and risk factors for mortality. Eur J Clin Microbiol Infect Dis 2008;27:969–76.
44. Macesic N, Morrissey CO, Cheng AC, et al. Changing microbial epidemiology in hematopoietic stem cell transplant recipients: increasing resistance over a 9-year period. Transpl Infect Dis 2014;16:887–96.
45. Bousquet A, Malfuson JV, Sanmartin N, et al. An 8-year survey of strains identified in blood cultures in a clinical haematology unit. Clin Microbiol Infect 2014; 20:O7–12.
46. Gudiol C, Bodro M, Simonetti A, et al. Changing aetiology, clinical features, antimicrobial resistance, and outcomes of bloodstream infection in neutropenic cancer patients. Clin Microbiol Infect 2013;19:474–9.
47. Blennow O, Ljungman P, Sparrelid E, et al. Incidence, risk factors, and outcome of bloodstream infections during the pre-engraftment phase in 521 allogeneic hematopoietic stem cell transplantations. Transpl Infect Dis 2014;16:106–14.
48. Montassier E, Batard E, Gastinne T, et al. Recent changes in bacteremia in patients with cancer: a systematic review of epidemiology and antibiotic resistance. Eur J Clin Microbiol Infect Dis 2013;32:841–50.
49. Bodro M, Gudiol C, Garcia-Vidal C, et al. Epidemiology, antibiotic therapy and outcomes of bacteremia caused by drug-resistant ESKAPE pathogens in cancer patients. Support Care Cancer 2014;22:603–10.
50. Chong Y, Yakushiji H, Ito Y, et al. Cefepime-resistant Gram-negative bacteremia in febrile neutropenic patients with hematological malignancies. Int J Infect Dis 2010;14(Suppl 3):e171–5.
51. Cornejo-Juarez P, Suarez-Cuenca JA, Volkow-Fernandez P, et al. Fecal ESBL Escherichia coli carriage as a risk factor for bacteremia in patients with hematological malignancies. Support Care Cancer 2016;24(1):253–9.

52. De Rosa FG, Motta I, Audisio E, et al. Epidemiology of bloodstream infections in patients with acute myeloid leukemia undergoing levofloxacin prophylaxis. BMC Infect Dis 2013;13:563.
53. Haeusler GM, Mechinaud F, Daley AJ, et al. Antibiotic-resistant Gram-negative bacteremia in pediatric oncology patients–risk factors and outcomes. Pediatr Infect Dis J 2013;32:723–6.
54. Lim CJ, Cheng AC, Kong DC, et al. Community-onset bloodstream infection with multidrug-resistant organisms: a matched case-control study. BMC Infect Dis 2014;14:126.
55. Marin M, Gudiol C, Ardanuy C, et al. Bloodstream infections in neutropenic patients with cancer: differences between patients with haematological malignancies and solid tumours. J Infect 2014;69:417–23.
56. Moghnieh R, Estaitieh N, Mugharbil A, et al. Third generation cephalosporin resistant Enterobacteriaceae and multidrug resistant gram-negative bacteria causing bacteremia in febrile neutropenia adult cancer patients in Lebanon, broad spectrum antibiotics use as a major risk factor, and correlation with poor prognosis. Front Cell Infect Microbiol 2015;5:11.
57. Papagheorghe R. Bloodstream infections in immunocompromised hosts. Roum Arch Microbiol Immunol 2012;71:87–94.
58. Rangaraj G, Granwehr BP, Jiang Y, et al. Perils of quinolone exposure in cancer patients: breakthrough bacteremia with multidrug-resistant organisms. Cancer 2010;116:967–73.
59. Rosa RG, Goldani LZ. Aetiology of bacteraemia as a risk factor for septic shock at the onset of febrile neutropaenia in adult cancer patients. Biomed Res Int 2014;2014:561020.
60. Sanz J, Cano I, Gonzalez-Barbera EM, et al. Bloodstream infections in adult patients undergoing cord blood transplantation from unrelated donors after myeloablative conditioning regimen. Biol Blood Marrow Transplant 2015;21:755–60.
61. Trecarichi EM, Pagano L, Candoni A, et al. Current epidemiology and antimicrobial resistance data for bacterial bloodstream infections in patients with hematologic malignancies: an Italian multicentre prospective survey. Clin Microbiol Infect 2015;21:337–43.
62. Trecarichi EM, Tumbarello M. Antimicrobial-resistant Gram-negative bacteria in febrile neutropenic patients with cancer: current epidemiology and clinical impact. Curr Opin Infect Dis 2014;27:200–10.
63. Zhang S, Wang Q, Ling Y, et al. Fluoroquinolone resistance in bacteremic and low risk febrile neutropenic patients with cancer. BMC Cancer 2015;15:42.
64. Miedema KG, Winter RH, Ammann RA, et al. Bacteria causing bacteremia in pediatric cancer patients presenting with febrile neutropenia–species distribution and susceptibility patterns. Support Care Cancer 2013;21:2417–26.
65. Cattaneo C, Antoniazzi F, Casari S, et al. P. aeruginosa bloodstream infections among hematological patients: an old or new question? Ann Hematol 2012; 91:1299–304.
66. Cattaneo C, Antoniazzi F, Tumbarello M, et al. Relapsing bloodstream infections during treatment of acute leukemia. Ann Hematol 2014;93:785–90.
67. Garza-Ramos U, Barrios H, Reyna-Flores F, et al. Widespread of ESBL- and carbapenemase GES-type genes on carbapenem-resistant Pseudomonas aeruginosa clinical isolates: a multicenter study in Mexican hospitals. Diagn Microbiol Infect Dis 2015;81:135–7.

68. Ammann RA, Laws HJ, Schrey D, et al. Bloodstream infection in paediatric cancer centres–leukaemia and relapsed malignancies are independent risk factors. Eur J Pediatr 2015;174:675–86.
69. Wattier RL, Dvorak CC, Auerbach AD, et al. Repeat blood cultures in children with persistent fever and neutropenia: Diagnostic and clinical implications. Pediatr Blood Cancer 2015;62:1421–6.
70. Aust C, Tolfvenstam T, Broliden K, et al. Bacteremia in Swedish hematological patients with febrile neutropenia: bacterial spectrum and antimicrobial resistance patterns. Scand J Infect Dis 2013;45:285–91.
71. Garcia-Vidal C, Ardanuy C, Gudiol C, et al. Clinical and microbiological epidemiology of Streptococcus pneumoniae bacteremia in cancer patients. J Infect 2012;65:521–7.
72. Gudiol C, Garcia-Vidal C, Arnan M, et al. Etiology, clinical features and outcomes of pre-engraftment and post-engraftment bloodstream infection in hematopoietic SCT recipients. Bone Marrow Transplant 2014;49:824–30.
73. Bassetti M, Righi E. Multidrug-resistant bacteria: what is the threat? Hematology Am Soc Hematol Educ Program 2013;2013:428–32.
74. Gudiol C, Calatayud L, Garcia-Vidal C, et al. Bacteraemia due to extended-spectrum beta-lactamase-producing Escherichia coli (ESBL-EC) in cancer patients: clinical features, risk factors, molecular epidemiology and outcome. J Antimicrob Chemother 2010;65:333–41.
75. Kang CI, Chung DR, Ko KS, et al. Risk factors for infection and treatment outcome of extended-spectrum beta-lactamase-producing Escherichia coli and Klebsiella pneumoniae bacteremia in patients with hematologic malignancy. Ann Hematol 2012;91:115–21.
76. Gudiol C, Tubau F, Calatayud L, et al. Bacteraemia due to multidrug-resistant Gram-negative bacilli in cancer patients: risk factors, antibiotic therapy and outcomes. J Antimicrob Chemother 2011;66:657–63.
77. Gudiol C, Ayats J, Camoez M, et al. Increase in bloodstream infection due to vancomycin-susceptible Enterococcus faecium in cancer patients: risk factors, molecular epidemiology and outcomes. PLoS One 2013;8:e74734.
78. Kim SH, Kwon JC, Choi SM, et al. Escherichia coli and Klebsiella pneumoniae bacteremia in patients with neutropenic fever: factors associated with extended-spectrum beta-lactamase production and its impact on outcome. Ann Hematol 2013;92:533–41.
79. Patel SJ, Oliveira AP, Zhou JJ, et al. Risk factors and outcomes of infections caused by extremely drug-resistant gram-negative bacilli in patients hospitalized in intensive care units. Am J Infect Control 2014;42:626–31.
80. Huh K, Kang CI, Kim J, et al. Risk factors and treatment outcomes of bloodstream infection caused by extended-spectrum cephalosporin-resistant Enterobacter species in adults with cancer. Diagn Microbiol Infect Dis 2014;78:172–7.
81. Nesher L, Rolston KV, Shah DP, et al. Fecal colonization and infection with Pseudomonas aeruginosa in recipients of allogeneic hematopoietic stem cell transplantation. Transpl Infect Dis 2015;17:33–8.
82. Tumbarello M, Sanguinetti M, Montuori E, et al. Predictors of mortality in patients with bloodstream infections caused by extended-spectrum-beta-lactamase-producing Enterobacteriaceae: importance of inadequate initial antimicrobial treatment. Antimicrob Agents Chemother 2007;51:1987–94.
83. Kim YJ, Jun YH, Kim YR, et al. Risk factors for mortality in patients with Pseudomonas aeruginosa bacteremia; retrospective study of impact of combination antimicrobial therapy. BMC Infect Dis 2014;14:161.

84. Girometti N, Lewis RE, Giannella M, et al. Klebsiella pneumoniae bloodstream infection: epidemiology and impact of inappropriate empirical therapy. Medicine (Baltimore) 2014;93:298–309.
85. Chopra T, Marchaim D, Veltman J, et al. Impact of cefepime therapy on mortality among patients with bloodstream infections caused by extended-spectrum-beta-lactamase-producing Klebsiella pneumoniae and Escherichia coli. Antimicrob Agents Chemother 2012;56:3936–42.
86. Ha YE, Kang CI, Cha MK, et al. Epidemiology and clinical outcomes of bloodstream infections caused by extended-spectrum beta-lactamase-producing Escherichia coli in patients with cancer. Int J Antimicrob Agents 2013;42:403–9.
87. Mayanja BN, Todd J, Hughes P, et al. Septicaemia in a population-based HIV clinical cohort in rural Uganda, 1996-2007: incidence, aetiology, antimicrobial drug resistance and impact of antiretroviral therapy. Trop Med Int Health 2010;15:697–705.
88. Crum-Cianflone NF, Burgi AA, Hale BR. Increasing rates of community-acquired methicillin-resistant Staphylococcus aureus infections among HIV-infected persons. Int J STD AIDS 2007;18:521–6.
89. Popovich KJ, Weinstein RA, Aroutcheva A, et al. Community-associated methicillin-resistant Staphylococcus aureus and HIV: intersecting epidemics. Clin Infect Dis 2010;50:979–87.
90. Delorenze GN, Horberg MA, Silverberg MJ, et al. Trends in annual incidence of methicillin-resistant Staphylococcus aureus (MRSA) infection in HIV-infected and HIV-uninfected patients. Epidemiol Infect 2013;141:2392–402.
91. Chacko J, Kuruvila M, Bhat GK. Factors affecting the nasal carriage of methicillin-resistant Staphylococcus aureus in human immunodeficiency virus-infected patients. Indian J Med Microbiol 2009;27:146–8.
92. Crum-Cianflone NF, Shadyab AH, Weintrob A, et al. Association of methicillin-resistant Staphylococcus aureus (MRSA) colonization with high-risk sexual behaviors in persons infected with human immunodeficiency virus (HIV). Medicine (Baltimore) 2011;90:379–89.
93. Giuliani M, Longo B, Latini A, et al. No evidence of colonization with community-acquired methicillin-resistant Staphylococcus aureus in HIV-1-infected men who have sex with men. Epidemiol Infect 2010;138:738–42.
94. Kotpal R, Krishna PS, Bhalla P, et al. Incidence and risk factors of nasal carriage of Staphylococcus aureus in HIV-infected individuals in comparison to HIV-uninfected individuals: a case-control study. J Int Assoc Provid AIDS Care 2014. [Epub ahead of print].
95. Farley JE, Hayat MJ, Sacamano PL, et al. Prevalence and risk factors for methicillin-resistant Staphylococcus aureus in an HIV-positive cohort. Am J Infect Control 2015;43:329–35.
96. Peters PJ, Brooks JT, McAllister SK, et al. Methicillin-resistant Staphylococcus aureus colonization of the groin and risk for clinical infection among HIV-infected adults. Emerg Infect Dis 2013;19:623–9.
97. Popovich KJ, Smith KY, Khawcharoenporn T, et al. Community-associated methicillin-resistant Staphylococcus aureus colonization in high-risk groups of HIV-infected patients. Clin Infect Dis 2012;54:1296–303.
98. Drapeau CM, Angeletti C, Festa A, et al. Role of previous hospitalization in clinically-significant MRSA infection among HIV-infected inpatients: results of a case-control study. BMC Infect Dis 2007;7:36.

99. Burkey MD, Wilson LE, Moore RD, et al. The incidence of and risk factors for MRSA bacteraemia in an HIV-infected cohort in the HAART era. HIV Med 2008;9:858–62.
100. Furuno JP, Johnson JK, Schweizer ML, et al. Community-associated methicillin-resistant Staphylococcus aureus bacteremia and endocarditis among HIV patients: a cohort study. BMC Infect Dis 2011;11:298.
101. Lee NE, Taylor MM, Bancroft E, et al. Risk factors for community-associated methicillin-resistant Staphylococcus aureus skin infections among HIV-positive men who have sex with men. Clin Infect Dis 2005;40:1529–34.
102. Tumbarello M, de Gaetano Donati K, Tacconelli E, et al. Risk factors and predictors of mortality of methicillin-resistant Staphylococcus aureus (MRSA) bacteraemia in HIV-infected patients. J Antimicrob Chemother 2002;50:375–82.
103. Cotton MF, Wasserman E, Smit J, et al. High incidence of antimicrobial resistant organisms including extended spectrum beta-lactamase producing Enterobacteriaceae and methicillin-resistant Staphylococcus aureus in nasopharyngeal and blood isolates of HIV-infected children from Cape Town, South Africa. BMC Infect Dis 2008;8:40.
104. Everett CK, Subramanian A, Jarisberg LG, et al. Characteristics of drug-susceptible and drug-resistant pneumonia in patients with HIV. Epidemiology 2013;3. pii: 122.
105. Fry AM, Facklam RR, Whitney CG, et al. Multistate evaluation of invasive pneumococcal diseases in adults with human immunodeficiency virus infection: serotype and antimicrobial resistance patterns in the United States. J Infect Dis 2003;188:643–52.
106. Adeleye A, Uju L, Idika N, et al. Cotrimoxazole resistance in Streptococcus pneumoniae isolated from sputum of HIV-positive patients. West Indian Med J 2008;57:497–9.
107. Munier AL, de Lastours V, Varon E, et al. Invasive pneumococcal disease in HIV-infected adults in France from 2000 to 2011: antimicrobial susceptibility and implication of serotypes for vaccination. Infection 2013;41:663–8.
108. Safari D, Kurniati N, Waslia L, et al. Serotype distribution and antibiotic susceptibility of Streptococcus pneumoniae strains carried by children infected with human immunodeficiency virus. PLoS One 2014;9:e110526.
109. Wilen M, Buwembo W, Sendagire H, et al. Cotrimoxazole resistance of Streptococcus pneumoniae and commensal streptococci from Kampala, Uganda. Scand J Infect Dis 2009;41:113–21.
110. Abebe W, Endris M, Tiruneh M, et al. Prevalence of vancomycin resistant Enterococci and associated risk factors among clients with and without HIV in Northwest Ethiopia: a cross-sectional study. BMC Public Health 2014;14:185.
111. Dhawan VK, Nachum R, Bhat N, et al. Vancomycin-resistant enterococcal colonization in nonhospitalized HIV-infected patients. West J Med 1998;169:276–9.
112. Chiller TM, Polyak CS, Brooks JT, et al. Daily trimethoprim-sulfamethoxazole prophylaxis rapidly induces corresponding resistance among intestinal Escherichia coli of HIV-infected adults in Kenya. J Int Assoc Physicians AIDS Care (Chic) 2009;8:165–9.
113. Morpeth SC, Thielman NM, Ramadhani HO, et al. Effect of trimethoprim-sulfamethoxazole prophylaxis on antimicrobial resistance of fecal Escherichia coli in HIV-infected patients in Tanzania. J Acquir Immune Defic Syndr 2008;47:585–91.

114. Vignesh R, Shankar EM, Murugavel KG, et al. Urinary infections due to multi-drug-resistant Escherichia coli among persons with HIV disease at a tertiary AIDS care centre in South India. Nephron Clin Pract 2008;110:c55–7.
115. Hoffmann C, Sahly H, Jessen A, et al. High rates of quinolone-resistant strains of Shigella sonnei in HIV-infected MSM. Infection 2013;41:999–1003.
116. Padmavathy K, Padma K, Rajasekaran S. Extended-spectrum beta-lactamase/AmpC-producing uropathogenic Escherichia coli from HIV patients: do they have a low virulence score? J Med Microbiol 2013;62:345–51.

Bacteremia due to Methicillin-Resistant *Staphylococcus aureus*

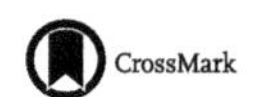

New Therapeutic Approaches

Marisa Holubar, MD, MS[a,*], Lina Meng, PharmD[b],
Stan Deresinski, MD[a]

KEYWORDS

- Methicillin • *Staphylococcus aureus* • MRSA • Bacteremia • Vancomycin
- Daptomycin • Ceftaroline • Endocarditis

KEY POINTS

- Vancomycin, optimally dosed, remains the initial antibiotic of choice for the treatment of patients with methicillin-resistant *Staphylococcus aureus* (MRSA) bacteremia and endocarditis due to isolates with vancomycin minimum inhibitory concentration ≤2 mg/mL. Daptomycin is an effective, although more costly alternative, and ceftaroline appears promising.
- Treatment options for persistent MRSA bacteremia or bacteremia due to vancomycin-intermediate or vancomycin-resistant strains include daptomycin, ceftaroline, and combination therapies.
- There is a critical need for high-level evidence from clinical trials to allow optimally informed decisions in the treatment of MRSA bacteremia and endocarditis.

INTRODUCTION

Resistance of *Staphylococcus aureus* to the first semisynthetic penicillin, methicillin, was reported within a year of its introduction into clinical medicine, mirroring the rapid identification of penicillin resistance less than a decade earlier. Methicillin-resistant *S aureus* (MRSA) subsequently increased in prevalence, but was largely confined to hospital settings until its emergence in the community in the last decade of the 20th century.

Financial Support: None reported.
Potential Conflicts of Interest: None.
[a] Division of Infectious Diseases and Geographic Medicine, Stanford University School of Medicine, 300 Pasteur Drive, Room L-134, Stanford, CA 94305-5105, USA; [b] Department of Pharmacy, Stanford Health Care, 300 Pasteur Drive, M/C 5616 Room H0301, Stanford, CA 94305-5105, USA
* Corresponding author.
E-mail address: mholubar@stanford.edu

Infect Dis Clin N Am 30 (2016) 491–507
http://dx.doi.org/10.1016/j.idc.2016.02.009 id.theclinics.com
0891-5520/16/$ – see front matter

The progressive emergence of MRSA led to the widespread use of vancomycin and, inevitably, reports of reduced susceptibility emerged, beginning with strain MU80 (vancomycin minimum inhibitory concentration [MIC] of 8 μg/mL) isolated in 1996 from the wound infection of a Japanese child receiving prolonged therapy with this glycopeptide antibiotic. This emergence represented the first identified vancomycin-intermediate *S aureus* (VISA; MIC 4–8 μg/mL) and was followed by the recognition of the emergence of heterogeneous intermediate reduced susceptibility (hVISA) strains, each resulting from cell wall alterations with sequestration of the glycopeptide. The first fully vancomycin-resistant (VRSA) strain (MIC >32 μg/mL) was identified in 2002, an occurrence that has fortunately remained rare.

This evolutionary history, together with the recognition of the frequent failure of vancomycin treatment of MRSA infections regardless of the MIC of the isolate, provides unequivocal evidence of the need for newer more effective therapies and therapeutic approaches (**Tables 1** and **2**).

GLYCOPEPTIDES AND SEMISYNTHETIC LIPOGLYCOPEPTIDES

Vancomycin

Optimization of vancomycin administration is a critical factor in improving outcomes of patients with MRSA infection, and recent information provides insight into this issue.

Table 1
Pharmacokinetic/pharmacodynamics profile of anti-infective agents for methicillin-resistant *Staphylococcus aureus*

Agent	MIC Breakpoint for *S aureus* (μg/mL)	PK-PD Indices Associated with Efficacy	Activity Against *S aureus*	% Protein Bound	Half-Life (h)	Excretion
Vancomycin	≤2	AUC/MIC	Bactericidal	50	5–11	80%–90% renal
Daptomycin	≤1	AUC/MIC	Bactericidal	90	8–9	89% renal, 6% feces
Ceftaroline	≤1	T > MIC	Bactericidal	20	2.7	88% renal, 6% feces
Dalbavancin	≤0.12	AUC/MIC	Bactericidal	93	346	33% renal, 20% feces
Oritavancin	≤0.12	AUC/MIC	Bactericidal	85	245	<5% renal, <1% feces
Telavancin	≤0.12	AUC/MIC	Bactericidal	90	6.6–9.6	76% renal, <1% feces
Tedizolid	≤0.5	AUC/MIC	Bacteriostatic	70–90	12	20% renal, 80% feces
Linezolid	≤4	AUC/MIC	Bacteriostatic	31	4–5	30% renal, 9% feces
Tigecycline	≤0.25	AUC/MIC	Bacteriostatic	71–89	42	33% renal, 59% feces

Abbreviations: AUC, area under the plasma concentration curve; T > MIC, time of drug concentration above MIC.

Data from Lexicomp Online, Pediatric and Neonatal Lexi-Drugs Online, Hudson, OH: Lexi-Comp, Inc; 2015; July 20, 2015; Micromedex Healthcare Series (Internet database). Greenwood Village, CO: Thomson Micromedex.

Although several studies have suggested that a vancomycin MIC = 2 μg/mL is associated with an increased risk of failure of treatment of these infections, a recent meta-analysis contradicted this conclusion.[1] Further confounding the understanding is the observation that a vancomycin MIC = 2 μg/mL is associated with an increased risk of failure of antibiotic therapy for methicillin-sensitive *S aureus* (MSSA) as well as MRSA infections, regardless of the administered antibiotic.[2] Finally, evidence is accumulating that the straightforward use of vancomycin trough concentration (Cmin) is an inaccurate means of achieving optimal dosing.

Although it has been generally accepted that the efficacy of vancomycin in bacteremia due to *S aureus* requires achievement of area under the plasma concentration-time curve (AUC) values greater than or equal to 400 times the MIC (AUC/MIC ≥400) and that this can be predicted by measured Cmin alone, recent evidence suggests these assumptions may be incorrect. Modeling studies have demonstrated that unadjusted extrapolation of AUC from serum trough concentrations underestimate AUC by up to 25% and that AUCs varied between patients with similar trough results by up to 30-fold.[3] Furthermore, the threshold for increased concentration-related nephrotoxicity was an AUC ≥700 mg h/L, and additional data indicate that a substantial increase in this risk occurs only at AUC ≥900 mg·h/L, thus bringing the effective treatment of infections due to isolates with MIC = 2 μg/mL more safely in line with the necessary vancomycin exposure. The increased accuracy of AUC estimations from serum vancomycin concentrations by the addition of Bayesian analysis may allow more precise individualized dosing, especially for targeting treatment of infections due to MRSA with an MIC = 2 μg/mL.[3]

The use of a loading dose and ongoing weight-based dosing are critical to rapid achievement of adequate serum concentrations, the importance of which has been demonstrated by the finding in patients with MRSA-associated septic shock that the highest survival rates were associated with an AUC_{24}/MIC well in excess of 400.[4]

Semisynthetic Lipoglycopeptides

Dalbavancin, oritavancin, and telavancin are semisynthetic lipoglycopeptides that are active in vitro against VISA. Telavancin and oritavancin are also active against VRSA and daptomycin nonsusceptible *S aureus*, while dalbavancin is not active against VRSA.[5]

The heptapeptide core common to all glycopeptides is responsible for impaired bacterial cell wall synthesis, inhibiting transglycosylation and transpeptidation by binding to C-terminal D-Ala-D-Ala. The addition of a lipophilic side chain anchors the molecule to the cell membrane and, in the cases of oritavancin and telavancin (but not dalbavancin), also alters cell membrane permeability by disrupting the bacterial membrane potential.

Oritavancin

A study of greater than 9000 MRSA isolates in the United States and Europe from 2008 to 2012 found that 94.6% were inhibited by oritavancin (MIC_{90} = 0.06 μg/mL).[5] Oritavancin is able to bind to D-Ala-D-Lac residues, and as a consequence, remains active against VRSA. The drug achieves very high concentrations within macrophages, a characteristic that may be of importance given the frequent intracellular residence of *S aureus*. Oritavancin therapy was associated with microbiological success in 47 (85%) of 55 patients with uncomplicated *S aureus* bacteremia, 47% of which were intravenous (IV) catheter associated.[5] The proportion due to MRSA (if any) was, however, not stated and, further complicating the analysis, the drug was administered in

Table 2
Dosing, pricing, and drug characteristics of anti-infective agents for methicillin-resistant *Staphylococcus aureus*

Agent	Dosing Regimens	Dose Adjustment	Advantages	Disadvantages, Adverse Effects	Average Daily Cost[a]
Vancomycin	25–30 mg/kg IV load, then 15 mg/kg IV every 8–12 h	Renal	Extensive clinical experience, inexpensive	Red man syndrome, nephrotoxicity (increased risk with higher doses, concurrent aminoglycosides, or pre-existing renal failure)	$15–$55
Daptomycin	6–10 mg/kg IV every 24 h	Renal	Strong evidence for wide range of MRSA infections	May be used in septic pulmonary emboli but not pneumonia; elevated CPK <1%: myopathy (increased risk in those on statins), eosinophilic pneumonia (onset 2–4 wk), peripheral neuropathy	$450–$750
Ceftaroline	600 mg IV every 8-12 h	Renal	Active against VISA, VRSA; exhibits a "see-saw" effect: inverse correlation between the MICs of ceftaroline and vancomycin	Positive Coombs test (without hemolysis ~11%)	$370–$550
Dalbavancin	1500 mg IV as a single dose	Renal	Activity against VISA, VRSA; rapidly bactericidal	Red man syndrome, ALT elevations	$5400 (1500 mg single dose)
Oritavancin	ABSSSI: 1200 mg IV as a single dose	Renal	Activity against VISA, some VRSA, and daptomycin nonsusceptible *S aureus*; in vitro bactericidal biofilm activity in both stationary and growth phases in *S aureus*	Artificially prolongs coagulation tests (INR, PT, aPTT) for ~48 h after administration: use is contraindicated with heparin IV	$3480 (1200 mg single dose)

Telavancin	cSSSI, HAP: 10 mg/kg IV every 24 h	Renal	Activity against VISA, VRSA, and MRSA strains that are resistant to vancomycin, linezolid, and daptomycin	Nephrotoxicity (boxed warning), red man syndrome, QTc prolongation; interferes with coagulation tests (INR, PT, aPTT, ACT) for ~18 h after administration: use is contraindicated with heparin IV. In those with CrCl ≤50 mL/min, decreased clinical response in cSSSI, increased mortality in HAP/VAP (boxed warning)	$430
Tedizolid	200 mg IV/PO daily	None	Excellent tissue penetration, 91% oral bioavailability	Animal and early clinical studies show potentially low to no MAO-mediated drug interactions, minimal myelosuppression or neuropathy (<21 d tedizolid treatment duration)	$300 (IV) $370 (PO)
Linezolid	600 mg IV/PO every 12 h	None	Excellent bone and tissue penetration, >99% oral bioavailability	Peripheral and optic neuropathy, reversible myelosuppression (after 14 d, increased risk in those with underlying hematologic abnormalities or renal insufficiency), serotonin syndrome due to MAO-mediated drug interactions	$190 (IV) $370 (PO)
Tigecycline	100 mg IV load, then 50 mg IV every 12 h	Hepatic	Widely distributed in tissues (Vd 500–700 L)	Controversial use in bacteremia due to low serum concentrations with standard dosing; nausea/vomiting, pancreatitis, hepatotoxicity, treatment-related mortality (US boxed warning)	$340

Abbreviations: ABSSSI, acute bacterial skin and skin structure infections; ACT, activated clotting time; ALT, alanine aminotransferase; aPTT, activated partial thromboplastin time; CPK, creatine phosphokinase; CrCl, creatinine clearance; cSSSI, complicated skin and skin structure infection; HAP, hospital-acquired pneumonia; INR, international normalized ratio; MAO, monoamine oxidase; PO, oral; PT, prothrombin time; VAP, ventilator associated pneumonia; Vd, volume of distribution.

[a] Average daily cost assumes patient is 70 kg.

Data from Lexicomp Online, Pediatric and Neonatal Lexi-Drugs Online, Hudson, OH: Lexi-Comp, Inc; 2015; July 20, 2015; Micromedex Healthcare Series (Internet database). Greenwood Village, CO: Thomson Micromedex.

doses ranging from 3 to 10 mg/kg daily (in contrast to recommended practice of a single 1200-mg dose.)

Dalbavancin

In a global surveillance program, 99.6% of 26,975 MRSA isolates were inhibited by dalbavancin at concentrations less than or equal to 0.12 μg/mL.[6] This teicoplanin analogue is not active against VRSA. In an examination of randomized clinical trials of patients with complicated skin and soft tissue infections (SSTI), an analysis of the subset with *S aureus* bacteremia found that bloodstream clearance occurred in 24 of 24 dalbavancin recipients and in 19 of 20 recipients of comparator agents.[7]

Telavancin

A study of almost 5000 MRSA isolates in the United States found that 100% were susceptible to 0.12 μg/mL or less of telavancin, as were isolates with vancomycin MICs of 2 to 4 μg/mL and daptomycin nonsusceptible strains. All 26 VISA strains collected between 2007 and 2008, 12 of which were also daptomycin nonsusceptible, were inhibited by telavancin (MIC ≤1 μg/mL). Separately, telavancin MICs of 13 VRSA isolates (MIC range, 2–8 μg/mL) were above the susceptibility breakpoint.[8]

In a retrospective analysis, all 9 clinically evaluable patients receiving telavancin for uncomplicated MRSA bacteremia were cured.[8] Fourteen patients, 11 of whom had endocarditis, received salvage therapy with telavancin after a median duration of persistent bacteremia of 13 days.[9] All 10 with follow-up cultures had clearance of MRSA of the bloodstream a median of 1 day (range, 1–3 days) after the therapeutic switch, although only 8 patients survived. A phase 3, multicenter, randomized, open-label, noninferiority trial of telavancin versus standard IV therapy in the treatment of patients with *S aureus* bacteremia and right-sided infective endocarditis is ongoing.[10]

DAPTOMYCIN

Daptomycin, a cyclic lipopeptide, is a large (1620-Da) molecule that inserts itself into the bacterial cell membrane in a calcium-dependent manner, disrupting cell membrane integrity and function.

Daptomycin nonsusceptibility in *S aureus* may emerge under the selective pressure exerted by its administration but may also occur in its absence, possibly as the result of similar pressure exerted by cationic host defense peptides.[11] The most commonly identified mutations associated with resistance occur in the *mprF* gene, which encodes a membrane protein important in phospholipid synthesis causing "gain-of-function" mutations that result in partial neutralization of the negatively charged bacterial cell membrane, thus reducing the binding affinity of the positively charged calcium-complexed daptomycin molecule.[12]

Daptomycin and vancomycin MICs may trend together, and a recent review estimated that between 38% and 83% of VISA isolates and 15% of hVISA isolates were nonsusceptible to daptomycin, although its activity against VRSA is maintained.[13] Although this has raised concern about the use of daptomycin salvage therapy in patients with persistent infection in the face of vancomycin administration, a recent retrospective analysis found that previous vancomycin exposure did not affect the efficacy of daptomycin.[14]

Although national guidelines recommend 6 mg/kg/d daptomycin dosing for uncomplicated MRSA bacteremia, they also indicate that 8 to 10 mg/kg/d dosing may be considered for complicated and/or persistent bacteremia, although the latter recommendation is not based on high-level evidence.[15] Higher doses, in addition to possibly enhancing the antibacterial effect, may also potentially prevent the emergence of resistance, especially in high burden infections. A recent review of persistent MRSA bacteremia cases, however, found that significant increases in daptomycin MICs occurred during therapy in 7 of 18 patients despite all 7 having received 8 to 10 mg/kg/d. The daptomycin MIC increase was associated with microbiological failure.[16]

Clinical evidence suggesting a benefit of higher doses of daptomycin is limited. A retrospective case series compared standard (mean 5 mg/kg/d) versus high (mean 8 mg/kg/d) dosing regimens in 53 patients with *S aureus* infections (mostly MRSA), including 37 with bacteremia or endocarditis. Although, in the entire cohort, high-dose recipients received therapy for a longer duration (mean of 13.5 days vs 19 days), there was no significant difference in outcomes in those with bacteremia or endocarditis.[17]

Treatment with high-dose daptomycin has been retrospectively compared with standard vancomycin administration in MRSA bacteremia. Kullar and colleagues[18] reviewed 70 patients with endocarditis, 54 due to MRSA, each with a baseline vancomycin MIC = 2 μg/mL, treated with daptomycin (median dose 9.8 mg/kg/d) alone or, in one-third, in combination with daptomycin that was added after a median of 4 days of vancomycin monotherapy. The investigators reported a clinical success rate of ~85%. However, details of the vancomycin dosing were not indicated, a problem with many relevant studies. Separately, Murray and colleagues reported 85 patients with MRSA bacteremia due to isolates with vancomycin MICs ≥1.5 μg/mL whose therapy was switched to daptomycin (median dose 8.4 mg/kg/d after median of 1.7 days of vancomycin) and compared their outcomes to 85 matched historical controls treated only with vancomycin (median trough 17.6 μg/mL).[19] Patients treated with daptomycin experienced less frequent clinical failure and had a lower 30-day mortality.[19]

FIFTH-GENERATION CEPHALOSPORINS: CEFTAROLINE

Ceftaroline fosamil received approval by the US Food and Drug Administration (FDA) in 2010. Another cephalosporin with MRSA activity, ceftobiprole medocaril, is not available in the United States, but has received approval in several European countries. The activity of ceftaroline against MRSA is the result of its high affinity for penicillin-binding proteins, but especially to an allosteric site of PBP2a near the transpeptidase domain. Binding to this site causes a conformational change that opens the active site of the molecule, allowing binding of a second ceftaroline molecule with consequent inhibition of its enzymatic activity. Resistance to ceftaroline results from *mecA* mutations that disrupt this allosteric mechanism, although additional mutations may contribute.[20]

A survey of 2013 MRSA bloodstream isolates collected at US medical centers from 2009 to 2013 found that 95.4% were susceptible (MIC ≤1 μg/mL), 4.6% had an MIC = 2 μg/mL (intermediate), whereas none were resistant to ceftaroline.[21] Ceftaroline is active in vitro against hVISA and VISA, as well as against at least one VRSA strain, and exhibits a "see-saw" effect, with an inverse correlation between the MICs of ceftaroline and vancomycin observed.[22]

Like other β-lactams, ceftaroline exerts time-dependent killing and has a relatively prolonged post-antibiotic effect against *S aureus*. Pharmacodynamic modeling found that $fT > MIC$ of 32.1% was associated with a 2 log_{10} decrease in CFUs, but if $fT > MIC$ is less than 50%, organism regrowth occurred at 96 hours.[23] As a consequence, it has been suggested that, in order to diminish the risk of resistance selection, the optimal pharmacodynamic target should be *f*T > MIC greater than 50%. This target is readily achieved in healthy volunteers for isolates with an MIC = 2 μg/mL after administration of the recommended dose of 600 mg every 12 hours infused over 1 hour.[24] This conclusion is of note because a dose of 600 mg every 8 hours has been used in several patients with MRSA bacteremia reported in the literature, but the added benefit resulting from this regimen remains to be demonstrated. A recent Monte Carlo analysis in adults with cystic fibrosis, however, found that 600 mg ceftaroline administered 1 hour every 8 hours was required to assure a >90% probability of attainment of ≥60% T>MIC.[25] This is presumably the consequence of the frequent increased renal clearance of drugs observed in cystic fibrosis patients.

In a phase 4 registry study of *S aureus* bacteremia secondary to either acute bacterial SSTIs or to community-acquired bacterial pneumonia, clinical success in those with MRSA infection was reported in 18 of 32.[26] For many patients (the proportion was not reported), however, ceftaroline was administered together with a second antibiotic.

Ceftaroline has been used as "salvage" therapy for patients with perceived failure of treatment of MRSA bacteremia with another antibiotic, but the definition of failure has been variable and, in some cases, difficult to discern. In one such study, ceftaroline therapy was reported to achieve clinical success in 101 of the 129 patients with *S aureus* (92.5% MRSA) bacteremia, 92.0% of whom had endocarditis.[27] An unstated proportion, however, received ceftaroline in combination with a second antibiotic.

The relative efficacy of continuing the initial therapy (most with vancomycin) or switching to ceftaroline in patients with ongoing MRSA bacteremia was evaluated in a small case-control study.[28] Microbiological cure was observed in 14 of 16 controls and in 16 of 16 cases, although the time to resolution of bacteremia was shorter after the switch to ceftaroline than it was for the total duration of vancomycin in controls.

Ceftaroline was administered to 31 patients after initial therapy with vancomycin or daptomycin; in 10 patients, it was given in combination with another antibiotic, most frequently daptomycin.[29] Nine of the patients had endocarditis, mostly involving the tricuspid valve. Overall, microbiological cure was achieved in 64.5% (not all patients had test of cure) and clinical success in 74.2%, and the median duration of bacteremia after the switch to ceftaroline monotherapy was 4 days (range, 1–8 days). Finally, after a change to ceftaroline therapy, blood cultures became negative in 1 to 5 days in 5 patients with persistent MRSA bacteremia, 2 of whom had endocarditis.[30] Switching from initial therapy to ceftaroline in 4 patients with endovascular infection was associated with clearance of bacteremia in all within 2 to 7 days.[31] Rapid clearance of bacteremia (day 0 of ceftaroline administration) in 2 of 3 patients occurred after a switch to ceftaroline therapy, while a third patient, who had been bacteremic for 28 days before a change to ceftaroline therapy, was still bacteremic on the day of death 7 days later.[32]

OXAZOLIDINONES

The oxazolidinones inhibit bacterial protein synthesis by binding to the 23S ribosomal RNA of the 50S ribosomal subunit, preventing the formation of the 70S initiation complex. Tedizolid, the second drug of this class to become available, has key structural differences that allow additional target binding site interactions, accounting for its greater potency (with MICs 2- to 8-fold lower than linezolid against staphylococci) and retained activity despite linezolid resistance in some instances.[33]

S aureus resistance to linezolid fortunately remains rare, having been detected in only 2 of 1454 isolates from 60 US centers; both carried *cfr*.[34] Most *cfr*-positive isolates, however, remain susceptible to tedizolid. Thus, 11 (85%) of 13 *S aureus* isolates were susceptible to tedizolid, whereas none of 17 with 23S rRNA mutations and only 1 (17%) of 6 with L3 or L4 modifications remained susceptible to this antibiotic.[35]

The FDA approved tedizolid in 2014 for use in acute bacterial SSTI caused by susceptible organisms, including MRSA. Published information regarding the use of tedizolid for the treatment of bacteremia is exceedingly limited. Bacteremia was present at enrollment in the ESTABLISH-1 and -2 trials of patients with SSTI in a small proportion of subjects.[35] In the 11 bacteremic patients assigned tedizolid, 4 infections were due to *S aureus* (2 MSSA and 2 MRSA), whereas in the 16 assigned linezolid, 9 were caused by *S aureus* (3 MSSA and 6 MRSA). All 11 tedizolid recipients and 11 of the 16 given linezolid responded to their assigned therapy.

The experience with linezolid may prove instructive in predicting the potential role of tedizolid in the treatment of MRSA bacteremia. A pooled analysis of 5 randomized trials found that clinical cure was achieved in 14 (56%) of 25 linezolid recipients, and in 13 (46%) of 28 of the subset with MRSA infection given vancomycin, a difference was not statistically significant.[36] In a prospective open randomized trial, clinical success at test of cure was achieved in 19 of 24 (79.2%) linezolid recipients and 16 of 21 (76.2%) of those given vancomycin.[37] In patients with persistent ($\geq$7 days) MRSA bacteremia while receiving vancomycin for at least 5 days, a switch to linezolid therapy (half also received a carbapenem) led to similar outcomes as seen in those in whom vancomycin was continued.[38]

Like linezolid, tedizolid is bacteriostatic, making its use in endocarditis problematic. When administered in a dose consistent with human exposure, tedizolid exerted only a modest bactericidal effect that was inferior to both vancomycin and daptomycin in a rabbit model of experimental endocarditis, a result similar to that previously observed with linezolid.[39]

TIGECYCLINE

The first of a new generation of tetracyclines, glycylcyclines, tigecycline inhibits bacterial protein synthesis, specifically by binding the 30S ribosomal subunit and blocking entry of amino-acyl tRNA to the A site of ribosome. Tigecycline is an analogue of minocycline that carries an added bulky side chain that sterically hinders the drug efflux and ribosomal protection mechanisms that cause resistance to the tetracyclines.[40]

The use of tigecycline in bacteremia is controversial because of its low serum levels with standard dosing.[41] In a pooled, retrospective data analysis of phase 3 clinical trials, 91 patients being treated with tigecycline had secondary bacteremia detected.[42] In the subset of patients with *S aureus* infection (n = 10), cure rates were 83.3% and 75% in the tigecycline and comparator arms, respectively.

COMBINATION THERAPY

Combinations with Vancomycin

Synergistic interactions between vancomycin and a wide variety of penicillinase-stable β-lactams, including semisynthetic penicillins, cephalosporins, β-lactam/β-lactamase inhibitor combinations, and carbapenems (but not the monobactam, aztreonam), have been demonstrated in vitro. With at least some β-lactams, this effect extends to isolates of hVISA, VISA and, at least in one case, VRSA. It has been suggested that synergy results from a reduction in cell wall thickness caused by β-lactam exposure with a reduction in sequestration of the glycopeptide, allowing increased access to its functional target.[43]

In a retrospective study of patients with MRSA bacteremia, microbiological eradication was achieved in 48 of 50 (96%) patients who received vancomycin together with a β-lactam (piperacillin-tazobactam in 34 of 50) and in 24 of 30 (80%) (P = .021) given vancomycin alone.[44] In the subset of patients with endocarditis, clearance of bacteremia was achieved in 11 of 11 and in 9 of 11 in the 2 groups, respectively. Separately, a hemodialysis patient with septic subclavian thrombophlebitis who failed treatment of relapsed MRSA bacteremia with ceftaroline plus daptomycin experienced clearance of bacteremia within 24 hours of a change to ceftaroline plus vancomycin.[45] In a pilot randomized study involving a total of 60 patients given vancomycin with or without flucloxacillin, combination therapy was associated with a reduction in mean duration of MRSA bacteremia from 3.00 to 2.94 days.[46] Thus, the mean time to resolution of bacteremia in those receiving vancomycin plus flucloxacillin was 65% (95% confidence interval, 41%–102%; P = .06) of that observed the patients given vancomycin alone. No differences in clinical endpoints were observed. In contrast to these experiences, there continues to be a lack of evidence of benefit of vancomycin combined with antibiotics other than β-lactams. Seah and colleagues[47] retrospectively reviewed the cases of 76 patients with persistent MRSA bacteremia for greater than 7 days after initiation of vancomycin therapy, 50 of whom continued to receive monotherapy with this glycopeptide, whereas 26 had one or more agents added to their regimen. These added antibiotics included rifampin plus fusidic acid in 12, rifampin alone in 3, rifampin plus trimethoprim-sulfamethoxazole and doxycycline plus trimethoprim-sulfamethoxazole in 2 each with 1 each receiving either rifampin plus gentamicin or rifampin plus ciprofloxacin. There was no evidence of benefit from combination therapy with these diverse agents; the median durations of bacteremia after initiation of combination therapy were 19 days and 14 days in the combination and continued vancomycin groups, respectively.

In a retrospective study, 35 patients with persistent (≥7 days) MRSA bacteremia while receiving vancomycin had their therapy altered.[48] In 12 cases, vancomycin was continued, with an aminoglycoside added in 6, rifampin in 4, and both an aminoglycoside and a rifampin added in 2, but bacteremia cleared within 72 hours in only 2 (17%).

Combinations with Daptomycin

Daptomycin plus β-lactams

In vitro synergy with daptomycin occurs in combination with any of a broad array of β-lactam antibiotics, although it is reported that β-lactams that preferentially bind PBP-1 are more potent in this regard.[49] When complexed with calcium at physiologic concentrations, daptomycin acts as a cation, allowing it to bind to the negatively charged bacterial cell membrane. β-Lactam antibiotic exposure increases membrane charge negativity, thus enhancing daptomycin binding and presumably accounting for synergy. In addition, the combination of daptomycin with a second antibiotic appears to slow the emergence of nonsusceptibility to the lipopeptide antibiotic.[50]

The combination of daptomycin and ceftaroline had superior bactericidal activity in an in vitro hollow fiber model compared with either agent alone against 2 MRSA isolates that were daptomycin nonsusceptible.[43] Examination of different potential clinical strategies of administration found that de-escalation from combination to monotherapy with either agent after 4 or 8 days was equivalent to continued combination therapy and superior to monotherapy from the start. In addition, a simulated daptomycin dose of 6 mg/kg/d was not inferior to a 10-mg/kg/d dose in the combination regimen.

Among patients with MRSA bacteremia enrolled in a daptomycin registry study, most of whom had received prior antibiotic therapy, clinical or microbiological success was observed in 18 of 22 (82%) who received daptomycin in combination with a β-lactam antibiotic and in 27 of 34 (79%) who received this lipopeptide antibiotic without a β-lactam (many, however, received other antibiotics), a difference that was not significant.[51] The use of daptomycin in combination with rifampin, gentamicin, or vancomycin was not associated with a significant difference in outcome when compared with monotherapy.

The efficacy of salvage therapy with daptomycin and ceftaroline in combination was examined in patients at 10 medical centers with persistent staphylococcal bacteremia.[52] Of the 26 infections, 22 were due to MRSA, including 2 VISA; 4 isolates were daptomycin nonsusceptible. Fourteen patients had endocarditis with 12 of these being left sided. The median duration of bacteremia before initiation of daptomycin plus ceftaroline was 10 days (range, 3–23 days), and this combination was a third- or fourth-line therapy in 69% of patients. Daptomycin monotherapy had failed in 12. The median duration of bacteremia after initiation of this combination therapy was 2 days (range, 1–6 days).

Seven patients with persistent or relapsed MRSA bacteremia who had sequentially failed vancomycin and daptomycin monotherapies cleared their bloodstreams a median of 1 day (range, 1–2 days) after the addition of a semisynthetic penicillin to daptomycin.[53]

Daptomycin plus trimethoprim-sulfamethoxazole

Trimethoprim-sulfamethoxazole given alone did not meet the test of noninferiority compared with vancomycin monotherapy in the treatment of patients with severe MRSA infections that included 91 patients with bacteremia,[54] but its role as part of combination regimens suggest possible benefit. The combination of daptomycin and trimethoprim-sulfamethoxazole was bactericidal against both daptomycin-susceptible and nonsusceptible strains of MRSA in an in vitro model of endocarditis using simulated vegetations.[55] In a retrospective review of patients with deep-seated MRSA infections, 75.0% initially received vancomycin before switching to daptomycin after a median of 4 days with the most frequent reason (60.7%) for change in therapy being a vancomycin MIC = 2 μg/mL. Daptomycin was then continued as monotherapy for a median of 5 days until the addition of trimethoprim-sulfamethoxazole. In the 20 patients still bacteremic at the time of addition of trimethoprim-sulfamethoxazole to daptomycin, subsequent bloodstream clearance occurred within a median of 2.5 days. The median time to clearance after the initiation of combination therapy in the 6 patients infected with a daptomycin-nonsusceptible strain was 6.5 days, whereas it was 2 days in those infected with a daptomycin-susceptible MRSA. Hyperkalemia was a frequent occurrence during combination therapy.

Daptomycin plus either ceftaroline or trimethoprim-sulfamethoxazole: A comparison

A retrospective analysis of 34 patients with MRSA bacteremia with a median duration of bacteremia while receiving primary or secondary treatment of 7 to 8 days had resolution of bloodstream infection when therapy was changed to daptomycin plus either ceftaroline or trimethoprim-sulfamethoxazole, after a median of 2 days in each case.[56]

Trimethoprim-sulfamethoxazole plus ceftaroline

Twenty-five patients with MRSA bacteremia (65% with endovascular infection) received combination therapy (trimethoprim-sulfamethoxazole in 23, daptomycin in 2) with ceftaroline after initial administration of another antibiotic, mostly vancomycin.[57] In those still bacteremic at the time of the switch, the median subsequent duration of bacteremia was 3 days, whereas it had been 9.5 days before the change. Although microbiologic success was achieved in 90%, only 31% were considered

Table 3
Approximate cost of combination therapy for methicillin-resistant *Staphylococcus aureus*

Weekly Cost (AWP 2016)	Cefazolin 1 g Q8H	Nafcillin 1 g Q4H	Ceftaroline 600 mg Q12H	Ceftaroline 600 mg Q8H	TMP/SMX 10 mg/kg/day
Daptomycin 700 mg Q24H (10 mg/kg)	$5400	$5800	$7800	$9000	$5500
Vancomycin 1g Q12H (15 mg/kg)	$230	$700	$2700	$4000	$350

Abbreviation: TMP/SMX, trimethoprim sulfamethoxazole.

Data from Lexicomp Online, Pediatric and Neonatal Lexi-Drugs Online, Hudson, OH: Lexi-Comp, Inc; 2015; July 20, 2015; Micromedex Healthcare Series (Internet database). Greenwood Village, CO: Thomson Micromedex.

Table 4
Investigational drugs with activity against methicillin-resistant *Staphylococcus aureus* in clinical trials

Antibiotic	Class	Status
Debio 1452 (prodrug of Debio 1450)	FabI inhibitor	Phase 1 completed
MRX-1	Oxazolidinone	Phase 1
Radezolid	Oxazolidinone	Phase 2 completed
LCB01-0371	Oxazolidinone	Phase 1
BC-3781	Pleuromutilin	Phase 2 completed
Fusidic acid (CEM-102)	EF-G blocker	Phase 2 completed (SSTI)
Omadacycline	Tetracycline	Phase 2 completed
Eravacycline	Tetracycline	Phase 3 (cIAI and cUTI)
Brilacidin	Mimics CDP	Phase 2
AFN-1252	*FabI* enoyl-(acyl carrier protein) reductase inhibitor	Phase 2 completed
CG400549	*FabI* enoyl-(acyl carrier protein) reductase inhibitor	Phase 2a completed
GSK1322322	Peptide deformylase inhibitor	Phase 2a completed
Delafloxacin	Fluoroquinolone	Phase 2 completed
Nemonoxacin	Fluoroquinolone	Phase 3 (CAP)
Finafloxacin	Fluoroquinolone	Phase 2 completed (cUTI)
GSK2140944	Type II topoisomerase inhibitor	Phase 1 completed
Avarofloxacin	Fluoroquinolone	Phase 2 completed
JNJ-32729463	Fluoroquinolone	Phase 2
WCK 2349	Type II topoisomerase inhibitor	Phase 1 completed
WCK 771	Type II topoisomerase inhibitor	Phase 1 completed
TD-1607	Cephalosporin-glycopeptide heterodimer	Phase 3
Iclaprim	Dihydrofolate reductase inhibitor	Phase 3
CBR-2092	Rifamycin-quinolone hybrid	Phase 1
WAP-8294A2	Cyclic lipodepsipeptide	Phase 1

Abbreviations: CAP, community-acquired pneumonia; cIAI, complicated intra-abdominal infections; cUTI, complicated urinary tract infections.

From Lexicomp Online, Pediatric and Neonatal Lexi-Drugs Online, Hudson, OH: Lexi-Comp, Inc; 2015; July 20, 2015; Micromedex Healthcare Series (Internet database). Greenwood Village, CO: Thomson Micromedex; with permission. Available at: http://www.pewtrusts.org/en/research-and-analysis/issue-briefs/2014/03/12/tracking-the-pipeline-of-antibiotics-in-development. Accessed June 30, 2015.

to be clinical successes, but the way in which this was defined is open to challenge. Thus, only 4 patients were considered by the investigators to be clinical failures, and in 2, this may have been the result of inadequate source control.

Combinations with Fosfomycin

Fosfomycin, which is not available in a parenteral formulation in the United States, has been demonstrated to be synergistic with daptomycin in vitro. Two patients with MRSA left-sided endocarditis were successfully treated with high-dose daptomycin plus fosfomycin after failure of initial therapy.[58] MRSA bloodstream infection cleared in a patient receiving vancomycin with persistent (>10 days) bacteremia 3 days after the addition of fosfomycin to the regimen.[59]

Sixteen patients with persistent (N = 14) or relapsed (N = 2) MRSA bacteremia who had received a median of 9.5 days of antibiotic therapy (mostly vancomycin, but daptomycin in 2 cases) were treated with the combination of imipenem and fosfomycin with bloodstream clearance within 72 hours in each case, and the clinical success rate was 69% (**Tables 3** and **4**).[60]

SUMMARY

The lack of high-level evidence precludes definitive conclusions regarding optimal treatment of MRSA bacteremia. However, based on the available data and experience, the following can be proposed:

- Vancomycin, appropriately dosed, remains the first-line therapy, with daptomycin an effective, although more costly, alternative.
- Laboratory data suggest that the administration of daptomycin in higher than approved doses may be superior to lower doses in terms of efficacy and reducing the risk of selection of resistance, but clinical data to support this hypothesis are largely lacking.
- Ceftaroline may be a promising alternative, but its broad spectrum of activity is an undesirable quality for use as definitive therapy in the absence of polymicrobial infection.
- Combinations of daptomycin or vancomycin with a β-lactam, or daptomycin with trimethoprim-sulfamethoxazole, may eventually prove to be more effective than monotherapy, particularly in "salvage" situations, but a definitive answer will require prospective randomized trials. In vitro modeling with daptomycin and ceftaroline suggests that, although the combination is superior to either agent alone, one or the other may be discontinued after 4 days without loss of efficacy; in addition, a simulated daptomycin dose of 6 mg/kg/d is not inferior to 10 mg/kg/d when used in combination.

REFERENCES

1. Kalil AC, Van Schooneveld TC, Fey PD, et al. Association between vancomycin minimum inhibitory concentration and mortality among patients with Staphylococcus aureus bloodstream infections. JAMA 2014;312(15):1552.
2. Cervera C, Castañeda X, De La Maria CG, et al. Effect of vancomycin minimal inhibitory concentration on the outcome of methicillin-susceptible Staphylococcus aureus endocarditis. Clin Infect Dis 2014;58(12):1668–75.
3. Neely MN, Youn G, Jones B, et al. Are vancomycin trough concentrations adequate for optimal dosing? Antimicrob Agents Chemother 2014;58(1): 309–16.

4. Zelenitsky S, Rubinstein E, Ariano R, et al. Vancomycin pharmacodynamics and survival in patients with methicillin-resistant Staphylococcus aureus-associated septic shock. Int J Antimicrob Agents 2013;41(3):255–60.
5. Zhanel GG, Calic D, Schweizer F, et al. New lipoglycopeptides. Drugs 2010; 70(7):859–86.
6. McCurdy SP, Jones RN, Mendes RE, et al. In vitro activity of dalbavancin against drug resistant *Staphylococcus aureus* from a global surveillance program. Antimicrob Agents Chemother 2015;59(8):5007–9.
7. Dunne M, Puttagunta S. Clearance of Staphylococcus aureus bacteremia in patients treated with dalbavancin. Poster session presented at: IDWeek 2013, October 2–6; San Francisco, CA.
8. Corey GR, Rubinstein E, Stryjewski ME, et al. Potential role for telavancin in bacteremic infections due to gram-positive pathogens: focus on Staphylococcus aureus. Clin Infect Dis 2014;60:787–96.
9. Ruggero MA, Peaper DR, Topal JE. Telavancin for refractory methicillin-resistant Staphylococcus aureus bacteremia and infective endocarditis. Infect Dis (Lond) 2015;47(6):379–84.
10. Theravance Biopharma Antibiotics, Inc. A phase 3 telavancin Staphylococcus aureus bacteremia trial. NCT02208063 [Internet]. Available at: https://clinicaltrials.gov/ct2/show/NCT02208063. Accessed June 30, 2015.
11. Bayer AS, Mishra NN, Sakoulas G, et al. Heterogeneity of mprF sequences in methicillin-resistant Staphylococcus aureus clinical isolates: role in cross-resistance between daptomycin and host defense antimicrobial peptides. Antimicrob Agents Chemother 2014;58(12):7462–7.
12. Bayer AS, Schneider T, Sahl H-G. Mechanisms of daptomycin resistance in Staphylococcus aureus: role of the cell membrane and cell wall. Ann N Y Acad Sci 2013;1277(1):139–58.
13. Humphries RM, Pollett S, Sakoulas G. A current perspective on daptomycin for the clinical microbiologist. Clin Microbiol Rev 2013;26(4):759–80.
14. Culshaw D, Lamp KC, Yoon MJ, et al. Duration of prior vancomycin therapy and subsequent daptomycin treatment outcomes in methicillin-resistant Staphylococcus aureus bacteremia. Diagn Microbiol Infect Dis 2015;83(2):193–7.
15. Liu C, Bayer A, Cosgrove SE, et al. Clinical practice guidelines by the Infectious Diseases Society of America for the treatment of methicillin-resistant Staphylococcus aureus infections in adults and children. Clin Infect Dis 2011;52(3): e18–55.
16. Gasch O, Camoez M, Domínguez MA, et al. Emergence of resistance to daptomycin in a cohort of patients with methicillin-resistant Staphylococcus aureus persistent bacteraemia treated with daptomycin. J Antimicrob Chemother 2014; 69(2):568–71.
17. Bassetti M, Nicco E, Ginocchio F, et al. High-dose daptomycin in documented Staphylococcus aureus infections. Int J Antimicrob Agents 2010;36(5):459–61.
18. Kullar R, Casapao AM, Davis SL, et al. A multicentre evaluation of the effectiveness and safety of high-dose daptomycin for the treatment of infective endocarditis. J Antimicrob Chemother 2013;68(12):2921–6.
19. Murray K, Zhao J, Davis S, et al. Early use of daptomycin versus vancomycin for methicillin-resistant staphylococcus aureus bacteremia with vancomycin minimum inhibitory concentration >1 mg/L: A matched cohort study. Clin Infect Dis 2013;56(11):1562–9.

20. Otero LH, Rojas-Altuve A, Llarrull LI, et al. How allosteric control of Staphylococcus aureus penicillin binding protein 2a enables methicillin resistance and physiological function. Proc Natl Acad Sci U S A 2013;110(42):16808–13.
21. Sader HS, Farrell DJ, Flamm RK, et al. Activity of ceftaroline and comparator agents tested against Staphylococcus aureus from patients with bloodstream infections in US medical centres (2009-13). J Antimicrob Chemother 2015;70(7): 2053–6.
22. Espedido BA, Jensen SO, van Hal SJ. Ceftaroline fosamil salvage therapy: an option for reduced-vancomycin-susceptible MRSA bacteraemia. J Antimicrob Chemother 2014;70(3):797–801.
23. MacGowan AP, Noel AR, Tomaselli S, et al. Pharmacodynamics of ceftaroline against Staphylococcus aureus studied in an in vitro pharmacokinetic model of infection. Antimicrob Agents Chemother 2013;57(6):2451–6.
24. Drusano GL. Pharmacodynamics of ceftaroline fosamil for complicated skin and skin structure infection: rationale for improved anti-methicillin-resistant Staphylococcus aureus activity. J Antimicrob Chemother 2010;65(Suppl 4):iv33–9.
25. Autry EB, Rybak JM, Leung NR, et al. Pharmacokinetic and pharmacodynamic analyses of ceftaroline in adults with cystic fibrosis. Pharmacotherapy 2016; 36(1):13–8.
26. Vazquez JA, Maggiore CR, Cole P, et al. Ceftaroline fosamil for the treatment of Staphylococcus aureus bacteremia secondary to acute bacterial skin and skin structure infections or community-acquired bacterial pneumonia. Infect Dis Clin Pract 2015;23(1):39–43.
27. Casapao AM, Davis SL, Barr VO, et al. Large retrospective evaluation of the effectiveness and safety of ceftaroline fosamil therapy. Antimicrob Agents Chemother 2014;58(5):2541–6.
28. Paladino JA, Jacobs DM, Shields RK, et al. Use of ceftaroline after glycopeptide failure to eradicate meticillin-resistant Staphylococcus aureus bacteraemia with elevated vancomycin minimum inhibitory concentrations. Int J Antimicrob Agents 2014;44(6):557–63.
29. Polenakovik HM, Pleiman CM. Ceftaroline for meticillin-resistant Staphylococcus aureus bacteraemia: case series and review of the literature. Int J Antimicrob Agents 2013;42(5):450–5.
30. Ho TT, Cadena J, Childs LM, et al. Methicillin-resistant Staphylococcus aureus bacteraemia and endocarditis treated with ceftaroline salvage therapy. J Antimicrob Chemother 2012;67(5):1267–70.
31. Lin JC, Aung G, Thomas A, et al. The use of ceftaroline fosamil in methicillin-resistant Staphylococcus aureus endocarditis and deep-seated MRSA infections: a retrospective case series of 10 patients. J Infect Chemother 2013;19(1):42–9.
32. Tattevin P, Boutoille D, Vitrat V, et al. Salvage treatment of methicillin-resistant staphylococcal endocarditis with ceftaroline: a multicentre observational study. J Antimicrob Chemother 2014;69(7):2010–3.
33. Rybak JM, Marx K, Martin CA. Early experience with tedizolid: clinical efficacy, pharmacodynamics, and resistance. Pharmacotherapy 2014;34(11):1198–208.
34. Flamm RK, Mendes RE, Hogan PA, et al. In vitro activity of linezolid as assessed through the 2013 LEADER surveillance program. Diagn Microbiol Infect Dis 2015; 81(4):283–9.
35. Burdette S, Trotman R. Tedizolid: the first once daily oxazoidinone class antibiotic. Clin Infect Dis 2015;61(8):1315–21.

36. Shorr AF, Kunkel MJ, Kollef M. Linezolid versus vancomycin for Staphylococcus aureus bacteraemia: pooled analysis of randomized studies. J Antimicrob Chemother 2005;56(5):923–9.
37. Wilcox MH, Tack KJ, Bouza E, et al. Complicated skin and skin-structure infections and catheter-related bloodstream infections: noninferiority of linezolid in a phase 3 study. Clin Infect Dis 2009;48(2):203–12.
38. Park HJ, Kim S-H, Kim M-J, et al. Efficacy of linezolid-based salvage therapy compared with glycopeptide-based therapy in patients with persistent methicillin-resistant Staphylococcus aureus bacteremia. J Infect 2012;65(6): 505–12.
39. Chan LC, Basuino L, Dip EC, et al. Comparative efficacy of tedizolid phosphate (prodrug of tedizolid), vancomycin and daptomycin in a rabbit model of methicillin-resistant Staphylococcus aureus endocarditis. Antimicrob Agents Chemother 2015;59(6):3252–6.
40. Chopra I, Roberts M. Tetracycline antibiotics: mode of action, applications, molecular biology, and epidemiology of bacterial resistance tetracycline antibiotics: mode of action, applications, molecular biology, and epidemiology of bacterial resistance. Microbiol Mol Biol Rev 2001;65(2):232–60.
41. Stein GE, Babinchak T. Tigecycline: an update. Diagn Microbiol Infect Dis 2013; 75(4):331–6.
42. Gardiner D, Dukart G, Cooper A, et al. Safety and efficacy of intravenous tigecycline in subjects with secondary bacteremia: pooled results from 8 phase III clinical trials. Clin Infect Dis 2010;50(2):229–38.
43. Barber KE, Werth BJ, Rybak MJ. The combination of ceftaroline plus daptomycin allows for therapeutic de-escalation and daptomycin sparing against MRSA. J Antimicrob Chemother 2015;70(2):505–9.
44. Dilworth TJ, Ibrahim O, Hall P, et al. β-Lactams enhance vancomycin activity against methicillin-resistant Staphylococcus aureus bacteremia compared to vancomycin alone. Antimicrob Agents Chemother 2014;58(1):102–9.
45. Barber KE, Rybak MJ, Sakoulas G. Vancomycin plus ceftaroline shows potent in vitro synergy and was successfully utilized to clear persistent daptomycin-non-susceptible MRSA bacteraemia. J Antimicrob Chemother 2015;70(1):311–3.
46. Davis JS, Sud A, O'Sullivan MV, et al. Combination of Vancomycin and β-Lactam Therapy for Methicillin-Resistant Staphylococcus aureus Bacteremia: A Pilot Multicenter Randomized Controlled Trial. Clin Infect Dis 2016;62(2):173–80.
47. Seah J, Lye DC, Ng T-M, et al. Vancomycin monotherapy vs. combination therapy for the treatment of persistent methicillin-resistant Staphylococcus aureus bacteremia. Virulence 2013;4(8):734–9.
48. Jang H, Kim S, Kim KH, et al. Salvage treatment for persistent methicillin-resistant Staphylococcus aureus bacteremia: efficacy of linezolid with or without carbapenem. Clin Infect Dis 2009;49(3):395–401.
49. Berti AD, Sakoulas G, Nizet V, et al. β-Lactam antibiotics targeting PBP1 selectively enhance daptomycin activity against methicillin-resistant Staphylococcus aureus. Antimicrob Agents Chemother 2013;57(10):5005–12.
50. Berti AD, Wergin JE, Girdaukas GG, et al. Altering the proclivity towards daptomycin resistance in methicillin-resistant Staphylococcus aureus using combinations with other antibiotics. Antimicrob Agents Chemother 2012;56(10):5046–53.
51. Moise PA, Amodio-Groton M, Rashid M, et al. Multicenter evaluation of the clinical outcomes of daptomycin with and without concomitant β-lactams in patients with Staphylococcus aureus bacteremia and mild to moderate renal impairment. Antimicrob Agents Chemother 2013;57(3):1192–200.

52. Sakoulas G, Brown J, Lamp KC, et al. Clinical outcomes of patients receiving daptomycin for the treatment of Staphylococcus aureus infections and assessment of clinical factors for daptomycin failure: a retrospective cohort study utilizing the Cubicin® Outcomes Registry and Experience. Clin Ther 2009;31(9): 1936–45.
53. Dhand A, Sakoulas G. Daptomycin in combination with other antibiotics for the treatment of complicated methicillin-resistant Staphylococcus aureus bacteremia. Clin Ther 2014;36(10):1303–16.
54. Paul M, Bishara J, Yahav D, et al. Trimethoprim-sulfamethoxazole versus vancomycin for severe infections caused by meticillin resistant Staphylococcus aureus: randomised controlled trial. BMJ 2015;350:h2219.
55. Claeys KC, Smith JR, Casapao AM, et al. Impact of the combination of daptomycin and trimethoprim-sulfamethoxazole on clinical outcomes in methicillin-resistant Staphylococcus aureus infections. Antimicrob Agents Chemother 2015;59(4):1969–76.
56. Zasowski E, Claeys K, Roberts K. Retrospective evaluation of daptomycin (DAP) plus ceftaroline fosamil (CPT) versus DAP plus sulfamethoxazole/trimethoprim (SMX/TMP) for methicillin-resistant Staphylococcus aureus (MRSA) bloodstream infections (BSI). Presented in poster session at the 25th European Congress of Clincial Microbiology and Infectious Diseases (ECCMID), Copenhagen, Denmark, April 25 – 28, 2015.
57. Fabre V, Ferrada M, Buckel WR, et al. Ceftaroline in combination with trimethoprim-sulfamethoxazole for salvage therapy of methicillin-resistant Staphylococcus aureus bacteremia and endocarditis. Open Forum Infect Dis 2014; 1(2):ofu046.
58. Miŕo JM, Entenza JM, Del Río A, et al. High-dose daptomycin plus fosfomycin is safe and effective in treating methicillin-susceptible and methicillin-resistant Staphylococcus aureus endocarditis. Antimicrob Agents Chemother 2012; 56(8):4511–5.
59. Linasmita P. Successful management of methicillin-resistant Staphylococcus aureus bacteremia unresponsive to Vancomycin by adding fosfomycin: a case report. J Med Assoc Thai 2012;95(7):960–3.
60. Del Rio A, Gasch O, Moreno A, et al. Efficacy and safety of fosfomycin plus imipenem as rescue therapy for complicated bacteremia and endocarditis due to methicillin-resistant Staphylococcus aureus: a multicenter clinical trial. Clin Infect Dis 2014;59(8):1105–12.

Drug-Resistant Tuberculosis

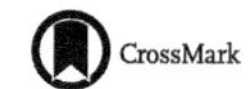

Challenges and Progress

Sebastian G. Kurz, MD, PhD[a,*], Jennifer J. Furin, MD, PhD[b], Charles M. Bark, MD[c]

KEYWORDS

- *Mycobacterium tuberculosis* • Drug-resistant tuberculosis • Antimicrobial resistance

KEY POINTS

- Antimicrobial resistance is a natural evolutionary process, which in the case of *Mycobacterium tuberculosis* is based on spontaneous chromosomal mutations, meaning that well-designed combination drug regimens provided under supervised therapy will prevent the emergence of drug-resistant strains.
- Unfortunately, limited resources, poverty, and neglect have led to the emergence of drug-resistant tuberculosis (DR-TB) throughout the world, particularly in the most vulnerable populations.
- The international community has responded with financial and scientific support, leading to new rapid diagnostics, new drugs and regimens in advanced clinical development, and an increasingly sophisticated understanding of resistance mechanisms and their application to all aspects of tuberculosis (TB) control and treatment.
- Although the obstacles are enormous, it is an exciting time based on optimism for substantial improvements for patients with DR-TB.
- Ultimately, for long-range success, the patient must remain in sight, for all new drugs and scientific advancements will be for naught if TB patients do not receive adequate, well-supervised care.

BACKGROUND

Treatment of drug-susceptible tuberculosis (TB) conducted under strong national TB programs (NTPs) using standard 4-drug therapy and directly observed therapy has led to relapse-free cure rates greater than 95% and dramatic national declines in TB

Funded by: NIH, Grant number(s): KL2TR000440.
[a] Division of Pulmonary, Critical Care and Sleep Medicine, Department of Medicine, Tufts University School of Medicine, 800 Washington Street, #257, Boston, MA 02111, USA; [b] Department of Global Health and Social Medicine, Harvard Medical School, 641 Huntington Avenue, Boston, MA 02115, USA; [c] Division of Infectious Diseases, Department of Medicine, MetroHealth Medical Center, Case Western Reserve University, 2500 MetroHealth Drive, Cleveland, OH 44109, USA
* Corresponding author.
E-mail address: SKurz1@tuftsmedicalcenter.org

Infect Dis Clin N Am 30 (2016) 509–522
http://dx.doi.org/10.1016/j.idc.2016.02.010 id.theclinics.com
0891-5520/16/$ – see front matter

incidence. This success has required consistent allocation of substantial money and resources. Conversely, poorly organized and underfunded NTPs result in unsupervised and inappropriate treatment, leading to treatment failure and the development of drug resistance, which is then spread to others.[1] The management of drug-resistant TB (DR-TB) is much more difficult than drug-susceptible TB, leading to epidemic spread of DR-TB in several countries. Drug resistance represents a major threat to global TB control with potential disastrous consequences[2]; this section explores new drugs and treatment regimens that are being developed to treat this deadly, communicable disease.[2]

Multidrug-resistant TB (MDR-TB) is defined as TB that is resistant to isoniazid (INH) and rifampin.[3] According to the Centers for Disease Control and Prevention (CDC), in 2014 there were 96 new cases of confirmed MDR-TB in the United States, representing 1.4% of the total 9421 new TB cases reported, and 88% of the MDR-TB patients were foreign-born.[4] Per the World Health Organization (WHO) Global Tuberculosis Report, there were an estimated 480,000 new cases of MDR-TB in the world in 2013, accounting for 3.5% of the total estimated 9 million TB cases.[3] Estimates are used because many of the countries with high MDR-TB incidence lack the resources and investment to accurately diagnose drug resistance on a national scale. Actual notifications were received for 136,412 people with MDR-TB or rifampicin-resistant TB, and of these, 96,617 (71%) were started on treatment. Treatment outcomes are available for 52,206 patients from 2011 with 48% reported as having successfully completed treatment. The WHO estimates that 210,000 of the 480,000 MDR-TB patients died. Although these numbers represent improvement, global control of MDR-TB remains dismal: less than one-third are diagnosed; about one-fifth are treated, and about 5% successfully complete treatment. The overwhelming majority of MDR-TB patients in the world are likely to have poor outcomes, causing great suffering and continued transmission.

A small subset, estimated at 9% of people with MDR-TB, have extensively drug-resistant TB (XDR-TB). XDR-TB is defined as MDR-TB with additional resistance to any fluoroquinolone and to at least 1 of 3 injectable agents (kanamycin, amikacin, or capreomycin). One hundred countries reported a case of XDR-TB in 2013, and of the 1269 patients reported in the 2011 cohort, only 284 (22%) completed their treatment successfully and 438 (35%) patients died.[3]

RESISTANCE MECHANISMS AND CURRENT APPROACHES TO TREATMENT

Soon after the discovery and initial use of streptomycin to treat TB in the 1940s, it became clear that single-drug treatment led to the rapid development of drug resistance, resulting in high failure rates.[5,6] This recognition led to the development of combination therapy using at least 2 active drugs to prevent resistance.[7] It was also noted that extension of therapy beyond seemingly successful treatment, with resolution of symptoms and microbiological clearance, was necessary to avoid relapse. The addition of INH, an agent with potent early bactericidal activity, led to effective combination therapy with high success rates after treatment for 18 to 24 months.[8] The introduction of rifampicin allowed a dramatic shortening of the treatment course to 6 to 9 months.[9] Ethambutol, an oral agent with relatively low toxicity, offered protection when drug resistance to INH or rifampicin was present. Finally, the addition of pyrazinamide (PZA) reliably allowed for shortening of treatment course to 6 months for most cases (for review, see Ref.[10]).

Although the phenomenon of drug resistance was quickly recognized, the underlying biological mechanisms were only recently elucidated. This scientific advancement has allowed for a progressive shift from culture-based, "phenotypic" drug-resistance testing to mutation-based genotypic resistance testing. It is noteworthy that all drug-resistance mutations found today are based on spontaneous chromosomal alterations. Mutations in drug target proteins are fairly restricted to confined gene loci and can easily be detected. Examples include the *rpoB* and *gyrA* genes, conferring resistance to rifampicin and fluoroquinolones, respectively. They can be quickly identified by semiautomated nuclear acid amplification tests (NAAT). A remarkable example that is revolutionizing TB diagnosis is the Xpert MTB/RIF (Cepheid), a fully-automated platform capable of NAAT testing for *Mycobacterium tuberculosis* and rifampicin resistance within 2 hours.[11] In contrast to target protein mutations, mutations in prodrug-activating enzymes are much more heterogeneous,[12] making them more difficult to capture in automated systems.

Standard Therapy for Drug-Susceptible Tuberculosis: Mechanisms and Resistance

INH has excellent early bactericidal activity resulting in a rapid drop in colony-forming units after beginning treatment.[13] It is a prodrug, which is activated by the catalase peroxidase KatG. The activated INH forms chemical entities with $NAD(P)^+$ coenzymes which inhibit the target protein InhA, an enoyl-acyl carrier protein, which takes part in mycolic acid synthesis. Mutations in the *katG* gene confer high-level INH resistance. The most common single-base mutation S315T leads to decreased INH substrate affinity at the expense of only modest reduction in overall catalase activity.[13] Other mutations, including missense and deletions, have been described. Alternatively, increased expression of *inhA* caused by alterations in the promoter region is associated with low-level INH resistance as well as cross-resistance to ethionamide.[14,15]

Rifampicin has excellent sterilizing activity, allowing for shorter treatment without relapse.[16] Rifampicin interferes with RNA synthesis by inhibition of the RNA polymerase RpoB. Resistance occurs spontaneously at a frequency of 1×10^{-7} to 1×10^{-8} bacilli via a single mutation in a well-defined region of the gene, which makes it detectable by molecular assays.[17] In contrast to INH, rifampicin monoresistance is uncommon,[18] making it a useful surrogate marker for MDR-TB.[11,19]

PZA is used for its sterilizing activity, which allowed for reduction in treatment length to 6 months. It is a prodrug that is activated by pyrazinamidase, coded for by *pncA*. The resultant pyrazinoic acid inhibits fatty acid synthetase 1.[20] Most described resistance mutations are found scattered over the *pncA* gene, which makes rapid molecular detection difficult.[21] Furthermore, the pH dependence of PZA activity makes culture-based phenotypic drug resistance testing challenging.

Ethambutol is primarily used to prevent acquired drug resistance in the setting of unknown INH resistance. It is usually discontinued once drug susceptibility is confirmed. Ethambutol inhibits the gene product of the *embCAB* cluster, which codes for an arabinosyl transferase necessary for arabinogalactan synthesis, a constituent of the mycobacterial cell wall.[22] Resistance mutations leading to overexpression or structural alteration have been identified.[23]

Current Treatment Regimen for Multidrug-Resistant Tuberculosis: Second-Line Agents

Treatment regimens for MDR-TB are complex. They rely on drugs with reduced efficacy and increased toxicity. Individual regimens are compiled in a stepwise approach, based on the WHO group scheme and taking drug susceptibility test results into account (**Table 1**). To start, a drug with preserved activity is picked from group 1. Because of limited activity, PZA and ethambutol should only be used as an adjunct to the regimen. Then, an injectable agent and a fluoroquinolone are added. Group 4

Table 1
World Health Organization group scheme of *Mycobacterium tuberculosis* drugs

Group 1	Group 2	Group 3	Group 4	Group 5
First-line drugs	Injectable drugs	Fluoroquinolones	Oral bacteriostatic second-line drugs	Drugs with unclear efficacy
Isoniazid, rifampicin, PZA, ethambutol	Kanamycin, amikacin, streptomycin, capreomycin, viomycin	Moxifloxacin, levofloxacin, gatifloxacin, ofloxacin	Pro-/ethionamide, cycloserine, terizidone, PAS, thiacetazone	Clofazimine, amoxicillin/clavulanate, clarithromycin, linezolid, imipenem

and 5 drugs are used to complement a regimen total of 4 drugs with the potential addition of PZA. The following paragraphs briefly describe mechanism and clinical utility of established second-line drugs.[24]

Aminoglycosides and the cyclic polypeptide *capreomycin* interfere with protein synthesis on the ribosomal level. High-resistance rates for streptomycin limit its use, and kanamycin or amikacin are the preferred agents. The most common resistance mutations affect the genes coding for 16S rRNA (*rrs*) and confer resistance to both kanamycin and amikacin.[25] The activity of capreomycin is only partly affected by these mutations and may still be of clinical use. Mutations in *tlyA*, which codes for a methyl rRNA transferase, results in loss of rRNA methylation and has been associated with capreomycin resistance.[26] There have been varying reports about different cross-resistance patterns among the aminoglycosides and cyclic peptides. A systematic molecular study revealed several different mutations conferring a heterogeneous pattern of cross-reactivity, which cautions against generalizations about cross-resistance without phenotypic testing.[27]

Levofloxacin, moxifloxacin, and gatifloxacin are the most studied *fluoroquinolones*. They target the DNA gyrase, which is necessary for uncoiling of the circular chromosome during replication. It is coded for by 2 genes, *gyrA* and *gyrB*. Resistance is caused by a single base substitution in a confined location known as quinolone-resistance-determining region.[28] Fluoroquinolones reach high tissue levels and have clinical efficacy similar to INH.[29] They have been included in MDR-TB regimens for decades, and because of their efficacy and favorable side effect profile, they remain a cornerstone of MDR-TB therapy.[30–32]

Cycloserine and its structural analogue *terizidone* have activity against gram-positive bacteria and mycobacteria. They inhibit peptidoglycan synthesis by interfering with Ala-racemase and $_D$Ala-$_D$Ala synthetase. Their use is limited by central nervous system toxicity caused by partial *N*-methyl-D-aspartate receptor agonism. Resistance mechanisms are not well defined. Overexpression of the target racemase AlaA, which serves as a cycloserine "sink," has been described as a major resistance mechanism in experimental mycobacteria.[33]

Ethionamide and *prothionamide* are thioamide drugs. Prodrug activation occurs by independent enzymes EthA and KatG. Like INH, ethionamide and prothionamide target InhA to inhibit fatty acid synthesis. Mutations in the *inhA* promoter region cause high-level ethionamide resistance in conjunction with low-level INH resistance as mentioned earlier.[15] Patient tolerance can be challenging because of gastrointestinal side effects, and they are associated with hypothyroidism.

β-Lactams are listed as group 5 drugs, agents with unclear benefit. Inconsistent reports exist about the early bactericidal activity of amoxicillin-clavulanate,[34,35] but clinicians have used it as adjunct therapy in the treatment of MDR-TB for some time.[36] *M tuberculosis* expresses a β-lactamase, BlaC, which was identified as the major determinant that renders *M tuberculosis* resistant to β-lactams,[37] but it is susceptible to inhibition by currently available β-lactamase inhibitors clavulanate, tazobactam, and sulbactam. The combination of carbapenems, which act as slow substrates, and β-lactamase inhibitors has been shown to have potent activity against otherwise drug-resistant strains.[38] Another reason for the preferred activity of carbapenems compared to other beta-lactams has been found in the way mcobacterial peptidoglycan is synthesized. Similar to other bacteria, peptidoglycan is an important constituent of the mycobacterial cell wall. It consists of longitudinal polysaccharide trunks, which bear branches of oligopeptide side-strands. These oligopeptides branches are cross-linked by transpeptidase enzymes to form a stable mesh. Recently, alternative cross-linking catalyzed by a different group of enzymes, the $_{L,\ D}$ transpeptidases, has been found to be the dominant type of peptidoglycan of *M tuberculosis*.[39] The $_{L,\ D}$ transpeptidases are effectively inhibited by carbapenems.[40] Case series of patients treated with the combination of meropenem and clavulanate as part of an MDR regimen demonstrated promising results.[41–43] One major drawback is the need for intravenous infusion of meropenem. Therefore, the introduction of the oral carbapenems tebipenem and biapenem, which were shown to have activity against a collection of 21 MDR and XDR isolates,[44] has raised considerable interest.

CLINICAL TRIALS

Given the poor performance of standard MDR-TB therapy along with its limited evidence base, there has been a substantial effort over the past decade to develop both new drugs and regimens specifically for DR-TB. Of note, most of the drugs used in the current treatment of MDR-TB have not been tested as single agents or in combination in randomized clinical trials. In addition to achieving relapse-free cure, an equally important part of therapeutic strategies for TB is preventing the development of drug resistance, and treatment of all forms of TB requires the use of combination regimens.[45] The classic approach to TB drug development, in which a single new drug is tested in combination with an optimized background regimen, has resulted in the approval of 2 new anti-TB drugs: bedaquiline and delaminid. *Bedaquiline* is an oral diarylquinoline, a new class of antimycobacterial drugs that inhibit ATP synthase.[46] In 2012, it was approved by the US Food and Drug Administration (FDA) for the treatment of MDR-TB.[47] The approval was based on a 2-stage phase 2b study. Phase 2b studies provide preliminary efficacy evidence and usually use sputum culture conversion to negative as the primary outcome (unlike phase 3 trials, which follow patients for relapse). The first phase conducted from 2007 to 2008 in South Africa enrolled 47 newly diagnosed MDR-TB patients treated with individualized therapy based on WHO guidelines and additionally randomized to receive bedaquiline versus placebo for a total of 8 weeks.[48] The study found significantly shorter times to sputum culture conversion at 8 weeks: 48% in the bedaquiline group versus 9% in the placebo group. There were no significant differences in severe adverse events, and absolute values for corrected QT interval were all less than 500 milliseconds. An earlier phase 2a trial had demonstrated an increase in corrected QT among patients taking bedaquiline.[49] The second phase of the phase 2b study enrolled 160 patients in Brazil, India, Latvia, Peru, the Philippines, Russia, South Africa, and Thailand. Patients were randomly assigned to receive either bedaquiline or placebo for 22 weeks, in addition to a 5-drug regimen.[50] Patients in the bedaquiline group had significantly shorter time to culture conversion compared with placebo (83 vs 125 days, $P<.001$), and higher rates of sputum culture conversion culture conversion: 79% versus 58% at 24 weeks ($P = .008$). Although the investigators reported no significant differences in adverse events, there were 10 deaths in 79 patients (13%) in the bedaquiline group compared with 2 of 81 patients (2%) in the placebo group. Nine of the 10 deaths occurred after completion of study drug; there was no association with QT prolongation, and none were considered to be related to bedaquiline.[50] The deaths led to the addition of a black-box warning regarding the increased risk of death as well as QT prolongation.[51] In addition, the CDC published provisional guidelines recommending that bedaquiline be used only for MDR-TB patients "when an effective regimen cannot otherwise be provided."[52] Preliminary reports suggest that in those situations, including XDR-TB, bedaquiline can be an effective addition to DR-TB regimens.[53]

Similar to bedaquiline, *delaminid* was studied as a single drug added to an optimized background regimen. Delaminid is derived from the nitroimidazole class of compounds that have been shown to inhibit mycolic acid synthesis. A phase 2b trial, with 2-month sputum culture conversion as the primary efficacy endpoint, enrolled 481 patients with pulmonary MDR-TB in 9 countries. Patients were randomized to receive either delaminid or placebo for 2 months in combination with a background regimen.[54] A significantly higher proportion of patients in the delaminid versus placebo group achieved culture conversion by 2 months (45.4% vs 29.6%, $P = .008$). Adverse events were similar in the groups, but there was a significant, dose-dependent increase in the frequency of QT prolongation with 3.8% of placebo, 9.9% of delaminid 100 mg group, and 13.1% of delaminid 200 mg group patients with QT prolongation.[54] A follow-up observational study found favorable outcomes, defined as cure or completion of treatment, in 75% of patients who received delaminid for 6 or more months compared with 55% who received 2 months or less.[55]

Another drug that has been successfully used and studied as a single-drug addition to the traditional DR-TB regimens is *linezolid*. Developed as an oxazolidinone, which inhibits protein synthesis by binding the 23S rRNA in the 50S ribosomal subunit of bacteria, linezolid demonstrated in vitro activity against *M tuberculosis*[56] and was adopted early on for the treatment of highly resistant TB.[57] A randomized trial of 41 patients with sputum culture-positive XDR-TB conducted in South Korea from 2008 to 2011 in which patients received linezolid at a dose of 600 mg daily in addition to an optimized background regimen found that 87% of patients had sputum culture conversion to negative during the first 6 months of linezolid treatment.[58] Notably, 82% of patients had significant adverse events, including 21 cases of peripheral neuropathy, 7 episodes of myelosuppression, 7 cases of optic neuropathy, and 1 case of rhabdomyolysis. In addition, *M tuberculosis* isolates from 4 patients developed linezolid resistance during treatment through acquired mutations in either 23S rRNA or ribosomal protein L3.[58] Two other oxazolidinones are under development for the treatment of TB with the hope of developing a potent drug with a lower side-effect profile. Sutezolid is a linezolid analogue and has undergone phase 1 and 2 testing, with the latter demonstrating bactericidal activity, although lower than standard therapy.[59] AZD5847 is a second-generation oxazolidinone that has recently undergone phase 2 testing with results expected in late 2015.

Although both bedaquiline and delaminid have been licensed using a "single-drug" approach, they still have limited safety and effectiveness data, and even less evidence for combinations of the 2 drugs.[60] Given the side-effect profiles, including QT prolongation, this is especially important and could limit their use in combination treatments.

Although single-drug studies are still ongoing, the experience with bedaquiline and delaminid highlights the limitations of this approach: decades are needed to identify therapeutic advances.[61]

Alternative Approaches to Drug-Resistant Tuberculosis Clinical Drug Development

Citing the practical challenges of implementing MDR-TB treatment based on WHO guidelines, the Damien Foundation, a nongovernmental organization based in Bangladesh, conducted a prospective observational study during which they used treatment outcomes and adverse drug reactions to guide adjustments in MDR-TB treatment with the goal of developing a well-tolerated, effective, and inexpensive regimen.[62] The study included 427 culture-confirmed MDR-TB patients in 6 successive cohorts of patient over 10 years, beginning in 1997. The final regimen, known as the "Bangladesh Regimen," consisted of an intensive phase, including kanamycin, clofazimine, gatifloxacin, ethambutol, high-dose INH, PZA, and prothionamide, given for 4 months (or until culture conversion), followed by a continuation phase of clofazimine, gatifloxacin, ethambutol, and PZA given for 5 months. Patients were followed for 2 years, and relapse-free cure was obtained in 170 of 206 patients (82.5%).[62] A follow-up study that included 515 patients treated with the same regimen demonstrated treatment success in 435 of 515 patients (84.5%).[63] To validate the remarkable outcomes of the Bangladesh regimen, the British Medical Research Council (MRC) is conducting a phase III randomized controlled clinical trial, called STREAM 1, to test this regimen against standard therapy.[64] The trial began in July 2012 in Ethiopia, Mongolia, South Africa, and Vietnam and completed enrollment in early 2015. It marks the first successful randomized clinical trial of a DR-TB regimen. The Bangladesh regimen also highlights the potential of drug repurposing. Initially synthesized in 1954 as a TB drug,[65] but primarily used since for the treatment of leprosy, *clofazimine* has made a surprising comeback as an important drug for the treatment DR-TB. Given promising retrospective data,[66] Tang and colleagues[67] conducted a prospective, randomized controlled study in China, enrolling 105 patient with sputum culture–positive MDR-TB to receive either a WHO-based regimen with or without the addition of clofazimine. Treatment success (cure or treatment completion) was significantly higher in the clofazimine group (74% vs 54%, $P = .04$). One unique side effect of clofazimine is a reddish-brown skin discoloration that is usually reversible with discontinuation; 94% of patients in the clofazimine group developed skin discoloration.

Given the limitations of studying single drugs and the success of the Bangladesh studies, a regimen-based approach is now favored in which new, old, and repurposed drugs are given in various combinations in order to identify a drug combination that can be used for treating TB and MDR-TB.[68,69] This approach has been supported by regulatory agencies, including the US FDA,[70] and is being adapted by several clinical trials as described in **Table 2**.[71,72] Some of the trials focus on finding a "universal regimen" that can be used for patients with pan-susceptible and drug-resistant forms of TB. The development of *pretomanid*, a new nitroimidazole, followed this approach. Unlike the phase 2b trials of bedaquiline and delaminid, which added a single drug to an optimized background regimen, pretomanid was investigated as part of a totally new TB regimen for both drug-susceptible TB and DR-TB. The regimen, consisting of pretomanid, PZA, and moxifloxacin, was studied in a randomized controlled phase 2b trial of 207 patients with drug-susceptible pulmonary TB.[73] In addition, there was an MDR-TB arm that received the same regimen. The combination, which was safe and well-tolerated with superior bactericidal activity, is now being tested in the phase 3 "STAND" trial enrolling patients with drug-susceptible TB and MDR-TB.[74] Other trial strategies focus on using novel methodologic strategies for identifying regimens based on early safety

Table 2
Current and planned phase III and pragmatic clinical trials of new regimens for drug-resistant tuberculosis

Trial Name	Trial Number	Description	Trial Group	Enrolllment Status
STREAM 1	ISRCTN78372190	4MCEZHKPro/ 5MCZE vs local regimen	MRC	Opened July 2012, results expected late 2017
STREAM 2	NCT02409290	4MCEZHKPro/ 5MCZE vs 4BLCEZHPro/ 5BLCEZ vs 2BLCZHK/4BLCZ vs local regimen	IUATLD/MRC	Opens Q3 2015
Trial 213	NCT01424670	6D + OBR vs Placebo + OBR	Otsuka Pharmaceuticals	Opened Sept 2011, results 2017
NIX-TB (XDR)	NCT02333799	6BPaLzd (single arm)	TB Alliance	Opened Feb 2015
STAND NC-006/ A5344	NCT02342886	6PaMZ (single arm for DR-TB)	TB Alliance/ACTG	Opened Feb 2015
Opti-Q	NCT01918397	L + OBR (high dose vs standard dose)	US NIH	Opened January 2015
NeXT	NCT02454205	LzdBLEthHZ (combination based on mutational analysis: given for 6–9 mo) vs local regimen	South Africa MRC	Opened June 2015
TB-PRACTECAL	—	6BPaLzdM vs 6BPaLzdC vs 6BPaLzd vs local regimen	Medecins Sans Frontiers (MSF)	Expected start Q3 2015
END-TB	—	Various combinations of Bdq-Pa_924, Lzd, Cfz, Lfx, Mfx, Pza	UNITAID-Partners In Health, MSF	Protocol development

Abbreviations: B, Bdq, bedaquiline; C, Cfz, clofazimine; D, delaminid; E, ethambutol; Eth, ethionamide; H, isoniazid; K, kanamycin; L, Lfx, levofloxacin; Lzd, linezolid; M, Mfx, moxifloxacin; OBR, optimized background regimen; Pa, pretomanid; Pro, prothianamide; Z, Pza, pyrazinamide.

and efficacy indicators. The PanACEA research group in using the Multi-Arm Multi-Stage design allowed for several different treatment regimens to be evaluated in a single trial.[75,76] These approaches have been adapted from clinical trials in cancer,[77] and it is hoped that they can not only identify full regimens instead of single drugs but also rapidly identify candidate regimens to move forward into phase III trials and thus shave years off the time it takes to advance programmatic use of new drugs.[78]

Although trials of new drugs and regimens for TB and DR-TB are advancing at a historic pace, the future control of DR-TB will require a clearer understanding of the mechanisms and impact of drug resistance to better inform trial design. Currently, the limited knowledge that exists about the clinical implications of drug-resistance mutations has led to a situation in which mechanisms of resistance play little role in regimen selection or design. For example, there have been limited data published showing there may be cross-resistance between bedaquiline and clofazimine,[79] which could have profound implications for DR-TB regimens that plan to use both drugs together. Understanding resistance goes beyond identifying specific mutations, such as *rpoB*, but rather takes a holistic approach that incorporates epistasis and bacterial fitness.[80] Epistasis is the phenomenon of multiple genetic interactions that create a phenotype, such that a single mutation can manifest in different ways depending on the modifying gene interactions of the genetic background.[81] Fitness is the concept that mutations can have a physiologic cost, affecting the growth rate or virulence of the mutated bacilli. In-depth understanding of these complex interactions is now possible with whole genome sequencing. The goal is to combine genetic and clinical information to create supranational surveillance for emerging resistance and guide the construction of future DR-TB regimens.

SUMMARY

Antimicrobial resistance is a natural evolutionary process, which in the case of *M tuberculosis* is based on spontaneous chromosomal mutations, meaning that well-designed combination drug regimens provided under supervised therapy will prevent the emergence of drug-resistant strains. Unfortunately, limited resources, poverty, and neglect have led to the emergence of DR-TB throughout the world, particularly in the most vulnerable populations. The international community has responded with financial and scientific support leading to new rapid diagnostics, new drugs and regimens in advanced clinical development, and an increasingly sophisticated understanding of resistance mechanisms and their application to all aspects of TB control and treatment. Although the obstacles are enormous, it is an exciting time based on optimism for substantial improvements for patients with DR-TB. Ultimately, for long-range success, the patient must remain in sight, for all new drugs and scientific advancements will be for naught if TB patients do not receive adequate, well-supervised care.

REFERENCES

1. Caminero JA. Multidrug-resistant tuberculosis: epidemiology, risk factors and case finding. Int J Tuberc Lung Dis 2010;14(4):382–90.
2. Antimicrobial resistance: tackling a crisis for the health and wealth of nations. Available at: http://amr-review.org/sites/default/files/AMR%20Review%20Paper%20-%20Tackling%20a%20crisis%20for%20the%20health%20and%20wealth%20of%20nations_1.pdf. Accessed March 7, 2016.
3. World Health Organization. Global tuberculosis report 2014. Geneva (Switzerland): World Health Organization; 2014.
4. Reported tuberculosis in the United States. Division of tuberculosis elimination, Centers for Disease Control and Prevention. Available at: http://www.cdc.gov/tb/statistics/. Accessed March 7, 2016.
5. Council MR. Streptomycin treatment of pulmonary tuberculosis. Br Med J 1948; 2(4582):769–82.
6. Jones D, Metzger HJ, Schatz A, et al. Control of gram-negative bacteria in experimental animals by streptomycin. Science 1944;100(2588):103–5.

7. PREVENTION of streptomycin resistance by combined chemotherapy; a Medical Research Council Investigation. Br Med J 1952;1(4769):1157–62.
8. Council MR. Long-term chemotherapy in the treatment of chronic pulmonary tuberculosis with cavitation. Tubercle 1962;43:201–67.
9. Short-course chemotherapy in pulmonary tuberculosis. A controlled trial by the British Thoracic and Tuberculosis Association. Lancet 1976;2(7995):1102–4.
10. Fox W, Ellard GA, Mitchison DA. Studies on the treatment of tuberculosis undertaken by the British Medical Research Council tuberculosis units, 1946-1986, with relevant subsequent publications. Int J Tuberc Lung Dis 1999;3(10 Suppl 2): S231–79.
11. Boehme CC, Nabeta P, Hillemann D, et al. Rapid molecular detection of tuberculosis and rifampin resistance. N Engl J Med 2010;363(11):1005–15.
12. Bottger EC, Springer B. Tuberculosis: drug resistance, fitness, and strategies for global control. Eur J Pediatr 2008;167(2):141–8.
13. Vilcheze C, Jacobs WR Jr. The mechanism of isoniazid killing: clarity through the scope of genetics. Annu Rev Microbiol 2007;61:35–50.
14. Zhang Y, Heym B, Allen B, et al. The catalase-peroxidase gene and isoniazid resistance of mycobacterium tuberculosis. Nature 1992;358(6387):591–3.
15. Banerjee A, Dubnau E, Quemard A, et al. inhA, a gene encoding a target for isoniazid and ethionamide in Mycobacterium tuberculosis. Science 1994; 263(5144):227–30.
16. Controlled trial of 2, 4, and 6 months of pyrazinamide in 6-month, three-times-weekly regimens for smear-positive pulmonary tuberculosis, including an assessment of a combined preparation of isoniazid, rifampin, and pyrazinamide. Results at 30 months. Hong Kong Chest Service/British Medical Research Council. Am Rev Respir Dis 1991;143(4 Pt 1):700–6.
17. Telenti A, Imboden P, Marchesi F, et al. Detection of rifampicin-resistance mutations in Mycobacterium tuberculosis. Lancet 1993;341(8846):647–50.
18. Somoskovi A, Parsons LM, Salfinger M. The molecular basis of resistance to isoniazid, rifampin, and pyrazinamide in mycobacterium tuberculosis. Respir Res 2001;2(3):164–8.
19. Watterson SA, Wilson SM, Yates MD, et al. Comparison of three molecular assays for rapid detection of rifampin resistance in mycobacterium tuberculosis. J Clin Microbiol 1998;36(7):1969–73.
20. Zimhony O, Cox JS, Welch JT, et al. Pyrazinamide inhibits the eukaryotic-like fatty acid synthetase I (FASI) of Mycobacterium tuberculosis. Nat Med 2000;6(9): 1043–7.
21. Miotto P, Cirillo DM, Migliori GB. Drug resistance in mycobacterium tuberculosis: molecular mechanisms challenging fluoroquinolones and pyrazinamide effectiveness. Chest 2015;147(4):1135–43.
22. Belanger AE, Besra GS, Ford ME, et al. The embAB genes of Mycobacterium avium encode an arabinosyl transferase involved in cell wall arabinan biosynthesis that is the target for the antimycobacterial drug ethambutol. Proc Natl Acad Sci U S A 1996;93(21):11919–24.
23. Telenti A, Philipp WJ, Sreevatsan S, et al. The emb operon, a gene cluster of Mycobacterium tuberculosis involved in resistance to ethambutol. Nat Med 1997;3(5):567–70.
24. World Health Organization. Guidelines for the programmatic management of drug-resistant tuberculosis—2011 update. Geneva (Switzerland): World Health Organization; 2011.

25. Shcherbakov D, Akbergenov R, Matt T, et al. Directed mutagenesis of Mycobacterium smegmatis 16s rRNA to reconstruct the in vivo evolution of aminoglycoside resistance in Mycobacterium tuberculosis. Mol Microbiol 2010;77(4):830–40.
26. Maus CE, Plikaytis BB, Shinnick TM. Mutation of tlyA confers capreomycin resistance in Mycobacterium tuberculosis. Antimicrob Agents Chemother 2005;49(2): 571–7.
27. Maus CE, Plikaytis BB, Shinnick TM. Molecular analysis of cross-resistance to capreomycin, kanamycin, amikacin, and viomycin in mycobacterium tuberculosis. Antimicrob Agents Chemother 2005;49(8):3192–7.
28. Alangaden GJ, Manavathu EK, Vakulenko SB, et al. Characterization of fluoroquinolone-resistant mutant strains of mycobacterium tuberculosis selected in the laboratory and isolated from patients. Antimicrob Agents Chemother 1995; 39(8):1700–3.
29. Dorman SE, Johnson JL, Goldberg S, et al. Substitution of moxifloxacin for isoniazid during intensive phase treatment of pulmonary tuberculosis. Am J Respir Crit Care Med 2009;180(3):273–80.
30. Yew WW, Kwan SY, Ma WK, et al. In-vitro activity of ofloxacin against mycobacterium tuberculosis and its clinical efficacy in multiply resistant pulmonary tuberculosis. J Antimicrob Chemother 1990;26(2):227–36.
31. Yew WW, Chan CK, Leung CC, et al. Comparative roles of levofloxacin and ofloxacin in the treatment of multidrug-resistant tuberculosis: preliminary results of a retrospective study from hong kong. Chest 2003;124(4):1476–81.
32. Ahuja SD, Ashkin D, Avendano M, et al. Multidrug resistant pulmonary tuberculosis treatment regimens and patient outcomes: an individual patient data meta-analysis of 9,153 patients. PLoS Med 2012;9(8):e1001300.
33. Caceres NE, Harris NB, Wellehan JF, et al. Overexpression of the D-alanine racemase gene confers resistance to D-cycloserine in Mycobacterium smegmatis. J Bacteriol 1997;179(16):5046–55.
34. Chambers HF, Kocagoz T, Sipit T, et al. Activity of amoxicillin/clavulanate in patients with tuberculosis. Clin Infect Dis 1998;26(4):874–7.
35. Donald PR, Sirgel FA, Venter A, et al. Early bactericidal activity of amoxicillin in combination with clavulanic acid in patients with sputum smear-positive pulmonary tuberculosis. Scand J Infect Dis 2001;33(6):466–9.
36. Nadler JP, Berger J, Nord JA, et al. Amoxicillin-clavulanic acid for treating drug-resistant mycobacterium tuberculosis. Chest 1991;99(4):1025–6.
37. Chambers HF, Moreau D, Yajko D, et al. Can penicillins and other beta-lactam antibiotics be used to treat tuberculosis? Antimicrob Agents Chemother 1995; 39(12):2620–4.
38. Hugonnet JE, Tremblay LW, Boshoff HI, et al. Meropenem-clavulanate is effective against extensively drug-resistant mycobacterium tuberculosis. Science 2009; 323(5918):1215–8.
39. Lavollay M, Arthur M, Fourgeaud M, et al. The peptidoglycan of stationary-phase Mycobacterium tuberculosis predominantly contains cross-links generated by L,D-transpeptidation. J Bacteriol 2008;190(12):4360–6.
40. Gupta R, Lavollay M, Mainardi JL, et al. The mycobacterium tuberculosis protein LdtMt2 is a nonclassical transpeptidase required for virulence and resistance to amoxicillin. Nat Med 2010;16(4):466–9.
41. Dauby N, Muylle I, Mouchet F, et al. Meropenem/clavulanate and linezolid treatment for extensively drug-resistant tuberculosis. Pediatr Infect Dis J 2011;30(9): 812–3.

42. De Lorenzo S, Alffenaar JW, Sotgiu G, et al. Efficacy and safety of meropenem-clavulanate added to linezolid-containing regimens in the treatment of MDR-/XDR-TB. Eur Respir J 2013;41(6):1386–92.
43. Payen MC, De Wit S, Martin C, et al. Clinical use of the meropenem-clavulanate combination for extensively drug-resistant tuberculosis. Int J Tuberc Lung Dis 2012;16(4):558–60.
44. Horita Y, Maeda S, Kazumi Y, et al. In vitro susceptibility of mycobacterium tuberculosis isolates to an oral carbapenem alone or in combination with beta-lactamase inhibitors. Antimicrob Agents Chemother 2014;58(11):7010–4.
45. Daley CL, Caminero JA. Management of multidrug resistant tuberculosis. Semin Respir Crit Care Med 2013;34(1):44–59.
46. Andries K, Verhasselt P, Guillemont J, et al. A diarylquinoline drug active on the ATP synthase of mycobacterium tuberculosis. Science 2005;307(5707):223–7.
47. FDA accelerated approval letter to janseen research and development. Food and Drug Administration. Available at: http://www.accessdata.fda.gov/drugsatfda_docs/appletter/2012/204384Orig1s000ltr.pdf. Accessed March 7, 2016.
48. Diacon AH, Pym A, Grobusch M, et al. The diarylquinoline TMC207 for multidrug-resistant tuberculosis. N Engl J Med 2009;360(23):2397–405.
49. Rustomjee R, Diacon AH, Allen J, et al. Early bactericidal activity and pharmacokinetics of the diarylquinoline TMC207 in treatment of pulmonary tuberculosis. Antimicrob Agents Chemother 2008;52(8):2831–5.
50. Diacon AH, Pym A, Grobusch MP, et al. Multidrug-resistant tuberculosis and culture conversion with bedaquiline. N Engl J Med 2014;371(8):723–32.
51. Sirturo (bedaquiline) tablets label. Food and Drug Administration. Available at: http://www.accessdata.fda.gov/drugsatfda_docs/label/2012/204384s000lbl.pdf. Accessed March 7, 2016.
52. Centers for Disease Control and Prevention. Provisional CDC guidelines for the use and safety monitoring of bedaquiline fumarate (sirturo) for the treatment of multidrug-resistant tuberculosis. MMWR Recomm Rep 2013;62(RR-09):1–12.
53. Guglielmetti L, Le Du D, Jachym M, et al. Compassionate use of bedaquiline for the treatment of multidrug-resistant and extensively drug-resistant tuberculosis: interim analysis of a French cohort. Clin Infect Dis 2015;60(2):188–94.
54. Gler MT, Skripconoka V, Sanchez-Garavito E, et al. Delamanid for multidrug-resistant pulmonary tuberculosis. N Engl J Med 2012;366(23):2151–60.
55. Skripconoka V, Danilovits M, Pehme L, et al. Delamanid improves outcomes and reduces mortality in multidrug-resistant tuberculosis. Eur Respir J 2013;41(6):1393–400.
56. Brickner SJ, Hutchinson DK, Barbachyn MR, et al. Synthesis and antibacterial activity of U-100592 and U-100766, two oxazolidinone antibacterial agents for the potential treatment of multidrug-resistant gram-positive bacterial infections. J Med Chem 1996;39(3):673–9.
57. Fortun J, Martin-Davila P, Navas E, et al. Linezolid for the treatment of multidrug-resistant tuberculosis. J Antimicrob Chemother 2005;56(1):180–5.
58. Lee M, Lee J, Carroll MW, et al. Linezolid for treatment of chronic extensively drug-resistant tuberculosis. N. Engl. J Med 2012;367(16):1508–18.
59. Wallis RS, Dawson R, Friedrich SO, et al. Mycobactericidal activity of sutezolid (PNU-100480) in sputum (EBA) and blood (WBA) of patients with pulmonary tuberculosis. PLoS One 2014;9(4):e94462.
60. Gruber K. Access sought to tuberculosis drug from nutraceutical company. Nat Med 2015;21(2):103.

61. Zumla AI, Schito M, Maeurer M. Advancing the portfolio of tuberculosis diagnostics, drugs, biomarkers, and vaccines. Lancet Infect Dis 2014;14(4):267–9.
62. Van Deun A, Maug AK, Salim MA, et al. Short, highly effective, and inexpensive standardized treatment of multidrug-resistant tuberculosis. Am J Respir Crit Care Med 2010;182(5):684–92.
63. Aung KJ, Van Deun A, Declercq E, et al. Successful '9-month Bangladesh regimen' for multidrug-resistant tuberculosis among over 500 consecutive patients. Int J Tuberc Lung Dis 2014;18(10):1180–7.
64. Nunn AJ, Rusen ID, Van Deun A, et al. Evaluation of a standardized treatment regimen of anti-tuberculosis drugs for patients with multi-drug-resistant tuberculosis (STREAM): study protocol for a randomized controlled trial. Trials 2014;15:353.
65. Barry VC, Belton JG, Conalty ML, et al. A new series of phenazines (rimino-compounds) with high antituberculosis activity. Nature 1957;179(4568):1013–5.
66. Dey T, Brigden G, Cox H, et al. Outcomes of clofazimine for the treatment of drug-resistant tuberculosis: a systematic review and meta-analysis. J Antimicrob Chemother 2013;68(2):284–93.
67. Tang S, Yao L, Hao X, et al. Clofazimine for the treatment of multidrug-resistant tuberculosis: prospective, multicenter, randomized controlled study in china. Clin Infect Dis 2015;60(9):1361–7.
68. Phillips PP, Nunn AJ. Challenges of phase III study design for trials of new drug regimens for the treatment of TB. Future Med Chem 2010;2(8):1273–82.
69. Wallis RS. Sustainable tuberculosis drug development. Clin Infect Dis 2013;56(1):106–13.
70. Guidance for industry: tuberculosis. Developing drugs for treatment. Draft guidance. Available at: http://www.fda.gov/downloads/drugs/guidancecomplianceregulatoryinformation/guidances/ucm373580.pdf. Accessed March 7, 2016.
71. Lienhardt C, Davies G. Methodological issues in the design of clinical trials for the treatment of multidrug-resistant tuberculosis: challenges and opportunities. Int J Tuberc Lung Dis 2010;14(5):528–37.
72. Critical path to TB drug regimens (CPTR) initiative. Available at: http://c-path.org/programs/cptr/. Accessed March 7, 2016.
73. Dawson R, Diacon AH, Everitt D, et al. Efficiency and safety of the combination of moxifloxacin, pretomanid (PA-824), and pyrazinamide during the first 8 weeks of antituberculosis treatment: a phase 2b, open-label, partly randomised trial in patients with drug-susceptible or drug-resistant pulmonary tuberculosis. Lancet 2015;385(9979):1738–47.
74. Global phase 3 "STAND" trial launched to test new tuberculosis drug regimen PAMZ to shorten, improve treatment. Available at: http://www.tballiance.org/newscenter/view-brief.php?id=1116. Accessed March 7, 2016.
75. Phillips PP, Gillespie SH, Boeree M, et al. Innovative trial designs are practical solutions for improving the treatment of tuberculosis. J Infect Dis 2012;205(Suppl 2):S250–7.
76. Panacea mams trial. Available at: http://panacea-tb.net/mams-study-has-completed-first-interim-analysis. Accessed March 7, 2016.
77. STAMPEDE trial. Available at: http://www.stampedetrial.org/. Accessed March 7, 2016.
78. Fauci AS, Group NTW. Multidrug-resistant and extensively drug-resistant tuberculosis: the National Institute of Allergy and Infectious Diseases research agenda and recommendations for priority research. J Infect Dis 2008;197(11):1493–8.

79. Hartkoorn RC, Uplekar S, Cole ST. Cross-resistance between clofazimine and bedaquiline through upregulation of mmpl5 in mycobacterium tuberculosis. Antimicrob Agents Chemother 2014;58(5):2979–81.
80. Trauner A, Borrell S, Reither K, et al. Evolution of drug resistance in tuberculosis: recent progress and implications for diagnosis and therapy. Drugs 2014;74(10): 1063–72.
81. Fenner L, Egger M, Bodmer T, et al. Effect of mutation and genetic background on drug resistance in mycobacterium tuberculosis. Antimicrob Agents Chemother 2012;56(6):3047–53.

Aminoglycoside Resistance

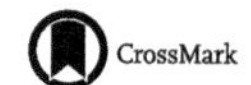

The Emergence of Acquired 16S Ribosomal RNA Methyltransferases

Yohei Doi, MD, PhD[a,*], Jun-ichi Wachino, PhD[b],
Yoshichika Arakawa, MD, PhD[b]

KEYWORDS

- Aminoglycoside • 16S ribosomal RNA • Posttranscriptional methylation
- Carbapenemease

KEY POINTS

- Aminoglycoside-producing Actinobacteria produce 16S ribosomal RNA methyltransferase (16S-RMTase) to protect themselves.
- High-level aminoglycoside resistance caused by production of acquired 16S-RMTase in pathogenic gram-negative bacteria was first reported in the early 2000s.
- Bacteria that produce 16S-RMTases frequently coproduce ESBL, and more recently, carbapenemase, especially NDM-1.
- Spread of 16S-RMTase-producing bacteria further compromises the already limited treatment options for infections caused by MDR/XDR pathogens.

INTRODUCTION

Antimicrobial resistance has been recognized as one of the most pressing public health and societal issues of our times. The problem is most acute in gram-negative bacteria, where strains resistant to multiple (multidrug-resistant [MDR]) or almost all (extensively drug-resistant [XDR]) available agents are emerging.[1] Of particular concern has been the spread of extended-spectrum β-lactamase (ESBL)-producing Enterobacteriaceae in the 1990s, which was followed closely by the emergence and rapid dissemination of carbapenemase-producing organisms.

Y. Doi was supported by research grants from the National Institutes of Health (R01AI104895, R21AI107302, and R21AI123747).
Potential Conflicts of Interest: Y. Doi has served on advisory boards for Shionogi, Meiji, Tetraphase, consulted for Melinta Therapeutics, received a speaker fee from Merck, and received research funding from Merck and The Medicines Company for studies unrelated to this work. The other authors report no potential conflicts of interest.
[a] Division of Infectious Diseases, University of Pittsburgh School of Medicine, S829 Scaife Hall, 3550 Terrace Street, Pittsburgh, PA 15261, USA; [b] Department of Bacteriology, Nagoya University School of Medicine, 65 Tsurumai-cho, Showa-ku, Nagoya, Aichi 466-8550, Japan
* Corresponding author.
E-mail address: yod4@pitt.edu

Infect Dis Clin N Am 30 (2016) 523–537
http://dx.doi.org/10.1016/j.idc.2016.02.011
id.theclinics.com
0891-5520/16/$ – see front matter

The three key classes of antimicrobial agents with gram-negative activity include β-lactams (especially β-lactam-β-lactamase inhibitor combinations, later-generation cephalosporins, and carbapenems), fluoroquinolones, and aminoglycosides. Aminoglycosides were identified through systematic screening of soil Actinobacteria that started in the 1940s. The first aminoglycoside streptomycin was discovered from *Streptomyces griseus* and successfully used for the treatment of tuberculosis and then infections with gram-negative bacteria. A typical aminoglycoside possesses an amino-containing or non-amino-containing sugars linked to six-membered rings with amino group substituents, hence the name aminoglycoside. Numerous aminoglycosides have since been identified or semisynthesized and used in clinical practice.

Aminoglycosides are grouped into 4,6-disubstituted 2-deoxystreptamine (DOS), 4,5-disubstituted DOS, and 4-monosubstituted DOS based on their chemical structures (**Figs. 1** and **2**). Representative 4,6-disubstituted DOS agents include gentamicin, tobramycin, and amikacin, which are widely used as intravenous or nebulized formulations for the treatment of infections caused by gram-negative bacteria (usually in combination with a β-lactam agent), gram-positive bacteria (for synergistic activity with a β-lactam or peptidoglycan), and atypical mycobacteria (again in combination with other active agents). 4,5-Disubstituted DOS agents, represented by neomycin, are limited in their utility by toxicity and are administered either orally or topically but not intravenously. Monosubstituted DOS agents are represented by apramycin, which is used in veterinary medicine.

MECHANISMS OF AMINOGLYCOSIDE RESISTANCE

Aminoglycosides bind to the aminoacyl-tRNA recognition site (A-site) of the 16S rRNA that constitutes the 30S ribosomal subunit, leading to inhibition of polypeptide synthesis and subsequent cell death. Resistance to aminoglycosides may occur based on several mechanisms: (1) enzymatic modification and inactivation of the aminoglycosides, mediated by aminoglycoside acetyltransferases, nucleotidyltransferases, or phosphotransferases and commonly observed across gram-positive and -negative bacteria[2,3]; (2) increased efflux; (3) decreased permeability; and (4) modifications of the 30S ribosomal subunit that interferes with binding of the aminoglycosides. For the latter, both mutations (nucleotide replacement) and posttranscriptional modifications have been associated with aminoglycoside resistance. Examples include point mutations in the 16S rRNA and the *rpsL* gene encoding the S12 protein in *Mycobacterium tuberculosis* leading to streptomycin resistance.[4] However, mutations within the 30S ribosomal subunit do not seem to be a common aminoglycoside resistance mechanism among fast-growing pathogenic bacteria in general.

However, posttranscriptional modification of the 16S rRNA is commonly observed among aminoglycoside-producing Actinobacteria, including *Streptomyces* spp and *Micromonospora* spp, which are naturally resistant to these metabolites of their own. This process is mediated by posttranscriptional methylation of either the N-7 position of nucleotide G1405 or the N-1 position of nucleotide A1408 on the 16S rRNA by various 16S rRNA methyltransferases (16S-RMTases) (**Fig. 3**).[5] Intrinsic N7-G1405 16S-RMTases are found in both *Streptomyces* spp and *Micromonospora* spp, whereas intrinsic N1-A1408 16S-RMTases have only been identified in *Streptomyces* spp.[6] N7-G1405 16S-RMTases confer resistance to 4,6-disubstituted DOS agents, such as gentamicin, tobramycin, and amikacin, but not 4,5-disubstituted and monosubstituted DOS agents. In contrast, N1-A1408 16S-RMTases are capable of conferring resistance all these groups.

4,6-Disubstituted 2-deoxystreptamines

Kanamycin group

	R^1	R^2	R^3	R^4
Kanamycin A	-OH	-OH	-OH	-H
Kanamycin B	$-NH_2$	-OH	-OH	-H
Tobramycin	$-NH_2$	-H	-OH	-H
Dibekacin	$-NH_2$	-H	-H	-H
Amikacin	-OH	-OH	-OH	-X
Arbekacin	$-NH_2$	-H	-H	-X

(*S*)
X=$COCH(OH)CH_2CH_2NH_2$

Gentamicin-group

Gentamicin

	R^1	R^2
Gentamicin C_1	$-NHCH_3$	$-CH_3$
Gentamicin C_{1a}	$-NH_2$	-H
Gentamicin C_2	$-NH_2$	$-CH_3$

Isepamicin
Netilmicin
Sisomicin

4,5-Disubstituted 2-deoxystreptamines

Neomycin (fradiomycin)

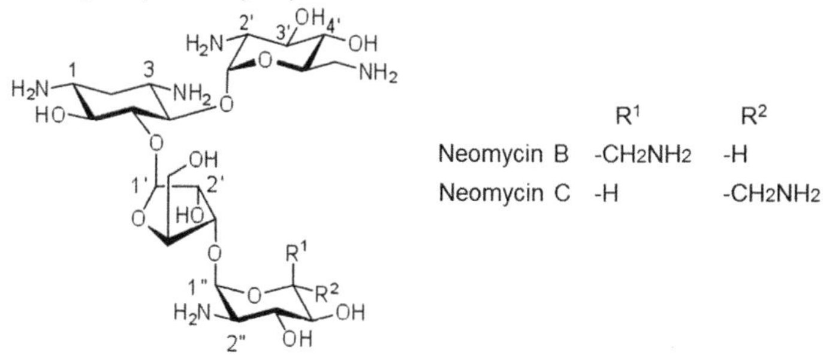

	R^1	R^2
Neomycin B	$-CH_2NH_2$	-H
Neomycin C	-H	$-CH_2NH_2$

Paromomycin
Lividomycin A
Ribostamycin

Other aminoglycosides

Apramycin

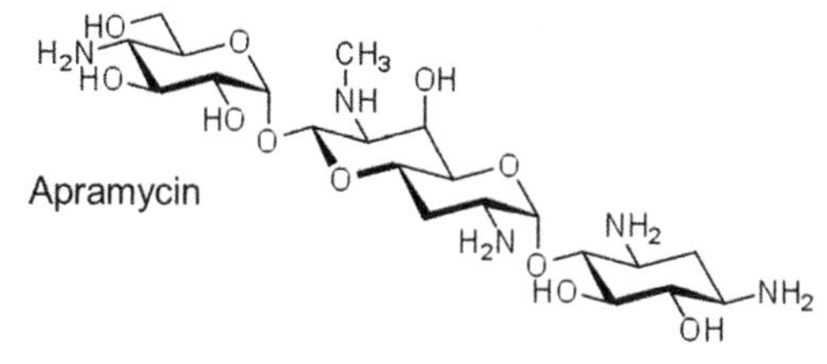

Fig. 1. Aminoglycosides whose activities are compromised by methylation of nucleotide G1405 or A1408 of 16S rRNA. (*From* Yonezawa M, Ida T, Umemura E, et al. Antibiotics and chemotherapy (kagakuryohou no ryouiki), 31:(1476)67–73, 2015, a review article written in Japanese; with permission.)

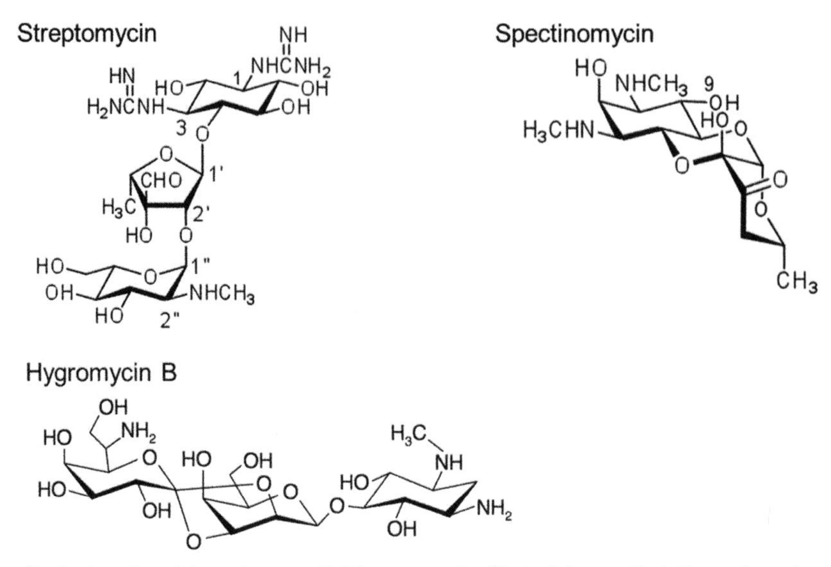

Fig. 2. Aminoglycosides whose activities are not affected by methylation of nucleotide G1405 or A1408 of 16S rRNA. (*From* Yonezawa M, Ida T, Umemura E, et al. Antibiotics and chemotherapy (kagakuryohou no ryouiki), 31:(1476)67–73, 2015, a review article written in Japanese; with permission.)

ACQUIRED 16S RIBOSOMAL RNA METHYLTRANSFERASES IN GRAM-NEGATIVE BACTERIA

The first 16S-RMTases mediating aminoglycoside resistance and reported from outside aminoglycoside-producing Actinobacteria were ArmA in *Klebsiella pneumoniae* and RmtA in *Pseudomonas aeruginosa*.[7,8] ArmA was first identified in an isolate of *K pneumoniae* from the urine of a patient admitted to a hospital in Paris in 2000,[7] but its nucleotide sequence could be found on a plasmid carried by a *Citrobacter freundii* clinical strain identified in Poland in 1996.[9,10] ArmA was subsequently

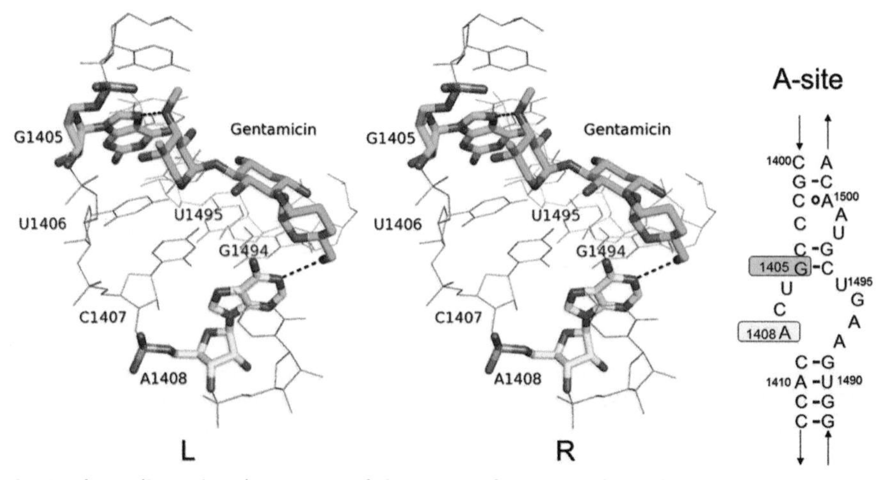

Fig. 3. Three-dimensional structure of the A-site of 16S rRNA bound to gentamicin.

confirmed to function as N7-G1405 16S-RMTase.[11] RmtA was identified in a sputum isolate of *P aeruginosa* in Japan in 1997.[8]

With the subsequent discovery of additional enzymes, a total of 9 N7-G1405 16S-RMTases, some with proven function (ArmA, RmtB, and RmtC) and others with putative function based on amino acid sequence similarity and resistance phenotype (ie, resistance to gentamicin, tobramycin, and amikacin but susceptibility to neomycin and apramycin), have been identified (**Table 1**). They include ArmA, RmtA, RmtB (which includes RmtB1 and RmtB2 alleles), RmtC, RmtD (which includes RmtD1 and RmtD2 alleles), RmtE, RmtF, RmtG, and RmtH (**Table 2**). These acquired N7-G1405 16S-RMTases share modest to high amino acid sequence similarities with each other.

In contrast, only a single acquired N1-A1408 16S-RMTase has been discovered to date. This enzyme, named NpmA, was identified from an *Escherichia coli* clinical strain in Japan in 2007.[12] NpmA confers a broader spectrum of aminoglycoside resistance that includes neomycin and apramycin in addition to gentamicin, tobramycin, and amikacin, and possesses an amino acid sequence that is distinct from those of the N7-G1405 16S-RMTases (see **Table 1**). NpmA has subsequently been shown to catalyze modification of nucleotide A1408.[13]

Reviewed next are the genetic context and epidemiology of the acquired 16S-RMTases that have been identified to date.

ArmA

The *armA* gene was initially identified on plasmid pCTX-M3 in *C freundii* and plasmid pIP1204 in *K pneumoniae*, both of which also carried an ESBL gene $bla_{CTX\text{-}M\text{-}3}$.[10,14] In these plasmids, *armA* is located downstream of insertion sequence IS*CR1*, which follows a class 1 integron comprising *dhfrA12* (trimethoprim resistance), *aadA2* (streptomycin resistance), and *sul1* (sulfonamide resistance). Typically, *mel* and *mph2* (macrolide resistance) are located downstream of *armA*. Although the incompatibility groups of the plasmids and the gene cassette contents of the class 1 integron may be variable, this overall genetic context of *armA* seems to be well conserved in the family Enterobacteriaceae and *Acinetobacter baumannii*.

armA is one of the most frequently encountered 16S-RMTase genes along with *rmtB*, and is widely distributed in Enterobacteriaceae and *A baumannii*. In Enterobacteriaceae, it has been found mostly in species, such as *K pneumoniae*, involved in health care–associated infections, but there are also reports of *armA* found in species implicated in food-borne and diarrheal illnesses, including *Salmonella enterica*[14,15] and *Shigella flexneri*.[14] In *A baumannii*, *armA* is often identified in

Table 1
Resistance phenotype of aminoglycosides conferred by acquired N7-G1405 and N1-A1408 16S-RMTases

	N7-G1405 16S-RMTase	N1-A1408 16S-RMTase
Aminoglycosides	RmtA through RmtH ArmA	NpmA
4,6-Disubstituted DOS (gentamicin, tobramycin, amikacin)	R	R
4,5-Disubstituted DOS (neomycin)	S	R
Monosubstituted DOS (apramycin)	S	R
No DOS ring (streptomycin)	S	S

Table 2
Overview of acquired N7-G1405 and N1-A1408 16S-RMTases

16S-RMTase	Common Species	Common Coresistance	Prevalence	Distribution
ArmA	*Klebsiella pneumoniae* *Acinetobacter baumannii*	CTX-M ESBL NDM carbapenemase OXA-23 carbapenemase	Very high in *A baumannii* High among NDM producers	Worldwide
RmtA	*Pseudomonas aeruginosa*	—	Low	Japan, Korea
RmtB	*Escherichia coli* *K pneumoniae*	CTX-M ESBL NDM carbapenemase	High in China High among NDM producers	Worldwide
RmtC	*K pneumoniae* *Proteus mirabilis*	NDM carbapenemase	High among NDM producers	India, United Kingdom
RmtD	*P aeruginosa* *K pneumoniae*	CTX-M ESBL KPC carbapenemase	Low	South America
RmtE	*E coli*	CMY-2 AmpC	Very low	United States
RmtF	*K pneumoniae*	NDM carbapenemase	High among NDM producers	India, United Kingdom
RmtG	*K pneumoniae*	CTX-M ESBL KPC carbapenemase	Low	South America
RmtH	*K pneumoniae*	CTX-M ESBL	Very low	Iraq
NpmA	*E coli* *K pneumoniae* *Enterobacter* spp	—	Very low	Japan, Saudi Arabia

Abbreviation: NDM, New Delhi Metallo-β-lactamase.

carbapenem-resistant strains that also carry the acquired carbapenemase gene *bla*$_{OXA-23}$, although these two genes are located on separate plasmids.[16] In a study of carbapenem-nonsusceptible *A baumannii* isolates collected from hospitals across the United States, 49% of the isolates carried *armA*, suggesting a high prevalence in this species (Doi Y, 2011, unpublished data).[17]

Another specific group of bacteria where *armA* seems to have high prevalence is Enterobacteriaceae producing NDM (New Delhi Metallo-β-lactamase)-type carbapenemase. NDM-1, the first NDM-type carbapenemase, was initially reported in *K pneumoniae* and *E coli* strains that were isolated from a patient who had traveled from New Delhi, India to Sweden in 2009.[18] NDM-producing Enterobacteriaceae has since spread worldwide rapidly causing many outbreaks, including recent ones in Denver and Chicago.[19,20] Soon after the discovery of NDM-1 it became clear that many Enterobacteriaceae strains producing NDM-1 or its variants were also highly resistant to 4,6-disubstituted DOS agents including gentamicin, tobramycin, and amikacin.[21] Investigations into the *bla*$_{NDM}$-carrying plasmids have revealed that *bla*$_{NDM}$ is frequently colocated with *armA*, or other 16S-RMTase genes (especially *rmtB*, *rmtC*, and *rmtF*), on the same plasmids.[22] Some of these plasmids additionally carry plasmid-mediated fluoroquinolone-resistance genes, such as *qnrB1*.[23] Acquisition of these MDR plasmids would therefore simultaneously confer resistance to most β-lactams including carbapenems, aminoglycosides, and fluoroquinolones, the three key groups of agents with activity against gram-negative bacteria. *armA* has also been found in *P aeruginosa* carrying another metallo-β-lactamase gene *bla*$_{IMP-1}$ in Korea,[24] and *K pneumoniae* or other Enterobacteriaceae carrying a *Klebsiella pneumoniae* carbapenemase (KPC)-type carbapenemase gene *bla*$_{KPC-2}$ in Italy and China.[25,26]

Finally, there seems to be a reservoir of *armA* in food animals. For instance, *armA* has been reported in *E coli* from chickens in China,[27] and *S enterica* in chicken meat at a supermarket in La Réunion Island.[28] However, the extent of spread of *armA* in food animals is unclear at this point.

RmtA

RmtA was first identified in Japan in a *P aeruginosa* clinical isolate that had been isolated in 1997 and showed high-level resistance to the 4,6-disubstituted DOS aminoglycosides.[8] The 6.2-kb genetic region including *rmtA* of *P aeruginosa* is located between two copies of a kappa-gamma element, a 262-bp possible mobile element.[29]

Compared with ArmA, the occurrence of RmtA has been sporadic so far, with a limited number of reports of *rmtA*-carrying *P aeruginosa* coming from Japan and Korea.[30,31] However, a plasmid carrying *bla*$_{NDM-1}$ and *rmtA* was reported in a *K pneumoniae* clinical strain that was isolated from a patient who was hospitalized in India and later sought care in Switzerland.[32] This association suggests that there may be an unrecognized reservoir of *rmtA* in India, where other 16S-RMTase genes are frequently found with *bla*$_{NDM-1}$.

RmtB

RmtB was first reported from a *Serratia marcescens* clinical strain that was isolated in Japan in 2002.[33] *rmtB* is located on a plasmid and downstream of a Tn*3*-like transposon, and *bla*$_{TEM-1}$. Although the sequences downstream of *rmtB* are variable, a fluoroquinolone efflux gene *qepA1* or its variants can sometimes be found adjacent to *rmtB*.

rmtB has revealed a worldwide distribution among Enterobacteriaceae, with reports of its identification coming from Asia, the Americas, Europe, the Middle East, Africa, and Oceania.[6,34–36] Like *armA*, *rmtB* is frequently associated with bla_{NDM-1} on the same plasmids.[37] Therefore, the ongoing spread of bla_{NDM-1}-carrying Enterobacteriaceae likely contributes significantly to further dissemination of *rmtB*.

Another unique feature of RmtB, as with ArmA, is its association with food animals, but RmtB seems to be more prevalent than ArmA in this ecological niche. Most reports come from China, with *rmtB* identified in high rates in *E coli* from pigs, farm workers and their environment,[38,39] chickens,[27] and pets.[40]

RmtC

RmtC was first reported in a *Proteus mirabilis* clinical strain that was isolated from a hospitalized patient in Japan in 2003.[41] Located on a nonconjugative plasmid, *rmtC* is adjacent to an IS*Ecp1*-like element, which also provides the promoter sequence for the expression *rmtC*.[42]

The second RmtC-producing isolate was reported from Australia in *P mirabilis*, which was isolated from the urine of a patient who had recently returned from India.[43] Then, 13 clonally related *S enterica* Virchow strains among the 2004 to 2008 culture collection at the Health Protection Agency in the United Kingdom were found to possess *rmtC*.[44] Remarkably, 4 of the 12 patients affected by these *S enterica* Virchow isolates reported recent travel to India. Soon thereafter, *rmtC* began to appear in conjunction with bla_{NDM-1}, just as had been observed with *armA* and *rmtB*. *rmtC* was found in 12 of 18 bla_{NDM-1}-carrying *E coli* isolates from the United Kingdom, India, and Pakistan.[45] In New Zealand, all 5 bla_{NDM-1}-carrying Enterobacteriaceae isolates referred to a national reference laboratory possessed *rmtC*, with all cases associated with recent health care contact in India.[46] In a survey at a hospital in India, 3.7% of Enterobacteriaceae isolates had *rmtC*, often along with bla_{NDM}.[47] *rmtC* has also been found among *K pneumoniae* clinical isolates in Nepal.[48] These data suggest that *rmtC* likely originated in the Indian subcontinent and *rmtC* is being incorporated by MDR/XDR Enterobacteriaceae, in particular those producing NDM-type carbapenemase.

RmtD

RmtD is unique in that it has only been reported from South America. First identified in *P aeruginosa* producing SPM-1 metallo-β-lactamase in Brazil,[49] *rmtD* (now also termed *rmtD1* because of the identification of its variant *rmtD2*) seems to have been mobilized by putative transposase IS*CR14* (formerly Orf494).[50] *rmtD1* and *rmtD2* have since been identified in various Enterobacteriaceae species in Brazil, Chile, and Argentina.[51,52] More recently, cocarriage of *rmtD1* or *rmtD2* with bla_{KPC-2} has been reported in *K pneumoniae* from Brazil.[53] Unlike with NDM-1-producing Enterobacteriaceae, *rmtD1* or *rmtD2* and bla_{KPC} are located on separate plasmids.

RmtE

Only two RmtE-producing strains have been reported to date, both *E coli*, one from a cow and another from a patient in the United States.[54,55] *rmtE* is located on a class 1 integron, but as an independent gene and not an integron gene cassette, on a large plasmid that also carries bla_{CMY-2} encoding an AmpC β-lactamase (cephalosporinase).[56]

RmtF

More so than any other acquired 16S-RMTases that have been identified to date, RmtF is very closely associated with NDM. The first RmtF-producing strain identified was *K pneumoniae* coproducing NDM-1 that was isolated from a patient in La Réunion Island.[57] *rmtF* has so far been found on class 1 integrons downsteam of bla_{NDM}.[58]

In a single hospital surveillance study in India, 3.4% of Enterobacteriaceae carried *rmtF*, 59% of them along with bla_{NDM}.[47] Isolates carrying *rmtF* have since been reported from Nepal, Australia, and Minnesota.[16,36,48,59]

RmtG

Like RmtD, RmtG is largely unique to South America. First identified in KPC-producing *K pneumoniae* clinical isolates in Brazil,[53] it has been found in Chile and Miami, all in *K pneumoniae*.[60,61] *rmtG* is flanked downstream by IS*Vsa3*, but this insertion sequence likely belongs to the site of insertion of the module carrying *rmtG* rather than the *rmtG*-containing module itself.[62] There are currently no data on the epidemiology of *rmtG*.

RmtH

RmtH was recently identified in an ESBL-producing *K pneumoniae* strain that was isolated from a US soldier who suffered wound infection from an explosion during deployment in Iraq.[63] *rmtH* is bracketed by two copies of IS*CR2*, which likely played a role in the initial mobilization of this unusual 16S-RMTase gene.

NpmA

NpmA was discovered in an *E coli* clinical strain that was isolated from a patient in Japan in 2003 and is the only acquired N1-A1408 16S-RMTases known to date.[12] Because of its unique site of action, NpmA confers resistance to 4,5-disubstituted and monosubstituted DOS agents (eg, neomycin and apramycin, respectively). *npmA* and its flaking sequences are bracketed by the two copies of IS*26*, suggesting their involvement in the mobilization of *npmA*. *K pneumoniae* and *Enterobacter* spp carrying *npmA* were recently reported from Saudi Arabia.[35]

PREVALENCE OF 16S RIBOSOMAL RNA METHYLTRANSFERASES

Prevalence data on acquired 16S-RMTases remain relatively scarce, and low prevalence rates of 1% or less have been reported among Enterobacteriaceae from Europe, Japan, and Argentina.[30,52,64–67] However, some studies, most of them single-center, have found alarmingly high rates of 16S-RMTase genes among Enterobacteriaceae. In Korea, rates of 2.8% to 11.4% have been reported among Enterobacteriaceae.[68,69] In China, of 680 and 337 unique *E coli* and *K pneumoniae* clinical isolates collected at a hospital between 2006 and 2008, 5.4% and 6.2% were positive for *rmtB* or *armA*, respectively.[70,71]

The prevalence rates may be even higher in India and Saudi Arabia. Of 1000 consecutive Enterobacteriaceae clinical isolates collected at a hospital in India between 2010 and 2011, a total of 14% carried at least one 16S-RMTase gene, including *armA*, *rmtB*, *rmtC*, and *rmtF*.[47] Of 330 unique Enterobacteriaceae clinical isolates collected at a hospital in Saudi Arabia in 2011, a total of 37% carried at least one 16S-RMTase gene.[35]

CLINICAL IMPLICATIONS

To date, no data are available on the impact of acquired 16S-RMTase production and clinical outcome of patients when they are treated with aminoglycosides, largely because aminoglycosides by themselves are not considered the first-line agents for either empiric or definitive therapy for infections from gram-negative bacteria in most clinical settings, and also because prevalence rates of 16S-RMTases are relatively low in developed countries.

Nonetheless, the real threat of 16S-RMTases is the loss of a potential treatment option for the salvage therapy for MDR/XDR gram-negative bacterial infections where treatment options are already limited. 16S-RMTase genes are increasingly identified along with other significant resistance genes, especially carbapenemase genes, in the same isolates. Given the extremely high level of aminoglycoside resistance conferred by the acquired 16S-RMTases, this precludes the use of key aminoglycosides (gentamicin, tobramycin, and amikacin) even when carbapenems have already been excluded from the treatment option. For instance, plazomicin, a new aminoglycoside agent that is under clinical development specifically for use against carbapenem-resistant Enterobacteriaceae, is not active against isolates that produce acquired 16S-RMTase. This is most prominently observed for NDM-producing Enterobacteriaceae that frequently coproduces 16S-RMTase.[72] Although most KPC-producing *K pneumoniae* remain susceptible to plazomicin at this point, increasing reports of KPC and 16S-RMTase coproduction are a cause for concern.[25,26,53,73]

SUMMARY

Antimicrobial resistance in gram-negative pathogens has become one of the most challenging issues faced in daily clinical practice. Especially troublesome is the global spread of carbapenem-resistant Enterobacteriaceae, which has accelerated since the appearance of KPC and NDM-type carbapenemases. Aminoglycoside resistance mediated by acquired 16S-RMTase is a relatively new mechanism that was described in the early 2000s, but it now seems to be converging with the carbapenemase epidemic, thereby facilitating the emergence of XDR and, in some instances, pandrug-resistant organisms. Although not first-line in many clinical scenarios, aminoglycosides remain an important class of agents with excellent bactericidal activity when the organisms of interest are resistant to other classes, especially β-lactams and fluoroquinolones. Therefore, the ongoing dissemination of 16S-RMTases among already MDR organisms is an unwelcome event.

REFERENCES

1. Magiorakos AP, Srinivasan A, Carey RB, et al. Multidrug-resistant, extensively drug-resistant and pandrug-resistant bacteria: an international expert proposal for interim standard definitions for acquired resistance. Clin Microbiol Infect 2012;18:268–81.
2. Ramirez MS, Tolmasky ME. Aminoglycoside modifying enzymes. Drug Resist Updat 2010;13:151–71.
3. Shaw KJ, Rather PN, Hare RS, et al. Molecular genetics of aminoglycoside resistance genes and familial relationships of the aminoglycoside-modifying enzymes. Microbiol Rev 1993;57:138–63.
4. Cooksey RC, Morlock GP, McQueen A, et al. Characterization of streptomycin resistance mechanisms among *Mycobacterium tuberculosis* isolates from patients in New York City. Antimicrob Agents Chemother 1996;40:1186–8.
5. Beauclerk AA, Cundliffe E. Sites of action of two ribosomal RNA methylases responsible for resistance to aminoglycosides. J Mol Biol 1987;193:661–71.
6. Wachino J, Arakawa Y. Exogenously acquired 16S rRNA methyltransferases found in aminoglycoside-resistant pathogenic gram-negative bacteria: an update. Drug Resist Updat 2012;15:133–48.

7. Galimand M, Courvalin P, Lambert T. Plasmid-mediated high-level resistance to aminoglycosides in Enterobacteriaceae due to 16S rRNA methylation. Antimicrob Agents Chemother 2003;47:2565–71.
8. Yokoyama K, Doi Y, Yamane K, et al. Acquisition of 16S rRNA methylase gene in *Pseudomonas aeruginosa*. Lancet 2003;362:1888–93.
9. Gniadkowski M, Schneider I, Palucha A, et al. Cefotaxime-resistant Enterobacteriaceae isolates from a hospital in Warsaw, Poland: identification of a new CTX-M-3 cefotaxime-hydrolyzing β-lactamase that is closely related to the CTX-M-1/MEN-1 enzyme. Antimicrob Agents Chemother 1998;42:827–32.
10. Golebiewski M, Kern-Zdanowicz I, Zienkiewicz M, et al. Complete nucleotide sequence of the pCTX-M3 plasmid and its involvement in spread of the extended-spectrum β-lactamase gene $bla_{CTX-M-3}$. Antimicrob Agents Chemother 2007;51:3789–95.
11. Liou GF, Yoshizawa S, Courvalin P, et al. Aminoglycoside resistance by ArmA-mediated ribosomal 16S methylation in human bacterial pathogens. J Mol Biol 2006;359:358–64.
12. Wachino J, Shibayama K, Kurokawa H, et al. Novel plasmid-mediated 16S rRNA m1A1408 methyltransferase, NpmA, found in a clinically isolated *Escherichia coli* strain resistant to structurally diverse aminoglycosides. Antimicrob Agents Chemother 2007;51:4401–9.
13. Dunkle JA, Vinal K, Desai PM, et al. Molecular recognition and modification of the 30S ribosome by the aminoglycoside-resistance methyltransferase NpmA. Proc Natl Acad Sci U S A 2014;111:6275–80.
14. Galimand M, Sabtcheva S, Courvalin P, et al. Worldwide disseminated *armA* aminoglycoside resistance methylase gene is borne by composite transposon Tn*1548*. Antimicrob Agents Chemother 2005;49:2949–53.
15. Du XD, Li DX, Hu GZ, et al. Tn*1548*-associated *armA* is co-located with *qnrB2*, *aac(6')-Ib-cr* and $bla_{CTX-M-3}$ on an IncFII plasmid in a *Salmonella enterica* subsp. *enterica* serovar Paratyphi B strain isolated from chickens in China. J Antimicrob Chemother 2012;67:246–8.
16. Wright MS, Haft DH, Harkins DM, et al. New insights into dissemination and variation of the health care-associated pathogen *Acinetobacter baumannii* from genomic analysis. MBio 2014;5:e00963–00913.
17. Adams-Haduch JM, Onuoha EO, Bogdanovich T, et al. Molecular epidemiology of carbapenem-nonsusceptible *Acinetobacter baumannii* in the United States. J Clin Microbiol 2011;49:3849–54.
18. Yong D, Toleman MA, Giske CG, et al. Characterization of a new metallo-β-lactamase gene, bla_{NDM-1}, and a novel erythromycin esterase gene carried on a unique genetic structure in *Klebsiella pneumoniae* sequence type 14 from India. Antimicrob Agents Chemother 2009;53:5046–54.
19. Epson EE, Pisney LM, Wendt JM, et al. Carbapenem-resistant *Klebsiella pneumoniae* producing New Delhi metallo-β-lactamase at an acute care hospital, Colorado, 2012. Infect Control Hosp Epidemiol 2014;35:390–7.
20. Epstein L, Hunter JC, Arwady MA, et al. New Delhi metallo-β-lactamase-producing carbapenem-resistant *Escherichia coli* associated with exposure to duodenoscopes. JAMA 2014;312:1447–55.
21. Kumarasamy KK, Toleman MA, Walsh TR, et al. Emergence of a new antibiotic resistance mechanism in India, Pakistan, and the UK: a molecular, biological, and epidemiological study. Lancet Infect Dis 2010;10:597–602.
22. Rahman M, Shukla SK, Prasad KN, et al. Prevalence and molecular characterisation of New Delhi metallo-β-lactamases NDM-1, NDM-5, NDM-6 and NDM-7

in multidrug-resistant Enterobacteriaceae from India. Int J Antimicrob Agents 2014;44:30–7.

23. Doi Y, Hazen TH, Boitano M, et al. Whole-genome assembly of *Klebsiella pneumoniae* coproducing NDM-1 and OXA-232 carbapenemases using single-molecule, real-time sequencing. Antimicrob Agents Chemother 2014;58: 5947–53.
24. Gurung M, Moon DC, Tamang MD, et al. Emergence of 16S rRNA methylase gene armA and cocarriage of bla_{IMP-1} in *Pseudomonas aeruginosa* isolates from South Korea. Diagn Microbiol Infect Dis 2010;68:468–70.
25. Mezzatesta ML, Gona F, Caio C, et al. Emergence of an extensively drug-resistant ArmA- and KPC-2-producing ST101 *Klebsiella pneumoniae* clone in Italy. J Antimicrob Chemother 2013;68:1932–4.
26. Luo Y, Yang J, Ye L, et al. Characterization of KPC-2-producing *Escherichia coli*, *Citrobacter freundii*, *Enterobacter cloacae*, *Enterobacter aerogenes*, and *Klebsiella oxytoca* isolates from a Chinese Hospital. Microb Drug Resist 2014;20: 264–9.
27. Du XD, Wu CM, Liu HB, et al. Plasmid-mediated ArmA and RmtB 16S rRNA methylases in *Escherichia coli* isolated from chickens. J Antimicrob Chemother 2009; 64:1328–30.
28. Granier SA, Hidalgo L, San Millan A, et al. ArmA methyltransferase in a monophasic *Salmonella enterica* isolate from food. Antimicrob Agents Chemother 2011;55: 5262–6.
29. Yamane K, Doi Y, Yokoyama K, et al. Genetic environments of the *rmtA* gene in *Pseudomonas aeruginosa* clinical isolates. Antimicrob Agents Chemother 2004; 48:2069–74.
30. Yamane K, Wachino J, Doi Y, et al. Global spread of multiple aminoglycoside resistance genes. Emerg Infect Dis 2005;11:951–3.
31. Jin JS, Kwon KT, Moon DC, et al. Emergence of 16S rRNA methylase *rmtA* in colistin-only-sensitive *Pseudomonas aeruginosa* in South Korea. Int J Antimicrob Agents 2009;33:490–1.
32. Poirel L, Schrenzel J, Cherkaoui A, et al. Molecular analysis of NDM-1-producing enterobacterial isolates from Geneva, Switzerland. J Antimicrob Chemother 2011; 66:1730–3.
33. Doi Y, Yokoyama K, Yamane K, et al. Plasmid-mediated 16S rRNA methylase in *Serratia marcescens* conferring high-level resistance to aminoglycosides. Antimicrob Agents Chemother 2004;48:491–6.
34. Al-Gallas N, Abbassi MS, Gharbi B, et al. Occurrence of plasmid-mediated quinolone resistance determinants and *rmtB* gene in *Salmonella enterica* serovar Enteritidis and *Typhimurium* isolated from food-animal products in Tunisia. Foodborne Pathog Dis 2013;10:813–9.
35. Al Sheikh YA, Marie MA, John J, et al. Prevalence of 16S rRNA methylase genes among β-lactamase-producing Enterobacteriaceae clinical isolates in Saudi Arabia. Libyan J Med 2014;9:24432.
36. Sidjabat HE, Townell N, Nimmo GR, et al. Dominance of IMP-4-producing *Enterobacter cloacae* among carbapenemase-producing Enterobacteriaceae in Australia. Antimicrob Agents Chemother 2015;59:4059–66.
37. Carattoli A, Villa L, Poirel L, et al. Evolution of IncA/C bla_{CMY-2}-carrying plasmids by acquisition of the bla_{NDM-1} carbapenemase gene. Antimicrob Agents Chemother 2012;56:783–6.

38. Chen L, Chen ZL, Liu JH, et al. Emergence of RmtB methylase-producing *Escherichia coli* and *Enterobacter cloacae* isolates from pigs in China. J Antimicrob Chemother 2007;59:880–5.
39. Deng Y, Zeng Z, Chen S, et al. Dissemination of IncFII plasmids carrying *rmtB* and *qepA* in *Escherichia coli* from pigs, farm workers and the environment. Clin Microbiol Infect 2011;17:1740–5.
40. Deng Y, He L, Chen S, et al. F33:A-:B- and F2:A-:B- plasmids mediate dissemination of *rmtB-bla*$_{CTX-M-9}$ group genes and *rmtB-qepA* in Enterobacteriaceae isolates from pets in China. Antimicrob Agents Chemother 2011;55:4926–9.
41. Wachino J, Yamane K, Shibayama K, et al. Novel plasmid-mediated 16S rRNA methylase, RmtC, found in a *Proteus mirabilis* isolate demonstrating extraordinary high-level resistance against various aminoglycosides. Antimicrob Agents Chemother 2006;50:178–84.
42. Wachino J, Yamane K, Kimura K, et al. Mode of transposition and expression of 16S rRNA methyltransferase gene *rmtC* accompanied by IS*Ecp1*. Antimicrob Agents Chemother 2006;50:3212–5.
43. Zong Z, Partridge SR, Iredell JR. RmtC 16S rRNA methyltransferase in Australia. Antimicrob Agents Chemother 2008;52:794–5.
44. Hopkins KL, Escudero JA, Hidalgo L, et al. 16S rRNA methyltransferase RmtC in *Salmonella enterica* serovar Virchow. Emerg Infect Dis 2010;16:712–5.
45. Mushtaq S, Irfan S, Sarma JB, et al. Phylogenetic diversity of *Escherichia coli* strains producing NDM-type carbapenemases. J Antimicrob Chemother 2011;66:2002–5.
46. Williamson DA, Sidjabat HE, Freeman JT, et al. Identification and molecular characterisation of New Delhi metallo-β-lactamase-1 (NDM-1)- and NDM-6-producing Enterobacteriaceae from New Zealand hospitals. Int J Antimicrob Agents 2012; 39:529–33.
47. Hidalgo L, Hopkins KL, Gutierrez B, et al. Association of the novel aminoglycoside resistance determinant RmtF with NDM carbapenemase in Enterobacteriaceae isolated in India and the UK. J Antimicrob Chemother 2013;68:1543–50.
48. Tada T, Miyoshi-Akiyama T, Dahal RK, et al. Dissemination of multidrug-resistant *Klebsiella pneumoniae* clinical isolates with various combinations of carbapenemases (NDM-1 and OXA-72) and 16S rRNA methylases (ArmA, RmtC and RmtF) in Nepal. Int J Antimicrob Agents 2013;42:372–4.
49. Doi Y, de Oliveira Garcia D, Adams J, et al. Coproduction of novel 16S rRNA methylase RmtD and metallo-β-lactamase SPM-1 in a panresistant *Pseudomonas aeruginosa* isolate from Brazil. Antimicrob Agents Chemother 2007;51:852–6.
50. Doi Y, Adams-Haduch JM, Paterson DL. Genetic environment of 16S rRNA methylase gene *rmtD*. Antimicrob Agents Chemother 2008;52:2270–2.
51. Fritsche TR, Castanheira M, Miller GH, et al. Detection of methyltransferases conferring high-level resistance to aminoglycosides in enterobacteriaceae from Europe, North America, and Latin America. Antimicrob Agents Chemother 2008;52:1843–5.
52. Tijet N, Andres P, Chung C, et al. *rmtD2*, a new allele of a 16S rRNA methylase gene, has been present in Enterobacteriaceae isolates from Argentina for more than a decade. Antimicrob Agents Chemother 2011;55:904–9.
53. Bueno MF, Francisco GR, O'Hara JA, et al. Coproduction of 16S rRNA methyltransferase RmtD or RmtG with KPC-2 and CTX-M group extended-spectrum β-lactamases in *Klebsiella pneumoniae*. Antimicrob Agents Chemother 2013;57:2397–400.
54. Davis MA, Baker KN, Orfe LH, et al. Discovery of a gene conferring multiple-aminoglycoside resistance in *Escherichia coli*. Antimicrob Agents Chemother 2010;54:2666–9.

55. Lee CS, Hu F, Rivera JI, et al. *Escherichia coli* sequence type 354 coproducing CMY-2 cephalosporinase and RmtE 16S rRNA methyltransferase. Antimicrob Agents Chemother 2014;58:4246–7.
56. Lee CS, Li JJ, Doi Y. Complete sequence of conjugative IncA/C plasmid encoding CMY-2 β-lactamase and RmtE 16S rRNA methyltransferase. Antimicrob Agents Chemother 2015;59:4360–1.
57. Galimand M, Courvalin P, Lambert T. RmtF, a new member of the aminoglycoside resistance 16S rRNA N7 G1405 methyltransferase family. Antimicrob Agents Chemother 2012;56:3960–2.
58. Mataseje LF, Boyd DA, Lefebvre B, et al, Canadian Nosocomial Infection Surveillance Program. Complete sequences of a novel bla_{NDM-1}-harbouring plasmid from Providencia rettgeri and an FII-type plasmid from *Klebsiella pneumoniae* identified in Canada. J Antimicrob Chemother 2014;69:637–42.
59. Lee CS, Vasoo S, Hu F, et al. *Klebsiella pneumoniae* ST147 coproducing NDM-7 carbapenemase and RmtF 16S rRNA methyltransferase in Minnesota. J Clin Microbiol 2014;52:4109–10.
60. Poirel L, Labarca J, Bello H, et al. Emergence of the 16S rRNA methylase RmtG in an extended-spectrum-β-lactamase-producing and colistin-resistant *Klebsiella pneumoniae* isolate in Chile. Antimicrob Agents Chemother 2014;58:618–9.
61. Hu F, Munoz-Price LS, DePascale D, et al. *Klebsiella pneumoniae* sequence type 11 isolate producing RmtG 16S rRNA methyltransferase from a patient in Miami, Florida. Antimicrob Agents Chemother 2014;58:4980–1.
62. Ramos PI, Picao RC, Almeida LG, et al. Comparative analysis of the complete genome of KPC-2-producing *Klebsiella pneumoniae* Kp13 reveals remarkable genome plasticity and a wide repertoire of virulence and resistance mechanisms. BMC Genomics 2014;15:54.
63. O'Hara JA, McGann P, Snesrud EC, et al. Novel 16S rRNA methyltransferase RmtH produced by *Klebsiella pneumoniae* associated with war-related trauma. Antimicrob Agents Chemother 2013;57:2413–6.
64. Galani I, Souli M, Panagea T, et al. Prevalence of 16S rRNA methylase genes in Enterobacteriaceae isolates from a Greek university hospital. Clin Microbiol Infect 2012;18:E52–4.
65. Bercot B, Poirel L, Ozdamar M, et al. Low prevalence of 16S methylases among extended-spectrum-β-lactamase-producing Enterobacteriaceae from a Turkish hospital. J Antimicrob Chemother 2010;65:797–8.
66. Bercot B, Poirel L, Nordmann P. Plasmid-mediated 16S rRNA methylases among extended-spectrum β-lactamase-producing Enterobacteriaceae isolates. Antimicrob Agents Chemother 2008;52:4526–7.
67. Sabtcheva S, Saga T, Kantardjiev T, et al. Nosocomial spread of *armA*-mediated high-level aminoglycoside resistance in Enterobacteriaceae isolates producing CTX-M-3 β-lactamase in a cancer hospital in Bulgaria. J Chemother 2008;20:593–9.
68. Kang HY, Kim KY, Kim J, et al. Distribution of conjugative-plasmid-mediated 16S rRNA methylase genes among amikacin-resistant Enterobacteriaceae isolates collected in 1995 to 1998 and 2001 to 2006 at a university hospital in South Korea and identification of conjugative plasmids mediating dissemination of 16S rRNA methylase. J Clin Microbiol 2008;46:700–6.
69. Park YJ, Lee S, Yu JK, et al. Co-production of 16S rRNA methylases and extended-spectrum β-lactamases in AmpC-producing *Enterobacter cloacae*, *Citrobacter freundii* and *Serratia marcescens* in Korea. J Antimicrob Chemother 2006;58:907–8.

70. Yu FY, Yao D, Pan JY, et al. High prevalence of plasmid-mediated 16S rRNA methylase gene *rmtB* among *Escherichia coli* clinical isolates from a Chinese teaching hospital. BMC Infect Dis 2010;10:184.
71. Yu F, Wang L, Pan J, et al. Prevalence of 16S rRNA methylase genes in *Klebsiella pneumoniae* isolates from a Chinese teaching hospital: coexistence of *rmtB* and *armA* genes in the same isolate. Diagn Microbiol Infect Dis 2009;64:57–63.
72. Livermore DM, Mushtaq S, Warner M, et al. Activity of aminoglycosides, including ACHN-490, against carbapenem-resistant Enterobacteriaceae isolates. J Antimicrob Chemother 2011;66:48–53.
73. Li JJ, Sheng ZK, Deng M, et al. Epidemic of *Klebsiella pneumoniae* ST11 clone coproducing KPC-2 and 16S rRNA methylase RmtB in a Chinese University Hospital. BMC Infect Dis 2012;12:373.

The Evolving Role of Antimicrobial Stewardship in Management of Multidrug Resistant Infections

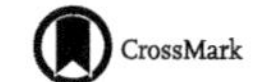

Debra A. Goff, PharmD[a,b], Thomas M. File Jr, MD, MSc[c,d,*]

KEYWORDS

- Antimicrobial stewardship • Antimicrobial resistance • Antibiotics

KEY POINTS

- It is crucial that antimicrobial stewardship programs (ASPs) be put into practice now to provide for optimal patient outcomes and preserve antimicrobials for future use.
- Strategies for improving antibiotic use and evidence for best practices in antibiotic stewardship will continue to evolve.
- The specific types of interventions implemented by institutions will depend on local circumstances and capabilities.
- It is vital that health care settings have ASPs so that patients, both present and future, will continue to have the benefit of life-saving antimicrobials.

INTRODUCTION

The discovery of potent antimicrobial agents was one of the greatest contributions to medicine in the 20th century. When introduced, they had an immediate and dramatic impact on the outcomes of infectious diseases (ID), making once lethal infections readily curable. Unfortunately, the emergence of antimicrobial-resistant pathogens now threatens these advances. Antimicrobial resistance is a serious health threat

Funding: None.
Conflict of Interest: Advisory boards The Medicines Company, Cempra, Actavis (Dr D.A. Goff). Recent research funding—Cempra; Pfizer; Consultant/Scientific Advisory Board Member—Actavis, Cempra, Genentech, Merck, Nabriva, Pfizer, Tetraphase (Dr T.M. File).
[a] Department of Pharmacy, The Ohio State University Wexner Medical Center, The Ohio State University, 368 Doan Hall, Columbus, OH 43210, USA; [b] College of Pharmacy, The Ohio State University, Columbus, OH, USA; [c] Infectious Disease Division, Summa Health System, 525 East Market Street, Akron, OH 44304, USA; [d] Infectious Disease Section, Internal Medicine, Northeast Ohio Medical University (NEOMED), 4029 Street, Rt. 44, PO Box 95, Rootstown, OH 44272, USA
* Corresponding author. Office: 75 Arch Street, Suite 506 (Main Office; Suite 105 for Research), Akron, OH 44304.
E-mail address: filet@summahealth.org

Infect Dis Clin N Am 30 (2016) 539–551
http://dx.doi.org/10.1016/j.idc.2016.02.012
id.theclinics.com
0891-5520/16/$ – see front matter

that affects the clinical outcome of patients as well as results in higher rates of adverse events and health care costs. The seriousness of the health impact of antimicrobial resistance is a major public health crisis.[1] Unfortunately, there are already patients every day who contract infections who cannot be treated with currently available antimicrobials. Antimicrobial resistance affects everybody and it has no geographic boundaries. As the world learned from the 2014 Ebola epidemic, every deadly pathogen is just a plane ride away.

What can be done to address this crisis? There is no question that antibiotic misuse is the most important modifiable factor that leads to antimicrobial resistance. The good news is that we do have a solution to this problem. Since their inception, antimicrobial stewardship programs (ASP) have proven highly successful in improving antibiotic use. These programs can improve patient outcomes, reduce adverse events (including *Clostridium difficile* infection), reduce readmission rates, and reduce antibiotic resistance.[2–6] The proven benefits of ASPs have led to increasing calls for their implementation in all hospitals.

This article explores the effect of ASPs toward optimizing antimicrobial use and the impact on antimicrobial resistance.

RESISTANCE AND THE NEED FOR ANTIMICROBIAL STEWARDSHIP

The primary goal of ASP is to optimize clinical outcomes while minimizing unintended consequences of antimicrobial use, including toxicity, the selection of pathogenic organisms (such as *Clostridium difficile* infection), and the emergence of resistance.[7] Thus, the appropriate use of antimicrobials is an essential part of patient safety and deserves careful oversight and guidance. There is a strong association between antimicrobial use and the emergence of resistance. Observational studies associate greater antibiotic prescribing with greater rates of antibiotic resistance.[8,9] Thus, overuse or inappropriate use of antimicrobials is primary drivers for antimicrobial resistance. However, according to the US Centers for Disease Control and Prevention, 20% to 50% of all antibiotics prescribed in US acute care hospitals are either unnecessary or inappropriate.[10,11]

Unlike other medications, the potential for spread of resistant organisms means that the misuse of antibiotics can adversely impact the health of patients who are not even exposed to them. The ability of antimicrobials to cause "collateral damage" is vastly underappreciated. As stated in the White House release dated March, 27, 2015, National Action Plan for Combating Antimicrobial-Resistant Bacteria, "the emergence of drug resistance in bacteria is reversing the gains of the past 80 years, with many important drug choices for the treatment of bacterial infections becoming increasingly limited.... The loss of antibiotics that kill or inhibit the growth of bacteria means that we can no longer take for granted quick and reliable treatment of rare or common bacterial infections, including bacterial pneumonia."[12] Within the first goal of the Action Plan is the recommendation for implementation of health care policies and ASPs that improve patient outcomes, and efforts to minimize the development of resistance by ensuring that each patient receives the right antibiotic at the right time at the right dose for the right duration. Over the next 5 years, the goals of this Action Plan include reducing the incidence of carbapenem-resistant Enterobacteriaceae (CRE) infections by 60%, *C difficile* infection (CDI) and methicillin-resistant *Staphylococcus aureus* bloodstream infections by 50%, MDR *P aeruginosa* by 35%, and invasive pneumococcal disease by 25%. ASPs are evolving from management of antimicrobial drug therapy to management of ID. Diagnostic accuracy is key for appropriate antimicrobial use. Filice and colleagues[13] found that, when the diagnosis was correct, 62% of antimicrobial courses were appropriate compared with 5% when the diagnosis was incorrect or indeterminate (*P*<.001) This big picture approach will be necessary to meet the disease based goals of the National Action plan.

ASPs can be implemented effectively in a wide variety of health care facilities; strategies and policies have been reviewed elsewhere.[1,7,14]

COLLABORATE FOR SUCCESS

Control of antimicrobial resistance with an effective stewardship programs requires a multifactorial collaborative effort, including physicians and pharmacists as the core members along with infection control, microbiology, administration, information technology, quality control, and other key stakeholders. Physicians are a key core member of an effective ASP. If available, an ID specialist is most effective in this role; however, smaller facilities may formulate an effective program with other physicians who have a strong knowledge of appropriate antimicrobial use. Hospitalists can be effective physician members of a stewardship program given their presence in inpatient care and their frequent use of antimicrobials.[15] ID specialists optimize treatment in the inpatient setting by recommending appropriate antibiotic choices, duration of therapy, and route of delivery.[16] Existing evidence suggests that, when recommendations by an ID specialist are followed, patients are more often correctly diagnosed, have shorter lengths of stay, receive more appropriate therapies, have fewer complications, and may use fewer antibiotics overall.[17]

Pharmacists, preferably with advanced training in ID, are also essential members of an ASP. The American Society of Health System Pharmacists states that, "Pharmacist have a responsibility to take prominent roles in ASP, in part, from pharmacists' understanding of and influence over antimicrobial use within the health system."[18] One role of the pharmacists is to ensure the optimal use of antimicrobials by assuring the 5 *D*s: right diagnosis, drug, dose, duration, and deescalation. Once appropriate therapy has been initiated, pharmacists can optimize therapy by applying pharmacokinetic pharmacodynamic principles such as extended-infusion β-lactam therapy. As shown in 1 study, patients who received extended-infusion cefepime for the treatment of MDR *P aeruginosa* infections had a lower mortality compared with those who receive standard 30-minute infusions (3% vs 20%; *P* = .03).[19]

Time to effective antimicrobial therapy is important to optimize patient outcomes. Pharmacists play a key role in applying microbiology rapid diagnostic test (RDT) results. One of the first studies to evaluate using a RDT for *S aureus* bacteremia in conjunction with ID pharmacist intervention showed mean time to optimal antimicrobial therapy was 1.7 days shorter (*P* = .002) after RDT implementation.[20] Two collateral benefits were observed; pharmacists were able to advocate and obtain ID consults in many cases and the mean hospital costs were $21,387 less per patient in the post-RDT group.

Ongoing education of the medical staff is another important role. The emergence of new resistance enzymes such as CRE, New Delhi Metallo-β-lactamase, and *Klebsiella pneumoniae* carbapenemases creates an "alphabet soup" of confusion for non-ID physicians. Pharmacists should provide timely education and guidance to health care providers for each new antimicrobial and emerging multidrug-resistant organisms (MDROs). The impact of MDRO on patient care extends beyond optimizing drug therapy. It also impacts infection control.

Even with ASPs, the most effective antimicrobials are of little value if health care providers do not wash their hands and thereby contribute to the spread of infection between patients. The need for meticulous attention to the fundamentals of infection control should not be understated. This was demonstrated in the 2011 *K pneumoniae* carbapenemase–producing *K pneumoniae* outbreak at the National Institutes for Health.[21] Despite isolation measures implemented at the beginning of hospitalization, silent transmission spawned a cluster that led to infections in 8 patients, 6 of whom died from the infection. Multidisciplinary meetings to keep everyone informed, involved physicians, nurses, pharmacists, infection preventionists, respiratory therapists, housekeepers, nutritionists, hospital administration, patient and environmental safety, and other staff.

As part of the ASP team, infection control preventionists play an important role in preventing the spread of MDRO. One of the most successful examples is the Israel nationwide intervention aimed at containing the spread of CRE. Nosocomial CRE acquisition in acute care declined from a monthly high of 55.5 to an annual low of 4.8 cases per 1000,000 patient-days ($P<.001$).[22]

As MDROs increase in the hospital setting, combination antimicrobial use increases. The collateral damage from exposure to multiple antibiotics is the development of CDI. A recent infection control survey of 571 US hospitals asked questions related to CDI prevention and found the use of ASP to prevent CDI is lacking in 48% of hospitals.[23]

The microbiologist provides essential data for ASPs. Hospital and unit specific antibiograms help to guide appropriate empiric antimicrobial therapy. New RDT are game changing in the management of patients. This new technology allows for the identification of organisms in hours versus 3 to 4 days using traditional methods. Multiple studies have documented the positive impact on patient care when RDT are used in conjunction with ASP.[24] Improvement in time to optimal therapy, shorter length of stay, and lower mortality has been reported.

COST OF RESISTANCE AND IMPACT OF ANTIMICROBIAL STEWARDSHIP PROGRAMS

Cost is the elephant in the room for ASP. Hospital administration often expects ID physicians to oversee ASP without any financial compensation. Pharmacists who are not ID trained are asked to perform stewardship intervention in addition to their current responsibilities without additional training, mentoring, or compensation. Without buy in from hospital administration and without appropriate financial support for ASP, it is unlikely that hospitals can perform stewardship at a high level. There is hope, however; the President's Council of Advisors on Science and Technology recommended that a regulatory requirement for antibiotic stewardship be in place by the end of 2017.[25]

Required programs that are linked to reimbursement are often what are needed to create change. It has been well-established that MDRO infections are associated with longer lengths of stays and higher costs of care compared with infections with susceptible organisms.[26]

Frequently, ASPs will need to recommend 2 or more antibiotics to treat patients infected with MDROs. New expensive antibiotics are often the most appropriate option, but the silo budget mentality in hospitals place tremendous pressure on the pharmacy department to use the least expensive antimicrobials. This penny wise–pound foolish approach may change with the new Centers for Medicare and Medicaid Services recommendation to document outcomes of antibiotic stewardship activities. Studies have shown delays in time to effective antibiotic therapy leads to increased costs and poor outcomes.[27]

Last, the recent CRE outbreak linked to colonized scopes has resulted in lawsuits from patients who acquired CRE infections after procedures.[28] This can be a significant financial loss to a hospital in addition to the negative publicity, loss of patient trust, and most important loss of life from a preventable infection.

EVIDENCE OF STEWARDSHIP ON THE IMPACT OF ANTIMICROBIAL RESISTANCE

There are 2 core strategies that provide the foundation for an ASP. These strategies are not mutually exclusive[7]:

1. Prospective audit with intervention and feedback. Prospective audit of antimicrobial use with direct interaction and feedback to the prescriber, performed by either an IDs physician or a clinical pharmacist with ID training, can result in reduced inappropriate use of antimicrobials.
2. Formulary restriction and preauthorization. Formulary restriction and preauthorization requirements can lead to immediate and significant reductions in antimicrobial use and cost and may be beneficial as part of a multifaceted response to a nosocomial outbreak of infection.

Several methods of improving prescribing of antimicrobial agents by ASP have been evaluated and include antimicrobial avoidance when not warranted (eg, avoid antibacterial agents for viral respiratory infections); appropriateness of initial antimicrobial choices and doses, which can be optimized by following existing guidelines; monitoring for drug–bug mismatches (eg, when the pathogen is resistant in vitro to the initially prescribed antimicrobial); reducing unnecessary prolongation of duration; and deescalation to a more narrow antimicrobial regimen from the empirical choice once a culture reveals the pathogen. No single intervention can solve the problem. Data are variable as to the impact each of the strategies have on reducing antimicrobial resistance.

The best strategies for the prevention and containment of antimicrobial resistance have not been established definitively. Often, multiple interventions have been made simultaneously, making it difficult to assess the benefit attributable to any 1 specific intervention. However, a comprehensive program that includes active monitoring of resistance, fostering of appropriate antimicrobial use, and collaboration with an effective infection control program to minimize secondary spread of resistance is considered to be optimal.

A recent Cochrane review evaluated 89 studies from 19 countries to determine effective interventions to improve antimicrobial prescribing practices for hospital inpatients.[29] Most of the interventions (80/95, 84%) targeted the choice of antibiotic prescribed (drug selected, timing of first dose, or route of administration). The remaining 15 interventions aimed to change exposure of patients to antibiotics by changing the decision to treat or the duration of treatment. Twelve studies evaluated antimicrobial resistance as an outcome. Interventions to change antimicrobial prescribing were associated with a decrease in CDI, resistant gram-negative bacteria, methicillin-resistant *S aureus*, and vancomycin-resistant enterococci. The metaanalysis indicated that restrictive interventions tended to have a more immediate effect on decreasing resistance of the restricted agent, but prospective audit and feedback seemed to be more effective for a long-term effect.

The effect of several studies on antimicrobial resistance is listed in **Table 1**. The studies listed assessed various interventions, which include antimicrobial restriction, deescalation, reduction of duration, and various forms of comprehensive antimicrobial stewardship with protocol adherence and audit and feedback. Five of the studies assessed the impact of antimicrobial restriction and subsequent development of antimicrobial resistance.[30–34] There has been robust evidence that reduction of resistance

Table 1
Antimicrobial stewardship interventions: impact on resistance as an outcome

Study/Design	Intervention	Resistance Outcome Assessed	Finding
de Man[30]/cross-over study in 2 neonatal ICUs; same hospital	*Antimicrobial restriction*: During the first 6 mo of the study unit A used an amoxicillin and cefotaxime regimen while unit B used a penicillin and tobramycin regimen. During the second 6 mo the units switched antibiotics	Colonization of cefotaxime or tobramycin resistant GNR at 6 mo	68% reduction in days of colonization with resistant bacteria
Lan[31]/Prospective, observational	*Restriction of ceftazidime*	Rate of ESBL *E coli* and *K pneumoniae* in ICU	Decrease in colonization and infection by ESBL-producing *E coli* or *K pneumoniae*
Lewis[32]/interrupted time analysis	*Restriction of ciprofloxacin*	Rate of ciprofloxacin resistant *P aeruginosa*	Significant decreasing trend observed in the percentage and the rate of isolates of *P aeruginosa* that were resistant to antipseudomonal carbapenems and ciprofloxacin.
Medina Presentado[33]/prospective	*Restriction of ciprofloxacin and ceftriaxone*; before/after design	Susceptibility of GNB	Reduction of resistant GNB in the after period—especially *Acinetobacter* spp and *P aeruginosa*
White[34]/observational	*ABX restriction*; before and after implementation of restriction of amikacin, ceftazidime, ciprofloxacin, fluconazole, ofloxacin	Susceptibility of Gram-negative blood isolates	Reduced resistance ($P<.01$)
Singh[46]/RCT	*Duration* and use of monotherapy vs standard duration based on CPIS	Antimicrobial Resistance and superinfection	Less resistance or superinfection with intervention (15% vs 37%; $P = .017$)
Chastre[47]/RCT	*Duration* 7 vs 14 d for VAP	Resistance, mortality, recurrence	Multidrug-resistant pathogens developed less with 8 d therapy ($P = .04$)

Kim[36]/prospective	*Deescalation* RCT for initial therapy of VAP; deescalation based on culture	Development of antimicrobial resistance	Nonsignificant more MRSA in deescalation arm; no difference GNB
Joffe[37]/second analysis of RCT of VAP invasive bronchitis vs endobronchial culture	*Deescalation* based on culture	Development of antimicrobial resistance	No difference observed
Leone[38]/prospective RCT	*Deescalation* of patients with sepsis	Development of superinfection	Increased superinfection in deescalation arm but no mention of resistance effect
Carling[39]/prospective	*Multidisciplinary* antimicrobial management program; before and after assessment	*C difficile* rates and resistance of Enterobacteriaceae	Significant reduction in both
Dortch[40]/prospective, observational	*Antimicrobial stewardship protocols*; observed effect	Rate of MDR gram-negative bacilli during implementation	MDR GNB decreased from 37.4% to 8.5%
Yong[41]/prospective, observational	*Antimicrobial Stewardship* intervention	Susceptibility of *Pseudomonas* before and after intervention	Reduced resistance of *Pseudomonas* to imipenem and gentamicin
Nowak[42]/observational, pre–post analysis	*Antimicrobial Stewardship Intervention*	Rates of infections owing to common nosocomial pathogens caused by resistant pathogens	Rates of MRSA and *C difficile* decreased
DiazGranados[43]/prospective audit	*Audit for AS in ICU;* baseline compared with intervention	ID physician and ID Pharmacist-recommendations and rounds	Lower rates of resistance ($P = .033$). audit and feedback were independently associated with appropriate antimicrobial selection and prevention of resistance

(*continued on next page*)

Table 1
(*continued*)

Study/Design	Intervention	Resistance Outcome Assessed	Finding
Niwa[44]/retrospective before/after intervention	*Assessment of comprehensive ASP* outcomes of extensive implementation of antimicrobial stewardship were evaluated from the standpoint of antimicrobial use density, treatment duration, duration of hospital stay	Occurrence of antimicrobial-resistant bacteria and medical expenses	Significant reduction in the antimicrobial consumption was observed in the second-generation cephalosporins, carbapenems, aminoglycosides, leading to a reduction in the cost of antibiotics by 11.7%. The appearance of MRSA and the proportion of MDR Gram-negative bacteria decreased significantly
Trienski[45]/observational evaluation	*Assessment of comprehensive ASP* prospective audit with intervention and feedback model with the clinical pharmacist and ID physician making formal rounds on selected patients in both critical care and medical/surgical units; interventions included deescalation, bug–drug mismatch, dose optimization, duration (refer to text)	Observation of resistance rates on basis of antibiograms	Observed a decrease in antimicrobial resistance rates of GNB in ICU

Abbreviations: ABX, antibiotics; ASP, antimicrobial stewardship program; CPIS, Clinical Pulmonary Infection Score; ESBL, extended spectrum beta-lactamase; GNB, gram-negative bacilli; ICU, intensive care unit; ID, infectious disease; MDR, multidrug-resistant; MRSA, methicillin-resistant *Staphylococcus aureus*; RCT, randomized clinical trial; VAP, ventilator-associated pneumonia.

to a restricted antimicrobial has been observed when that agent is restricted for use; however, an unintended consequence may be development of resistance of alternative agents that replace the restricted agents—squeezing the balloon.[35]

Three studies assessed deescalation and observed no effect on antimicrobial resistance within the time frame of the investigation.[36–38] Although there is a general perception that "deescalation" is appropriate and a primary principle of antimicrobial stewardship and while prior national guidelines and numerous papers contend that deescalation is beneficial for patients and the health system (eg, reduction of cost and resistance), there is very little high-level evidence to support this. As stated in a recent Cochrane review of antimicrobial deescalation for adults with sepsis, "There is no adequate or direct evidence on whether de-escalation of antimicrobial agents is effective and safe for adults with sepsis.... Appropriate studies are needed to investigate the potential benefits proposed by de-escalation treatment."[29] Subsequent to this Cochrane Review, Leone and colleagues[38] reported the first randomized, controlled trial to specifically assess deescalation, defined as narrowing the spectrum of the initial antimicrobial therapy, in patients with sepsis in the intensive care unit. Of 116 patients included in the analysis, 59 were assigned randomly to the deescalation group and 57 to the continuation of appropriate antimicrobial therapy group (pneumonia was the cause of infection in 58% and 40% patients in the deescalation and continuation arms, respectively; $P = .06$). Deescalation was associated with an increased number of antimicrobial days (the primary study outcome) as well as risk of superinfection; but there was no mention of an effect on resistance. The authors concluded that deescalation was not noninferior to the continuation of appropriate empirical antimicrobial therapy. There was no impact on mortality or length of intensive care stay. Despite the randomized, controlled trial design, there were several limitations of the study, including nonblinding, a misbalance of type of infection (more lung infections in the deescalation arm), nonreporting the number of healthcare-associated pneumonia versus ventilator-associated pneumonia, and nonreporting of the appropriateness of the initial antimicrobial therapy. Furthermore, in a post hoc analysis of the 56 patients with pneumonia there was no difference in outcomes measured. In light of the absence of mortality difference and the presence 'serious' flaws of this randomized, controlled trial, we believe deescalation should remain recommended for the potential benefits to reduce antimicrobial use and resistance.

Most of the remaining studies assessed a comprehensive ASP often with audit and feedback and specific antibiotic stewardship protocols.[39–45] Many of the programs described in these studies combined some form of restriction (eg, reserved specific antimicrobials for ID or intensive care use) with a prospective audit and feedback process. Several studies used computer systems to identify various bug–drug relationships or for implementation of specific protocols for a particular syndrome (eg, pneumonia or urinary tract infection). At Summa Health System, patients are prospectively evaluated daily (5 days a week) by an ID physician and a dedicated ID-trained doctor of pharmacy using a software program to identify patients on various aspects and courses of antimicrobial agents.[45] Stewardship rounds on the general wards and intensive care units are conducted and various recommendations concerning antimicrobial therapy are communicated to the prescribing service. The goal of ASP is to limit antimicrobial use by optimizing the antimicrobial selection, dosing, route, and duration of therapy. The most common interventions recommended are deescalation, change of regimen based on microbiology results (especially for drug–bug mismatches), dosing adjustments including dose optimization on the basis of a minimum inhibitory concentration, discontinuation of antimicrobials, and ID consult. In addition to showing a reduction in antimicrobial use and cost, we have observed a reduction of 30-day readmission rates (from 16.7% to 6.5% for all cause readmissions; $P = .05$) and antimicrobial resistance to most Gram-negative bacilli as listed in our yearly antibiograms.[5,45]

Duration of therapy is important; each additional day of unnecessary antibiotics increases a patients' risk of acquiring CDI.[46,47] The appropriate duration of therapy for intraabdominal infections is unclear. Traditionally duration of antimicrobial therapy has been 7 to 14 days. A shorter course could decrease the risk of antimicrobial resistance. A recent study in surgery patients with complicated intraabdominal infection and adequate source control found patient outcomes after short course antibiotic therapy (approximately 4 days) were similar to those after a longer course of antibiotics (approximately 8 days).[48]

USE OF NEW ANTIMICROBIALS

After an extended period in which few new systemic antibiotics were approved for use in the United States, the last few years have seen an increase in newly approved antimicrobials, and government policies, and professional society advocacy are combining to increase the development of additional agents. In the past year several new approvals have focused on gram-positive infections (dalbavancin, ortivancin, tedizolid) and 2 on gram-negative infections (ceftolozane-tazobactam and ceftazadime-avibactam). Other agents in late stage development include delafloxacin, eravacycline, omadacycline, solithromycin, surotomycin, and plazomicin. The appropriate use of these new agents will be facilitated by effective stewardship. Many clinicians accept at face value the misperception that use of newer agents does not accord with practicing stewardship; this idea represents a false dichotomy. In reality, the concepts of use of new drugs and stewardship can be very compatible. There has been a common perception in the past that as new agents became available, we were going to restrict them and never use them because we wanted to save them. But that may not be best for our patients. We have patients who are at high risk and so are good candidates for use of these new agents as initial therapy. Appropriate selection and timely administration of initial therapy is critically important and has a major impact on outcomes, including risk for death. Given the effectiveness of newer—and sometimes more expensive—agents against pathogens that have developed resistance to established agents, the use of newer agents in appropriately selected patients is compatible with good clinical care and antimicrobial stewardship. Oversight of treatment of newer agents by ASPs can assure appropriate use. As stated in the past by Dennis Maki, MD, "The development of new antibiotics without having mechanisms to insure their appropriate use is much like supplying your alcoholic patient with finer brandy."[49]

The development of rapid molecular tests able to quickly identify or rule out the presence of MDROs will also have great value in helping clinicians individualize newer antimicrobial therapy to optimal effect.

SUMMARY

In light of the serious threat of emerging antimicrobial-resistant pathogens, it is crucial that ASPs be put into practice now to provide for optimal patient outcomes and preserve antimicrobials for future use. Strategies for improving antibiotic use and evidence for best practices in antibiotic stewardship will continue to evolve. The specific types of interventions implemented by institutions will depend on local circumstances and capabilities. Nevertheless, it is vital that health care settings have ASP so that patients, both present and future, will continue to have the benefit of life-saving antimicrobials.

REFERENCES

1. Centers for Disease Control and Prevention. Antibiotic resistance threats in the US, 2013. Available at: www.cdc.gov/AntibioticResistanceThreats/index.html. Accessed June 1, 2015.
2. File TM Jr, Srinivasan A, Bartlett JB. Antimicrobial stewardship: importance for patient and public health. Clin Infect Dis 2014;59(S3):S93–6.
3. Srinivasan A. Implementing a strategy for monitoring inpatient antimicrobial use among hospitals in the United States. Clin Infect Dis 2014;58:401–6.
4. Goff DA, Bauer KA, Reed EE, et al. Is the "low hanging fruit" worth picking for antimicrobial stewardship programs? Clin Infect Dis 2012;55:587–92.
5. Pasquale TR, Trienski TL, Tan MJ, et al. Evaluation of the impact of an antimicrobial stewardship program in patients with acute bacterial skin and skin structure infections (ABSSSI) at a teaching hospital. Am J Health Syst Pharm 2014;71: 1136–9.
6. Malani AN, Richards PG, Kapila S, et al. Clinical and economic outcomes from a community hospital's antimicrobial stewardship program. J Infect Control 2013; 41:145–8.
7. Dellit TH, Owens RC, McGowan JE Jr, et al. Infectious Diseases Society of America and the Society for Healthcare Epidemiology of America guidelines for developing an institutional program to enhance antimicrobial stewardship. Clin Infect Dis 2007;44:159–77.
8. Neuhauser MM, Weinstein RA, Rydman R. Antibiotic resistance among gram-negative bacilli in US intensive care units: implications for fluoroquinolone use. JAMA 2003;289(7):885–8.
9. Costelloe C, Metcalfe C, Lovering A. Effect of antibiotic prescribing in primary care on antimicrobial resistance in individual patients: systematic review and meta-analysis. BMJ 2010;340:c2096.
10. Centers for Disease Control and Prevention (CDC). Core elements of hospital antibiotic stewardship programs. Atlanta (GA): US Department of Health and Human Services, CDC; 2014. Available at: http://www.cdc.gov/getsmart/healthcare/implementation/core-elements.html. Accessed June 1, 2015.
11. Bartlett JG. A call to arms: the imperative for antimicrobial stewardship. Clin Infect Dis 2011;53(Suppl 1):S4–7.
12. Available at: https://www.whitehouse.gov/the-press-office/2015/01/27/fact-sheet-president-s-2016-budget-proposes-historic-investment-combat-a. Accessed June 1, 2015.
13. Filice GA, Drekonja DM, Thurn JR, et al. Diagnostic errors that lead to inappropriate antimicrobial use. Infect Control Hosp Epidemiol 2015;36(8):949–56.
14. Cosgrove SE, Hermsen ED, Rybak MJ, et al. Guidance for the knowledge and skills required for antimicrobial stewardship leaders. Infect Control Hosp Epidemiol 2014;35:1444–51.
15. Rosenberg DJ. Infections, bacterial resistance, and antimicrobial stewardship: the emerging role for hospitalists. J Hop Med 2012;7(Suppl 1):S34–43.
16. Schmitt S, McQuillen DP, Nahass R, et al. Infectious diseases specialty intervention is associated with decreased mortality and lower healthcare costs. Clin Infect Dis 2014;58:22–8.
17. Nilhom H, Holmsrand L, Ahl J. An audit-based infections disease specialist-guided antimicrobial stewardship program profoundly reduced antibiotic use without negatively affecting patient outcomes. Open Forum Infect Dis 2015;2(2):ofv042.

18. ASHP Statement on the pharmacist's role in antimicrobial stewardship and infection prevention and control. Am J Health Syst Pharm 2010;67:575–7.
19. Bauer KA, West JE, O'Brien JM, et al. Extended-infusion cefepime reduces mortality in patients with Pseudomonas aeruginosa infections. Antimicrob Agents Chemother 2013;57(7):2907–12.
20. Bauer K, West J, Balada-Llasat JM, et al. An antimicrobial stewardship program's impact with rapid polymerase chain reaction methicillin-resistant *Staphylococcus aureus/S. aureus* blood culture test in patients with *S. aureus* bacteremia. Clin Infect Dis 2010;51(9):1074–80.
21. Palmore TN, Henderson DK. Managing transmission of carbapenem-resistant Enterobacteriaceae in healthcare settings: a view from the trenches. Clin Infect Dis 2013;57(11):1593–9.
22. Schwaber MJ, Carmeli Y. An ongoing national intervention to contain the spread of carbapenem-resistant Enterobacteriaceae. Clin Infect Dis 2014;58:697–703.
23. Saint S, Fowler KE, Krein SL, et al. Clostridium difficile infection in the United States: a national study assessing preventive practices used and perceptions of practice evidence. Infect Control Hosp Epidemiol 2015;36(8):969–71.
24. Bauer KA, Perez K, Forrest G, et al. Review of rapid diagnostic tests used by antimicrobial stewardship. Clin Infect Dis 2014;59(8):S134–45.
25. CMS sets the table for regulation requiring antibiotic stewardship programs. Available at: http://www.ahcmedia.com/articles/134561-cms-sets-the-table-for-regulation-requiring-antibiotic-stewardship-programs. Accessed May 30, 2015.
26. Tansarli GS, Karageorgopoulos DE, Kapaskelis A, et al. Impact of antimicrobial multidrug resistance on inpatient care cost: an evaluation of the evidence. Expert Rev Anti Infect Ther 2013;11(3):321–31.
27. Huang AM, Newton D, Kunapuli A, et al. Impact of rapid organism identification via matrix-assisted laser desorption/ionization time-of-flight combined with antimicrobial stewardship team intervention in adult patients with bacteremia and candidemia. Clin Infect Dis 2013;57(9):1237–45.
28. Terhune C. New lawsuits filed against scope maker in deadly UCLA superbug outbreak. Available at: http://www.latimes.com/business/la-fi-ucla-superbug-patients-20150317-story.html. Accessed June 2, 2015.
29. Davey P, Brown E, Charani E, et al. Interventions to improve antibiotic prescribing practices for hospital inpatients. Cochrane Database Syst Rev 2013;(4):CD003543.
30. de Man P, Verhoeven BAN, Verbrugh HA, et al. An antibiotic policy to prevent emergence of resistant bacilli. Lancet 2000;355:973–8.
31. Lan CK, Hsueh PR, Wong WW, et al. Association of antibiotic utilization measures and reduced incidence of infections with extended-spectrum beta-lactamase-producing organisms. J Microbiol Immunol Infect 2003;36(3):182–6.
32. Lewis GJ, Fang X, Gooch M, et al. Decreased resistance of Pseudomonas aeruginosa with restriction of ciprofloxacin in a large teaching hospital's intensive care and intermediate care units. Infect Control Hosp Epidemiol 2012;33(4):368–73.
33. Medina Presentado JC, Paciel López D, Berro Castiglioni M, et al. Ceftriaxone and ciprofloxacin restriction in an intensive care unit: less incidence of *Acinetobacter spp.* and improved susceptibility of *Pseudomonas aeruginosa*. Rev Panam Salud Publica 2011;30(6):603–9.
34. White AC Jr, Atmar RL, Wilson J. Effects of requiring prior authorization for selected antimicrobials: expenditures, susceptibilities, and clinical outcomes. Clin Infect Dis 1997;25:230–9.

35. Rahal JJ, Urban C, Segal-Maurer S. Nosocomial antibiotic resistance in multiple gram-negative species: experience at one hospital with squeezing the resistance balloon at multiple sites. Clin Infect Dis 2002;34(4):499–503.
36. Kim JW, Chung J, Choi SH, et al. Early use of imipenem and vancomycin followed b de-escalation versus conventional antimicrobials without de-escalation for patients with hospital-acquired pneumonia. in a medical ICU: a randomize trial. Crit Care 2012;16:R28.
37. Joffe AR, Muscedere J, Marshall JC, et al. The safety of targeted antibiotic therapy for ventilator-associated pneumonia: a multicenter observational study. J Crit Care 2008;23:82–90.
38. Leone M, Bechis C, Baumstarck K, et al. De-escalation versus continuation of empirical antimicrobial treatment in severe sepsis: a multicenter non-blinded randomized noninferiority trial. Intensive Care Med 2014;40:1399–408.
39. Carling P, Fung T, Killion A, et al. Favorable impact of a multidisciplinary antibiotic management program conducted during 7 years. Infect Control Hosp Epidemiol 2003;24:699–706.
40. Dortch MJ, Fleming SB, Kauffmann RM, et al. Infection reduction strategies including antibiotic stewardship protocols in surgical and trauma intensive care units are associated with reduced resistant gram-negative healthcare-associated infections. Surg Infect (Larchmt) 2011;12(1):15–25.
41. Yong MK, Buising KL, Cheng AC. Improved susceptibility of Gram-negative bacteria in an intensive care unit following implementation of a computerized antibiotic decision support system. J Antimicrob Chemother 2010;65:1062–9.
42. Nowak MA, Nelson RE, Breidenbach JL, et al. Clinical and economic outcomes of a prospective antimicrobial stewardship program. Am J Health Syst Pharm 2012; 69:1500–8.
43. DiazGranados CA. Prospective audit for antimicrobial stewardship in intensive care: impact on resistance and clinical outcomes. Am J Infect Control 2012;40: 526–9.
44. Niwa T, Shinoda Y, Suzuki A, et al. Outcome measurement of extensive implementation of antimicrobial stewardship in patients receiving intravenous antibiotics in a Japanese university hospital. Int J Clin Pract 2012;66:999–1008.
45. Trienski TL, File TM Jr. Antimicrobial stewardship program at an academic medical center. Abstract 83 OR, Annual Meeting MAD-ID (Making a Difference in Infectious Diseases). Orlando (FL), May 7–9, 2015.
46. Singh N, Rogers P, Atwood CW, et al. Short-course empiric antibiotic therapy for patients with pulmonary infiltrates in the intensive care unit. A proposed solution for indiscriminate antibiotic prescription. Am J Respir Crit Care Med 2000;162:505–11.
47. Chastre J, Wolff M, Fagon JY, et al. Comparison of 8 vs 15 days of antibiotic therapy for ventilator-associated pneumonia in adults: a randomized trial. JAMA 2003; 290(19):2588–98.
48. Sawyer RG, Claridge JA, Nathens AB, et al. Trial of short-course antimicrobial therapy for intraabdominal infection. N Engl J Med 2015;372:1996–2005.
49. Fishman N. Antimicrobial stewardship. Am J Med 2006;119:S53–61.

Index

Note: Page numbers of article titles are in **boldface** type.

Infect Dis Clin N Am 30 (2016) 553–565
http://dx.doi.org/10.1016/S0891-5520(16)30036-8
0891-5520/16/$ – see front matter

I

L

N

O

R

S

W

Printed and bound by CPI Group (UK) Ltd, Croydon, CR0 4YY

12/05/2025

01866863-0001